AF342145

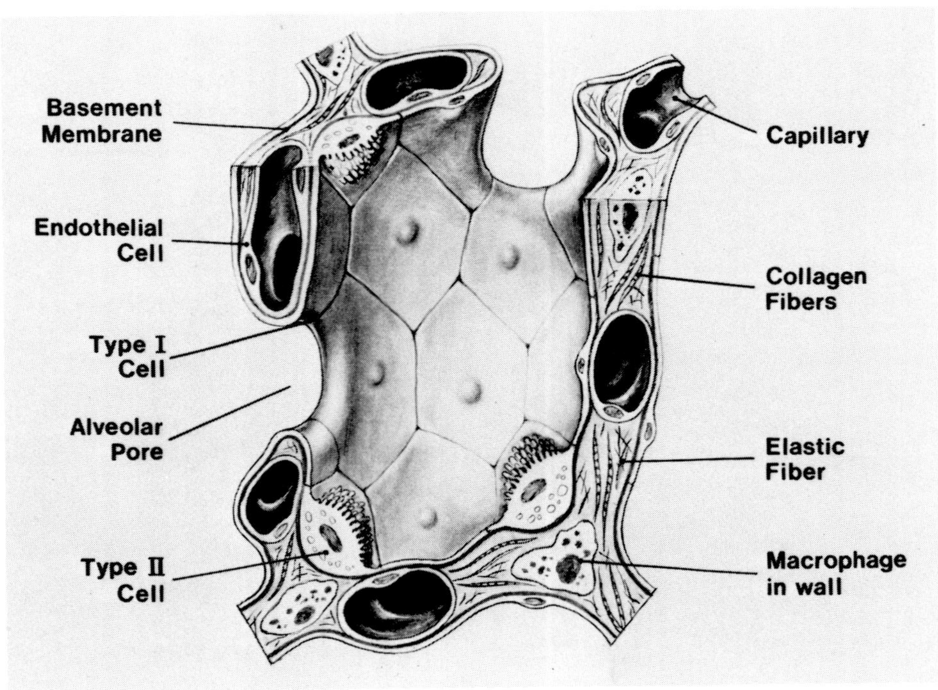

FIGURE: Microanatomy of a pulmonary alveolus.

Interstitial Lung Diseases in Children

Volume III

Editors

Lourdes R. Laraya-Cuasay
Professor, Clinical Pediatrics
Director, Pediatric Pulmonary and
Cystic Fibrosis Division
UMDNJ-Robert Wood Johnson Medical School
New Brunswick, New Jersey

Walter T. Hughes
Director, Infectious Diseases
Chairman, Department of Child
Health Sciences
St. Jude Children's Research Hospital
Memphis, Tennessee

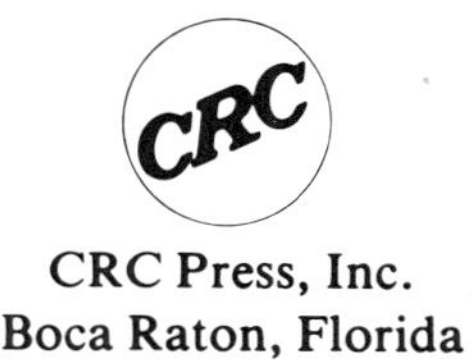

CRC Press, Inc.
Boca Raton, Florida

Library of Congress Cataloging-in-Publication Data

Interstitial lung diseases in children.

Includes bibliographies and index.
1. Interstitial lung diseases in children.
I. Laraya-Cuasay, Lourdes R.   II. Hughes, Walter T.
(Walter Thompson), 1930-   . [DNLM: 1. Pulmonary
Fibrosis—in infancy & childhood. WF 600 I6175]
RJ436.I56I56   1988   618.92′24   87-18185
ISBN 0-8493-4300-3 (set)
ISBN 0-8493-4301-1 (vol. 1)
ISBN 0-8493-4302-X (vol. 2)
ISBN 0-8493-4303-8 (vol. 3)

This book represents information obtained from authentic and highly regarded sources. Reprinted material is quoted with permission, and sources are indicated. A wide variety of references are listed. Every reasonable effort has been made to give reliable data and information, but the author and the publisher cannot assume responsibility for the validity of all materials or for the consequences of their use.

All rights reserved. This book, or any parts thereof, may not be reproduced in any form without written consent from the publisher.

Direct all inquiries to CRC Press, Inc., 2000 Corporate Blvd., N.W., Boca Raton, Florida, 33431.

© 1988 by CRC Press, Inc.

International Standard Book Number 0-8493-4300-3 (set)
International Standard Book Number 0-8493-4301-1 (vol. 1)
International Standard Book Number 0-8493-4302-X (vol. 2)
International Standard Book Number 0-8493-4303-8 (vol. 3)

Library of Congress Card Number 87-18185
Printed in the United States

Lovingly Dedicated to

**Ramon, R. Peter, Catherine Anne,
Margaret Rose, and Joseph Paul**

Nancy N. Huang, M.D.

**Jeanette, Carla, Christopher,
and Gregory**

PREFACE

This book was conceived back in the early 1970s in the busy X-ray reading room at St. Christopher's Hospital for Children in Philadelphia, Pennsylvania. During X-ray rounds, Dr. John A. Kirkpatrick and I would discuss the various possible entities with which the streaky densities or infiltrates found in chest radiographs correlated. Clinicopathological and radiological correlations were conducted on patients on whom open lung biopsies or autopsies were performed. Drs. James Arey and Dale Huff were most cooperative and patient with queries. Great emphasis was placed on very accurate history taking. In my pursuit of the meaning of these "interstitial densities", I covered many possible etiologies, so that sharing the product of this search with interested physicians and allied health professionals with interest in pediatric lung disease seemed to be a likely consequence. The medical literature on interstitial lung disease in infants, children, and adolescents were found in various journals and books, most of which were not usually read by pediatricians. Compiling these pieces of information for easy reference for my colleagues was a needed task.

An overview and the different etiologies in interstitial lung diseases in infants, children, and adolescents are presented. The etiologies are categorized into known and unknown, and further classified into infectious and noninfectious causes. A registry for interstitial lung diseases in children is a major need to be able to study this problem in greater depth. If after referring to this book, the reader is able to realize the varied etiologies of streaky lung densities described in chest radiographs, and how normal or benign the chest radiographs could look despite major and potentially fatal pathologies, then our goal would have been achieved.

Lourdes R. Laraya-Cuasay, M.D.

ACKNOWLEDGMENTS

The guidance of my former mentors, Drs. Walter T. Hughes, William W. Waring, and Nancy N. Huang, and the continued encouragement and support of Drs. John A. Kirkpatrick, George C. Polgar, Faustino Niguidula, James Arey, Judy Palmer, and Daniel Schidlow are appreciated.

I thank the contributors for their splendid cooperation and the editors, Barbara Brownlee and James V. McCabe, for their patience and thoroughness throughout the years that this book was being written. The prompt attention of the librarians doing the medical search at UMDNJ-Robert Wood Johnson Medical School is most appreciated.

Special thanks to Joseph Paul Cuasay for typing my manuscripts.

Lourdes R. Laraya-Cuasay, M.D.

THE EDITORS

Lourdes R. Laraya-Cuasay, M.D., is Professor of Clinical Pediatrics at the University of Medicine and Dentristy of New Jersey Robert Wood Johnson Medical School (formerly Rutgers Medical School) and Director of the Pediatric Pulmonary and Cystic Fibrosis Programs in the Robert Wood Johnson University Hospital in New Brunswick, New Jersey. She is a Fellow of the American College of Chest Physicians and of the American Lung Association/American Thoracic Society. She received her medical degree from the University of Santo Tomas College of Medicine and Surgery in Manila, Philippines. She trained in Pediatrics at the Santo Tomas University Hospital, Children's Hospital of Louisville, Tulane Division of Charity Hospital of New Orleans, and at the Children's Hospital of Philadelphia. Her pediatric pulmonology and cystic fibrology training was at Saint Christopher's Hospital for Children in Philadelphia, Pennsylvania from 1969 to 1972. She served as attending staff, Associate Director of the Pediatric Pulmonary Fellowship Program and the Pediatric Pulmonary and Cystic Fibrosis Center at Saint Christopher's Hospital for Children until 1977. Thereafter, she became Associate Professor of Pediatrics at Thomas Jefferson University School of Medicine. Her interests are in the sequelae of respiratory viral and mycoplasmal infections in patients with cystic fibrosis and in those with chronic lung disorders other than cystic fibrosis, and in the various causes of interstitial lung disease in infants, children, and adolescents with normal or compromised immunity.

Walter Thomson Hughes, M.D., is Chairman of the Department of Child Health Sciences and Director of the Division of Infectious Diseases, St. Jude Children's Research Hospital, and Professor of Pediatrics at the University of Tennessee Center for Health Sciences.

Dr. Hughes received his M.D. degree from the University of Tennessee College of Medicine. He completed an internship at the Knoxville General Hospital and a pediatric residency at the Le Bonheur Children's Hospital at the University of Tennessee. Following his residency, he spent two years in infectious diseases research at the Walter Reed Army Medical Center and the Ft. Dietrick laboratories in Maryland. His first academic appointment was at the University of Louisville School of Medicine where he worked with Dr. Alex Steigman in clinical studies of the more common infections of children. In 1969 he moved to St. Jude Children's Research Hospital, an institute dedicated primarily to research in childhood cancer, to concentrate on infections of the immunosuppressed host. In 1977 Dr. Hughes joined the faculty at The Johns Hopkins University School of Medicine as Eudowood Professor of Pediatrics and Director of the Division of Infectious Diseases. Here he continued research and became actively involved in teaching clinical aspects of infectious diseases. In 1981 he returned to St. Jude Children's Research Hospital, but contunues to hold the faculty appointment of Lecturer in Pediatrics at the Johns Hopkins University. Currently Dr. Hughes' research is aimed at methods to prevent, diagnose, and treat *Pneumocystis carinii* pneumonitis. He has published over 250 scientific papers dealing primarily with infectious diseases in the immunosuppressed host.

CONTRIBUTORS

Rosalind S. Abernathy, M.D.
Associate Professor
Department of Pediatrics
University of Arkansas for Medical
  Sciences
Little Rock, Arkansas

Brad E. Alpert, M.D.
Assistant Professor
Pediatric Pulmonary Section
St. Christopher's Hospital for Children
Philadelphia, Pennsylvania

H. Jorge Baluarte, M.D.
Chief and Professor
Section for Pediatric Nephrology
St. Christopher's Hospital for Children
Philadelphia, Pennsylvania

Michael R. Bye, M.D.
Assistant Professor of Pediatrics
Director, Pediatric Pulmonary Medicine
Albert Einstein College of Medicine
Bronx, New York

Lawrence J. Ettinger, M.D.
Associate Professor
Department of Pediatrics
UMDNJ-Robert Wood Johnson Medical
  School
New Brunswick, New Jersey

Bonnie Hepburn, M.D.
Associate Professor
Department of Medicine
UMDNJ-Robert Wood Johnson Medical
  School
New Brunswick, New Jersey

Bettina C. Hilman, M.D.
Professor
Department of Pediatrics
Louisiana State University
Shreveport, Louisiana

Walter T. Hughes, M.D.
Director
Division of Infectious Diseases
St. Jude Children's Research Hospital
Memphis, Tennessee

Lourdes R. Laraya-Cuasay, M.D.
Professor of Clinical Pediatriacs
Director, Pediatric Pulmonary and Cystic
  Fibrosis Division
Department of Pediatrics
UMDNJ-Robert Wood Johnson Medical
  School
New Brunswick, New Jersey

Stephen T. Lawless, M.D.
Fellow
Department of Pediatric Critical Care
Children's Hospital of Pittsburgh
Pittsburgh, Pennsylvania

Hsiu-San Lin, M.D., Ph.D.
Professor
Radiation Oncology Center
Mallinckrodt Institute of Radiology
Washington University School of
  Medicine
St. Louis, Missouri

Marina I. Liscano, M.D.
Pulmonary Fellow
Department of Pediatrics
UMDNJ-Robert Wood Johnson Medical
  School
New Brunswick, New Jersey

David J. Riley, M.D.
Professor
Department of Medicine
UMDNJ-Robert Wood Johnson Medical
  School
New Brunswick, New Jersey

Daniel V. Schidlow, M.D.
Chief, Section of Pediatric Pulmonary
  Medicine
St. Christopher's Hospital for Children
Associate Professor of Pediatrics
Temple University School of Medicine
Philadelphia, Pennsylvania

**Patrick R. M. Thomas, M.B.,
  M.R.C.P., F.R.C.R.**
Associate Professor
Radiation Oncology Center
Mallinckrodt Institute of Radiology
Washington University School of
  Medicine
St. Louis, Missouri

INTERSTITIAL LUNG DISEASES IN CHILDREN

Volume I

Clinical Aspects of Interstitial Lung Disease in Children
Genetic Aspects of Interstitial Lung Disease
Cells and Extracellular Matrix of the Alveolar Wall
Pulmonary Immunology
Pulmonary Functions in Children with
Interstitial Lung Disease
Radiology of Interstitial Lung Disease in Children
The Role of Lung Biopsy in Interstitial
Lung Diseases in Children
Nutrition and the Lung
Effects of Infection on Function and
Development of the Lung
Neonatal Pneumonia
Bacterial Pneumonia of Infants and Children
Chlamydia Pneumonitis

Volume II

Varicella-Zoster Virus Pneumonia
Viral Infections of the Lungs
Infectious Mononucleosis
Mycoplasma Pneumoniae Pneumonia
Pneumonitis in Rickettsial Infections
Pneumonitis in Acquired Immune Deficiency Syndrome (AIDS)
Pneumonitis in Bone Marrow Transplant Recipients
Pneumonitis Accompanying Sepsis
Pulmonary Tuberculosis in Children
Pulmonary Candidiasis
Disseminated Histoplasmosis, Coccidioidomycosis,
and Cryptococcosis
Nocardiosis
Pneumocystis Carinii Pneumonia
Pulmonary Disease of Parasitic Cause
Cardiovascular Causes of Interstitial Lung Disease
Bronchopulmonary Dysplasia
Acute Lung Injury in Children Due to
Chemical and Physical Agents

Volume III

Radiation Pneumonitis
Drug-Induced Interstitial Pneumonitis in Children
Gastroesophageal Reflux and Interstitial Pneumonia
Metabolic, Degenerative, and Unclassified
Conditions Associated with Interstitial Lung Disease
Neurocutaneous Syndromes with
Interstitial Lung Disease
Sarcoidosis
Hypersensitivity Pneumonitis
Idiopathic Pulmonary Hemosiderosis
Pulmonary Involvement in Systemic Cancer
Noninfectious Pulmonary Manifestations of
Renal Disease in Children
Interstitial Lung Disease in
Childhood Rheumatic Disorders
The Interstitial Pneumonias
Lymphoproliferative Disorders of the Lung
Future Therapy of Interstitial Lung Disease

TABLE OF CONTENTS

Volume III

Chapter 30

RADIATION PNEUMONITIS

Patrick R.M. Thomas and Hsiu-San Lin

TABLE OF CONTENTS

I. INTRODUCTION

The effects of radiation on the lung were first described in 1922 by Groover et al.[1] Radiation pneumonitis in clinical or subclinical manifestations is almost an inevitable consequence of radiotherapy for cancer of the lung, breast, esophagus, or Hodgkin's disease. In childhood, the condition is less common due to the relatively fewer indications for radiation in pediatric oncology. However, the mediastinum in lymphoma or dumbbell neuroblastoma and substantial lung volumes in small round cell tumors of the chest may be irradiated. Whole lung irradiation may be indicated for the treatment of metastatic disease to the chest. Radiation pneumonitis is considered as the most important dose-limiting factor in total body irradiation in preparing patients for bone marrow transplantation and in upper hemi-body irradiation for osseous metastasis.

II. ETIOLOGY AND PREDISPOSING FACTORS

The incidence of pneumonitis is related primarily to the total dose of radiation. In addition the use of certain chemotherapeutic agents, particularly dactinomycin, doxorubicin, and bleomycin, potentiates the radiation effects. Wara et al.[2] have estimated that a 5% incidence of clinically evident radiation pneumonitis occurs with 770 ret* and 50% with 972 ret. However, with dactinomycin the 5% incidence falls to 520 ret with 50% at 749 ret. In this study the irradiated volume did not appear to be a factor. However, a recent study in breast cancer patients suggested that volume was the most significant factor.[3] There is also evidence to show that dose per fraction can be important.[4] When single large doses are given, the dose rate becomes an important factor.[5,6]

A sudden steroid withdrawal is a well known predisposing factor.[7] In pediatrics this can occur in patients treated with combination chemotherapy including steroids and mantle radiotherapy. Conversely there is much experimental data in mice that has shown steroid administration to be beneficial in preventing death from pneumonitis.[8,9] Previous radiotherapy is also a contributory factor to the development of pneumonitis as has been shown in Hodgkin's disease with mediastinal irradiation[10] and in Wilms' tumor with whole lung radiotherapy.[11]

III. CLINICAL SYMPTOMS

There are two main types of radiation pneumonitis — the acute and chronic manifestations. These are usually distinct clinical entities but sometimes the definition may not be so clear and occasionally the acute phase can merge into the chronic.

The acute variety is typified by a relatively sudden onset of cough, dyspnea, and intermittent fever. This can occur any time between 2 weeks and 6 months following therapy. The physical examination may be noncontributory but sometimes tachypnea will be noticed and in severe cases the patient can be cyanosed and show signs of consolidation over the area concerned. Radiographic changes are discussed in Chapter 6.

Spontaneous recovery occurs in all but the most severe cases. However, radiographic abnormalities (Chapter 6) will usually appear despite the absence of clinical symptoms and signs. Frequently these radiologic changes persist indefinitely without any clinical manifestations.

The symptomatic chronic phase of radiation pneumonitis is much rarer than and is usually

---

* The ret (Rad Equivalent Therapy) calculates a nominal standard dose (NSD) of radiation based on the formula — dose in rad = NSD × (No. of fractions)$^{0.24}$ × (elapsed days)$^{0.11}$. It is a method for comparing different dose fractionation schedules.

preceded by acute pneumonitis. However, the occasional patient will develop problems with a history of minimal or no preceding dysfunction.[12] The interval is usually 6 months to 1 year following radiotherapy and the clinical manifestations consist of chronic pulmonary insufficiency due to the fibrosis with repeated infections leading to cor pulmonale and occasionally death.

IV. DIFFERENTIAL DIAGNOSIS

The diagnosis of radiation pneumonitis should usually be made without undue difficulty if the treatment volumes are known accurately. This is because the radiological changes are entirely confined to the treated area (Chapter 6). However, recurrent tumor or an infective process may easily mimic these changes.

The treatment of pneumonitis with more radiation is unfortunate and can be fatal so the differentiation between reaction and recurrence is important.[13] In addition to the volume the timing of the appearance of the radiological abnormalities after radiation and progression of disease elsewhere may be suggestive. Lymphangitic spread usually involves the bases and is symptomatic out of proportion to the radiologic changes.[12]

Possible infective changes may sometimes also provide a diagnostic dilemma,[14] especially if the onset of symptoms and signs are rapid. The treatment of infective pneumonitis by corticosteroids can be disastrous and a lung biopsy may be required for differentiation or confirmation.

V. PATHOLOGY

As the early phase of radiation pneumonitis is almost always self limiting, very little human histopathological information is available. Animal data suggest that the earliest and most significant damage is to the surfactant-secreting type II pneumocytes.[15] There are three distinct chronologic phases; early up to 2 months, intermediate from 2 to 9 months, and late from 9 months.[13] In the early phase there are endothelial changes with increased capillary permeability and edema accompanying the type II pneumocyte damage. In the intermediate phase there is proliferation of the latter with repair of capillaries and decreased permability. The third phase is usually an attempted return to normality with a large increase of collagen.

Human data is sketchy but confirms the above. The late phase has the most information but the histologic changes are relatively nonspecific. Dense fibrosis, thickening of the alveolar walls and reduction in capillaries are frequent.[9]

VI. TREATMENT

Mild early pneumonitis requires recognition, reassurance, and symptomatic measures only. Frequently the first two are sufficient but physical activity should be limited. Antipyretics and antitussive drugs may be required.

When such measures fail and, in severe cases, from the outset the use of corticosteroids may be dramatic. There is experimental evidence that the use of prednisone reduced the mortality of mice after thoracic irradiation.[8] In humans the effects can be dramatic with considerable improvement in dyspnea within 12 hr when high dosages (prednisone 100 mg orally daily) are used.[13] After satisfactory response the dosage can be reduced slowly to about 30 mg daily. Because of the likely recurrence of symptomatology, tapering of the dosage must be done with considerable caution, starting after at least 2 weeks. Usually a patient will be on corticosteroids for months.

The late phase of pneumonitis is radiation fibrosis and there is no known medication. Surgery, including pneumonectomy, may be indicated in unilateral disease.

VII. SUMMARY

Radiation pneumonitis is a well recognized clinical syndrome related to the dose, dose per fraction and volume of lung irradiation. Predisposing factors include chemotherapy and steroid withdrawal. The pathology corresponds to the clinical phases. Treatment consists of steroid administration for severe pneumonitis in the acute phase. There is no effective therapy for the symptomatic chronic fibrotic phase.

REFERENCES

1. **Groover, T. A., Christie, A. C., and Merritt, E. A.,** Observations on the use of the cooper filter in the Roentgen treatment of deep seated malignancies, *South. Med. J.,* 15, 440, 1922.
2. **Wara, W. M., Phillips, T. L., Margolis, L. W., and Smith, V.,** Radiation pneumonitis: a new approach to the deviation of time-dose factors, *Cancer,* 32, 547, 1973.
3. **Rothwell, R. I., Kelly, S. A., and Joslin, C. A. F.,** Radiation pneumonitis in patients treated for breast cancer, *Radiother. Oncol.,* 4, 9, 1985.
4. **Chabora, B. M., Lattin, P. B., Rosen, G., Chu, F. C. H., and Herskovic, A.,** Whole lung irradiation in the pediatric age group: low dose vs. conventional fractionation with multidrug chemotherapy, *Int. J. Rad. Oncol. Biol. Phys.,* 2, 465, 1977.
5. **Depledge, M. H. and Barrett, A.,** Dose-rate dependence of lung damage after total body irradiation in mice, *Int. J. Rad. Biol. Phys.,* 41, 325, 1982.
6. **Barrett, A., Depledge, M. H., and Powles, R. L.,** Interstitial pneumonitis following bone marrow transplantation after low dose rate total body irradiation, *Int. J. Rad. Oncol. Biol. Phys.,* 9, 1029, 1983.
7. **Castellino, R. A., Glatstein, E., Rurbow, M. M., Rosenberg, S., and Kaplan, H. S.,** Latent radiation injury of lungs or heart activated by steroid withdrawal, *Ann. Int. Med.,* 80, 593, 1974.
8. **Phillips, T. L., Wharam, M. D., and Margolis, L. W.,** Modification of radiation injury to normal tissues by chemotherapeutic agents, *Cancer,* 35, 1678, 1975.
9. **Gross, N. J.,** Radiation pneumonitis in mice, *J. Clin. Invest.,* 66, 504, 1980.
10. **Kaplan, H. S. and Stewart, J. R.,** Complications of intensive megavoltage radiotherapy for Hodgkin's disease, *N.C.I. Monogr.,* 36, 439, 1973.
11. **Tefft, M.,** Radiation related toxicities in National Wilms' Tumor Study Number 1, *Int. J. Rad. Oncol. Biol. Phys.,* 2, 455, 1977.
12. **Lipshitz, H. Z. and Southard, M. E.,** Complications of radiation therapy: the thorax, *Semin. Roentgenol.,* 9, 41, 1974.
13. **Gross, N. J.,** Pulmonary effects of radiation therapy, *Ann. Int. Med.,* 86, 81, 1977.
14. **Paris, T. M., Knight, J. G., Hess, C. E., and Constable, W. C.,** Severe radiation pneumonitis precipitated by withdrawal of corticosteroids, *Am. J. Roentgenol.,* 132, 284, 1979.
15. **Penney, D. P., Shapiro, D. L., Rubin, P., Finkelstein, J., and Siemann, D. W.,** Effects of radiation on the mouse lung and potential induction of radiation pneumonitis, *Virchow. Arch. B Cell Pathol.,* 37, 327, 1981.

Chapter 31

DRUG-INDUCED INTERSTITIAL PNEUMONITIS IN CHILDREN

Marina I. Liscano and Lawrence J. Ettinger

TABLE OF CONTENTS

I. INTRODUCTION

Pulmonary toxicity has been recognized as a potentially serious and life-threatening complication of several chemotherapeutic agents and other commonly used drugs. Although these toxicities are infrequent and sporadic, bleomycin and the nitrosoureas may result in dose-related, potentially life-threatening, pulmonary toxicity.[1]

Interstitial pneumonitis and pulmonary fibrosis are the major pulmonary toxicities, resulting in abnormal pulmonary function manifested by a restrictive pattern and a decrease in diffusing capacity (DLCO).[2] The pathophysiology has not been defined in man, but has been described in mice following bleomycin administration.[1] Ad described by Adamson and Bowden[3] the first pathologic finding is the development of endothelial blebs in the alveolar capillary endothelium. This is followed by the development of interstitial fibrinous edema, a mononuclear cell response, and hyaline membranes. Electron microscopic studies in man have shown a decrease in type I pneumocytes and a subsequent change in type II pneumocytes, including proliferation, delamellation, and migration into alveolar sacs. Finally, the alveolar septae become thickened, collagen fibers are noted adjacent to fibroblasts, and a dense proliferation of fibrous tissue and a decrease in the number of alveolar septae occur. In several animal species, these changes have been observed initially in the subpleural region with later extension into the bronchiolar areas. Pleural thickening may accompany the pneumonitis.[1] Although pulmonary toxicity is thought to be the result of a direct toxic effect in most cases, immunologic and hypersensitivity mechanisms may also play a role in certain cases.[2,4,5] These toxicities may occur during therapy or following discontinuation of the implicated drug.

The clinical, radiographic, and pathologic findings are similar for most of the drugs that cause pulmonary toxicity. The characteristic clinical features include fever, nonproductive cough, dyspnea, and basilar rales.[4,6] Radiographic studies may or may not show any positive findings at the initial presentation of symptomatology. Typical radiographic findings include diffuse alveolar and/or interstitial infiltrates. Since lung tissue responds in only a limited number of ways to various insults, histologic examination of tissue may not be diagnostic of a specific etiology, but must be interpreted in the context of the clinical setting and prior therapy. The final common expression usually seen from these agents is pulmonary fibrosis, a pathologic state that may also be seen with other conditions. Nevertheless, histologic examination of lung tissue is frequently indicated to confirm the clinical impression so that therapy can be directed to the suspected etiology. In addition, the biopsy can rule out other potential causes of pneumonitis, such as viral infections and *Pneumocystis carinii* pneumonia that may complicate the course of many of these patients who are being treated for malignancies or who are immunosuppressed for other disorders, and infiltration by leukemia, lymphoma, or other malignancies.[4,5,7]

The incidence of pulmonary toxicity from various chemotherapeutic agents is difficult to ascertain since such toxicity may occur late, most patients have received multiple chemotherapeutic agents, many of these patients have received pulmonary and/or mediastinal irradiation, and other disease and/or infectious complications can result in pulmonary pathology.[1,4] Even less information is available in the pediatric population.[8]

II. DRUGS IMPLICATED IN PULMONARY TOXICITY

A. Antineoplastic Agents

Busulfan (Myleran) was the first anticancer drug implicated in the development of pulmonary fibrosis in adults. Since the main therapeutic role of busulfan is in the treatment of chronic myelogenous leukemia, an uncommon form of leukemia in children, its use in children is limited.

Table 1
DRUGS REPORTED TO CAUSE
PULMONARY TOXICITY

I. Antineoplastic Agents
    A. Alkylating Agents
        1. Busulfan
        2. Chlorambucil
        3. Cyclophosphamide
        4. Melphalan
        5. Uracil Mustard
    B. Antibiotics
        1. Bleomycin
        2. Mitomycin-C
        3. Neocarzinostatin
    C. Nitrosoureas
        1. BCNU
        2. CCNU
        3. Chlorozotocin
        4. Methyl-CCNU
    D. Antimetabolites
        1. Azathioprine
        2. Cytosine arabinoside
        3. 6-Mercaptopurine
        4. Methotrexate
    E. Miscellaneous Agents
        1. Procarbazine
        2. Vinblastine
        3. VM-26
        4. Neocarzinostatin

II. Nonantineoplastic Agents
    A. Amiodarone
    B. Carbamazepine
    C. Cephalosporins
    D. Ergotamine
    E. Gold Salts
    F. Nitrofurantoin
    G. Penicillamine
    H. Sulfazalazine
    I. Tocainide

Pulmonary toxicity is most commonly seen in children treated with bleomycin and nitro-soureas. The incidence of toxicity is related to increasing cumulative doses with these agents. Many other chemotherapeutic agents, as well as other drugs, have been implicated in causing pulmonary toxicity (Table 1). A description of the clinical manifestations of these drug-induced pneumonitides follows.

1. Bleomycin

Bleomycin is a mixture of cytotoxic glycopeptide antibiotics isolated from *Streptomyces verticillus*. Its main use in pediatric oncology is against Hodgkin's disease[5,9] and malignant germ cell tumors.[10] The incidence of pulmonary toxicity varies widely across reports. The incidence of fatal bleomycin pulmonary toxicity is about 1 to 2%. An additional 2 to 3% of patients experience nonlethal pulmonary fibrosis. Other large reviews report the incidence of bleomycin-induced morbidity as high as 11%.[1] The incidence of toxicity is dose-related. At a total dose of less than 150 U, no life-threatening pulmonary disease occurred in 1,035 treated patients.[11] At total doses of bleomycin ≤400 to 500 U, there is a constant low incidence of pulmonary toxicity. This incidence significantly increases at doses ≥500 U.[1]

A 10% death rate due to pulmonary insufficiency has been documented in patients receiving a total dose $\geqslant$550 U.[12] Other risk factors include old age, pulmonary radiotherapy, pre-existing lung disease, and high inspired oxygen concentrations.[1,5,13-15]

The clinical manifestations of bleomycin-induced pulmonary toxicity include fever, non-productive hacking cough, and dyspnea.[1,5,11,13] Physical findings include tachypnea and fine crackling bibasilar rales.[1,11]

Pulmonary function tests may reveal arterial hypoxemia, a restrictive pattern, and decreased DLCO.[1,5,11,13,14] The earliest manifestation on chest radiograph is fine reticular bibasilar infiltrates that may progress to bibasilar alveolar and interstitial infiltrates, progressive lower lobe involvement, and lobar consolidation.[1] Microscopic examination reveals fibroblastic proliferation in alveolar septa and metaplasia of alveolar epithelium that is generally of greater severity than with other drugs.[4]

Careful monitoring of all patients receiving bleomycin and withdrawal of drug at the onset of symptomatology, radiographic abnormalities, or significant changes in pulmonary function is prudent and may prevent progressive pulmonary disease. Limiting the total dose of bleomycin to 400 U in adults will also lessen the risk of significant morbidity and mortality.

Although steroids have been used in the treatment of pulmonary toxicity, there is no known effective therapy for interstitial fibrosis. Patients who have the rare hypersensitivity type of bleomycin pulmonary toxicity manifested by fever, diffuse infiltrates, and eosinophilia may respond to steroids.[1]

2. The Nitrosoureas

The nitrosoureas are a group of synthetic alkylating agents that are a major cause of pulmonary toxicity.[16] In pediatric malignancies, BCNU (*bis*-chloroethylnitrosourea, carmustine) and CCNU (chloroethylcyclohexylnitrosourea, lomustine) are most commonly utilized in the therapy of primary brain tumors and non-Hodgkin's lymphomas.[17,18] The other nitrosoureas, such as methyl-CCNU (semustine), chlorozotocin, and streptozotocin, are infrequently administered to pediatric patients.

The incidence of pulmonary toxicity is dependent upon the cumulative dose received and the time since the administration of the agent.[1] Thus, the incidence of BCNU related pulmonary toxicity may be 20 to 30% in patients receiving a mean cumulative dose of 1000 to 1400 mg/m^2 (range 240 to 2400 mg/m^2).[1,19,20] Approximately 50% of patients develop pulmonary toxicity at total cumulative doses of 1500 mg/m^2.[18] The duration of time since exposure to the nitrosourea is also related to the incidence of toxicity. Patients receiving a smaller dose generally have a brief survival, whereas patients receiving larger doses have had remission or control of their malignancy, thus allowing for prolonged survival, administration of larger doses of chemotherapy, and a greater chance of developing toxicity. Nevertheless, the appearance of pulmonary symptomatology has been reported with a duration of treatment as short as 1 month and as long as 54 months.[6,16] Younger patients may be at increased risk of developing pulmonary toxicity since they can generally tolerate more nitrosourea than older patients.[1]

Exposure to high concentrations of inspired oxygen, concomitant pulmonary irradiation, combined therapy with cyclophosphamide, and pre-existing lung disease have all been implicated as risk factors in the development of nitrosourea-related pulmonary toxicity.[1,16,20]

The clinical presentation is usually manifested by the gradual onset of dyspnea, non-productive cough, and tachypnea.[1,4,15,16] Physical examination may be normal or bibasilar rales may be heard on auscultation. The chest radiograph may be normal or abnormal with decreased lung volume, bibasilar interstitial infiltrates with a reticulonodular pattern, and less commonly a pneumothorax may be present.[1] Pulmonary function studies show hypoxemia, a restrictive ventilatory pattern, and a decreased DLCO.[1,15,18] Histologically, fibroblastic proliferation of alveolar septae, metaplasia of alveolar epithelium, disappearance of type I pneumocytes, and proliferation of type II pneumocytes is seen.[13,15,16]

Discontinuation of the implicated drug at the earliest sign of pulmonary toxicity is the only proven effective therapy. Nevertheless, reported mortality rates range from 24 to 80%. There is no evidence that corticosteroids are of therapeutic benefit in the treatment or prevention of pulmonary toxicity.[1]

3. Busulfan

Busulfan (Myleran) is an alkylating agent that is commonly used in the long-term management of patients with chronic myelogenous leukemia.[21] It was the first chemotherapeutic agent to be associated with pulmonary toxicity.[22] An interstitial pneumonitis, "busulfan lung", has been recognized as an infrequent but serious and often fatal, complication of the long-term use of busulfan.[11,13] No clear relationship between the total dose of busulfan and the incidence of pulmonary toxicity exists. However, there may be a threshold phenomenon since pulmonary toxicity has not been reported at total doses of busulfan under 500 mg.[1]

A characteristic feature of busulfan lung is the long interval between the initiation of busulfan therapy and the onset of pneumonitis, with a mean time to presentation of 4 years and a range up to 8 to 10 years.[11,13]

The presentation includes an insidious onset of dyspnea, dry cough, and fever. Weakness and weight loss may occur. Tachypnea and bibasilar rales are characteristic. Cyanosis may be seen at presentation in the more severe cases.[1,11,13,23] The chest radiograph shows a diffuse intra-alveolar or interstitial process, or a combination of both.[13] Hypoxemia is commonly present, DLCO is decreased, and a restrictive ventilatory defect has sometimes been seen.[1]

Histological changes include atypia of the alveolar and bronchiolar epithelium with a background of interstitial and intra-alveolar edema and fibrosis. It is postulated that the cytotoxic drug effect on the alveolar epithelium results in the edema and fibrosis. The alveolar epithelial atypia is manifested by hyperplasia of type II pneumocytes, which are exfoliated into the sputum of patients with busulfan lung and may be helpful in the diagnosis.[13]

The clinical course is variable; however, most patients with busulfan-induced pulmonary toxicity have died of a progressive respiratory death.[1,11,13] In a few cases, improvement has been noted following cessation of busulfan.[1,11] The role of corticosteroids in reversing or stabilizing the pneumonitis is not clear, but it is probably generally not helpful.[1,11,23]

4. Cyclophosphamide

Cyclophosphamide (Cytoxan) is the most commonly utilized alkylating agent in children with neoplastic disease. It has therapeutic efficacy against a wide-spectrum of pediatric malignancies, including leukemias, lymphomas, sarcomas, germ cell tumors, neuroblastoma, and brain tumors. It is also used in the treatment of nonmalignant disorders, such as nephritis and collagen vascular disease.

In most of the reported cases of cyclophosphamide associated pulmonary toxicity, the patient had been treated with other drugs in addition to cyclophosphamide, had received pulmonary irradiation, or had prolonged oxygen exposure.[1] Thus, a definitive causal relationship is difficult to establish. Despite the widespread use of this drug, reported pulmonary toxicity is a rare event.[1,4,11,13] There does not appear to be a relationship between the dose or schedule of administration of cyclophosphamide or the duration of treatment and the development of pulmonary toxicity.[1,5] The onset of symptomatology may be as early as 1 month after instituting therapy or as late as 6 years after the discontinuation of cyclophosphamide.[1,14,15]

The clinical presentation includes dyspnea, nonproductive cough, and fever. The onset of symptomatology may be insidious, subacute or acute.[1,13,14] Physical findings may include tachypnea and fine rales. A radiograph of the chest typically demonstrates bilateral interstitial or interstitial and alveolar infiltrates. On rare occasions, the infiltrate may have a fibronodular appearance.[1] Pulmonary function tests demonstrate hypoxemia, a restrictive ventilatory pattern, and a decreased DLCO.[1] Histologic examination reveals a drug-induced alveolitis that results in a fibroblastic proliferation and eventual intra-alveolar fibrosis. Atypical type II pneumocytes are also a prominent pathologic finding.[13]

Recovery may occur following the discontinuation of cyclophosphamide and is usually seen within 1 to 8 weeks. The role of corticosteroids has not been defined.[1,11,13,14] Clinical improvement precedes radiographic improvement. Pulmonary function tests may also show marked improvement.[1] Nevertheless, one half of patients who developed pulmonary toxicity succumb to this complication.[1,13,14]

Although the relationship is ill-defined, cyclophosphamide may predispose patients to the development of pulmonary toxicity when they subsequently receive bleomycin, azathioprine, BCNU, or oxygen.[14]

5. Methotrexate

Methotrexate is a folate antagonist commonly used in pediatrics in the treatment of acute lymphocytic leukemia, non-Hodgkin's lymphoma, and osteosarcoma.[24] It is also used to treat various dermatologic and immunologic disorders.[23]

Three types of methotrexate related pulmonary toxicity have been described: a delayed type causing pulmonary parenchymal disease, an immediate type resulting in noncardiogenic pulmonary edema, and a syndrome of acute pleuritic chest pain.[1]

The delayed type of toxicity is the most common, although relatively unusual. The usual complaints of dyspnea, nonproductive cough, and fever may be present for days or weeks prior to seeking medical attention.[1,11] Headache and malaise have been described as common prodromal symptoms.[1,11,14] Tachypnea, crepitant rales, cyanosis in 50%, and skin eruptions in 16% of patients are the typical physical findings.

Radiograph of the chest may be normal at presentation. However, interstitial infiltrates located in the lung bases and mid-lung zones are typical. If disease progression occurs, alveolar infiltrates may develop and predominate. Hilar or mediastinal lymphadenopathy, pleural effusion, and unilateral infiltrates have been reported.[1,11,25]

Pulmonary function tests indicate hypocapnea, hypoxemia, restrictive ventilatory defect, and decreased DLCO. Residual abnormalities of pulmonary function may persist even after apparent clinical recovery.[1,11,25]

Histologic examination of the lung reveals diffuse alveolar damage with prominent hyaline membranes, and hyperplasia of the alveolar epithelium with desquamation and fibrosis. Interstitial infiltrates are composed predominantly of lymphocytes, but may also contain plasma cells and eosinophils.[11,25] The latter findings suggest that a hypersensitivity reaction may be the cause of this type of methotrexate-induced pulmonary toxicity.[7,8,11,13,25]

Pulmonary toxicity has been reported following the oral, intramuscular, intravenous, and intrathecal routes of administration.[1,11,15] There is no clear-cut relationship between dosage and the incidence of pulmonary toxicity. However, toxicity may be schedule-dependent since daily or weekly administration schedules are more likely to result in toxicity than administration every 2 to 4 weeks.[1] There is no correlation with age or presence of underlying disease. Patients may present from 12 days to 5 years after treatment with methotrexate.[1,14] The onset of methotrexate toxicity can be very abrupt or quite insidious.

The clinical course is generally self-limited and recovery from methotrexate-induced pulmonary toxicity commonly occurs, whether or not specific therapy is utilized or treatment with methotrexate is discontinued. However, the use of corticosteroids may lead to more rapid recovery, whereas the continued use of methotrexate may delay recovery.[1,13]

Methotrexate has also been associated with the development of noncardiogenic pulmonary edema and the syndrome of pleuritic chest pain. Noncardiogenic pulmonary edema has been described in three patients and has occurred within 6 to 12 hr following methotrexate administration.[1] The development of pleuritic chest pain has been reported in patients with trophoblastic tumors and osteogenic sarcoma. The etiology was not clear in most of these patients and did not always recur upon rechallenge with methotrexate.[1]

6. Cytosine Arabinoside

Cytosine arabinoside (ara-C) is a pyrimidine nucleoside analog which interferes with DNA synthesis. It is most efficacious in the treatment of acute nonlymphocytic leukemia and acute lymphocytic leukemia.[26] Unexplained fatal pulmonary edema observed at autopsy in patients with leukemia treated with ara-C has suggested a possible role of ara-C in causing increased alveolar capillary permeability.[27] Patients who had received ara-C within 30 days of their death showed significantly more frequent severe and moderate pulmonary edema and unexplained pulmonary edema than did patients who either had not received ara-C or had received it more than 30 days before death. Respiratory insufficiency was commonly seen prior to death in this group of patients, manifesting as tachypnea, hypoxemia, and the acute development of pulmonary infiltrates. Such toxicity was not necessarily fatal.

7. Other Antineoplastic Agents

Virtually all antineoplastic agents have been reported to cause pulmonary toxicity in at least several cases. As new agents are placed into clinical trials and then added to the armamentarium of the oncologist, the list continues to grow. Among other agents that have been implicated in the development of pulmonary toxicity are alkylating agents such as melphalan (Alkeran), chlorambucil (Leukeran), and uracil mustard, the antibiotic mitomycin-C (Mutamycin), other antimetabolites such as 6-mercaptopurine (Purinethol) and azathioprine (Imuran), and various miscellaneous agents including procarbazine hydrochloride (Matulane), VM-26 (Teniposide), vinblastine (Velban), and neocarzinostatin (Zinostatin).[1,5,14] The clinical manifestations of these agents are similar to those described above. The toxicity seen with procarbazine may be secondary to a hypersensitivity phenomenon.

B. Nonantineoplastic Agents

Although antineoplastic agents account for the majority of drug-induced causes of pulmonary toxicity, nonantineoplastic agents have also been implicated in causing such toxicity. The clinical manifestations are similar to those reported for the antineoplastic agents.

1. Nitrofurantoin

Of the nonantineoplastic agents, nitrofurantoin (Furadantin) is most commonly associated with pulmonary toxicity. Nitrofurantoin is a synthetic antimicrobial agent that is used in the treatment of urinary tract infections. Its use is associated with acute, subacute, and chronic hypersensitivity-related pulmonary reactions.[28,29]

Acute reactions are commonly manifested by fever, chills, cough, chest pain, and dyspnea. Eosinophilia is frequently seen. A radiograph of the chest may reveal pulmonary infiltration and consolidation or pleural effusion. Hypoxemia is a common feature. The acute reactions usually occur within the first week of treatment and are reversible with cessation of therapy. Such resolution may be dramatic. It has been suggested that this toxicity is hypersensitivity-related.[5]

Fever and eosinophilia are observed less often in patients with subacute toxicity. Recovery is slower than in patients with the acute toxicity, perhaps taking several months. Symptomatology may become more severe if nitrofurantoin is continued despite symptomatology.

Chronic toxicity is insidious in onset and is associated with the chronic use of nitrofurantoin. The insidious onset of malaise, dyspnea on exertion, and cough are common manifestations. Pulmonary function studies reveal a restrictive pattern and a decrease in DLCO. A diffuse interstitial pattern is seen on a radiograph of the chest. Pathologically, nonspecific interstitial pneumonitis and/or fibrosis is common.[28,29] If nitrofurantoin is promptly withdrawn after the first clinical signs of pulmonary toxicity appear, the chances for recovery are good. However, pulmonary function may be permanently impaired even after cessation of nitrofurantoin, especially if its use is not discontinued early.

2. Penicillamine

Penicillamine (Cuprimine) is a chelating agent indicated in the treatment of Wilson's disease, cystinuria, and in selected patients with severe, active rheumatoid arthritis. It has been associated with an allergic alveolitis, obliterative bronchiolitis, interstitial pneumonitis, and pulmonary fibrosis.[30]

3. Amiodarone

Amiodarone is an antiarrhythmic drug which has been reported to cause pulmonary fibrosis when used chronically.[31-34] In one report, it was suggested that the mechanism of toxicity was hypersensitivity. The pathologic findings include nonspecific alveolar wall fibrosis. Withdrawal of amiodarone, and perhaps the use of corticosteroid therapy, are very important for recovery.

4. Other Nonantineoplastic Agents

A spectrum of other nonantineoplastic agents have been implicated in the development of pulmonary toxicity. In general, the reports of toxicity for these drugs are limited. Included in the implicated agents are the cephalosporins,[35] carbamazepine,[36] sulfazalazine,[37] tocainide,[38] ergotamine,[39] and gold salts.[40,41]

ACKNOWLEDGMENT

The authors thank Ms. Kathleen Bardon for her secretarial assistance.

REFERENCES

1. **Ginsberg, S. J. and Comis, R. L.,** The pulmonary toxicity of antineoplastic agents, in *Toxicity of Chemotherapy*, Perry, M. C. and Yarbro, J. W., Eds., Grune & Stratton, New York, 1984, 227.
2. **Brettner, A., Heitzman, E. R., and Woodin, W. G.,** Pulmonary complications of drug therapy, *Radiology*, 96, 31, 1970.
3. **Adamson, I. Y. R. and Bowden, D. H.,** The pathogenesis of bleomycin-induced pulmonary fibrosis in mice, *Am. J. Pathol.*, 77, 185, 1974.
4. **Muggia, F. M., Louie, A. C., and Sikic, B. I.,** Pulmonary toxicity of antitumor agents, *Cancer Treat. Rev.*, 10, 221, 1983.
5. **Kercsmar, C. M. and Boat, T. F.,** Lung diseases caused by chemotherapeutic agents, in *Disorders of the Respiratory Tract in Children*, 4th ed., Kendig, E. L., Jr. and Chernick, V., Eds., W.B. Saunders, Philadelphia, 1983.
6. **Klein, D. S. and Wilds, P. R.,** Pulmonary toxicity of antineoplastic agents: anaesthetic and postoperative implications, *Can. Anaesth. Soc. J.*, 30, 399, 1983.
7. **Sostman, H. D., Putman, C. E., and Gamsu, G.,** Diagnosis of chemotherapy lung, *Am. J. Roentgenol.*, 136, 33, 1981.
8. **Platzker, A. C. G., Hindman, B., and Pysher, T. J.,** Interstitial pneumonitis and pleural effusion in a one-year-old child with an abdominal tumor, *J. Pediatr.*, 98, 497, 1981.
9. **Bonadonna, G. and Santoro, A.,** ABVD chemotherapy in the treatment of Hodgkin's disease, *Cancer Treat. Rev.*, 9, 21, 1982.
10. **Einhorn, L. H. and Williams, S. D.,** Chemotherapy of disseminated testicular cancer, a random prospective study, *Cancer*, 46, 1339, 1980.
11. **Sostman, H. D., Matthay, R. A., and Putman, C. E.,** Cytotoxic drug-induced lung disease, *Am. J. Med.*, 62, 608, 1977.

12. **Blum, R. H., Carter, S. K., and Agre, K.,** A clinical review of bleomycin — a new antineoplastic agent, *Cancer,* 31, 903, 1973.
13. **Willson, J. K. V.,** Pulmonary toxicity of neoplastic drugs, *Cancer Treat. Rep.,* 62, 2003, 1978.
14. **Batist, G. and Andrews, J. L., Jr.,** Pulmonary toxicity of antineoplastic drugs, *JAMA,* 246, 1449, 1981.
15. **Weiss, R. B. and Muggia, F. M.,** Cytotoxic drug-induced pulmonary disease: update 1980, *Am. J. Med.,* 68, 259, 1980.
16. **Weiss, R. B., Poster, D. S., and Penta, J. S.,** The nitrosoureas and pulmonary toxicity, *Cancer Treat. Rev.,* 8, 111, 1981.
17. **Anderson, J. R., Wilson, J. F., Jenkin, R. D. T., Meadows, A. T., Kersey, J., Chilcote, R. R., Coccia, P., Exelby, P., Kushner, J., Siegel, S., and Hammond, D.,** Childhood non-Hodgkin's lymphoma, the results of a randomized therapeutic trial comparing a 4-drug regimen (COMP) with a 10-drug regimen (LSA2-L2), *N. Engl. J. Med.,* 308, 559, 1983.
18. **Aronin, P. A., Mahaley, M. S., Jr., Rudnick, S. A., Dudka, L., Donohue, J. F., Selker, R. G., and Moore, P.,** Prediction of BCNU pulmonary toxicity in patients with malignant gliomas. An assessment of risk factors, *N. Engl. J. Med.,* 303, 183, 1980.
19. **Selker, R. G., Jacobs, S. A., Moore, P. B., Wald, M., Fisher, E. R., Cohen, M., and Bellot, P.,** 1-3-Bis (2-chloroethyl)-1-nitrosourea (BCNU) induced pulmonary fibrosis, *Neurosurgery,* 7, 560, 1980.
20. **Durant, J. R., Norgard, M. J., Murad, T. M., Bartolucci, A. A., and Langford, K. H.,** Pulmonary toxicity associated with bischloroethylnitrosourea (BCNU), *Ann. Intern. Med.,* 90, 191, 1979.
21. **Bolin, R. W., Robinson, W. A., Sutherland, J., and Hamman, R. F.,** Busulfan versus hydroxyurea in long-term therapy of chronic myelogenous leukemia, *Cancer,* 50, 1683, 1982.
22. **Oliner, H., Schwartz, R., Rubio, F., Jr., and Dameshek, W.,** Interstitial pulmonary fibrosis following busulfan therapy, *Am. J. Med.,* 31, 134, 1961.
23. **Oakhill, A., Green, I. D., Knowlson, G. T., Cameron, A. H., Shah, K. J., Hill, F. G. H., and Mann, J. R.,** Busulphan lung in childhood, *J. Clin. Pathol.,* 34, 495, 1981.
24. **Bleyer, W. A.,** Methotrexate: clinical pharmacology, current status and therapeutic guidelines, *Cancer Treat. Rev.,* 4, 87, 1977.
25. **Iyer, R., Ravindranath, Y., Kulkarni, R., Philippart, A., Reed, J. O., Brough, A. J., and Zuelzer, W. W.,** Bilateral interstitial pneumonia in acute lymphoblastic leukemia, *Am. J. Hematol.,* 1, 225, 1976.
26. **Capizzi, R. L., Powell, B. L., Cooper, M. R., Stuart, J. J., Muss, H. B., Richards, F., II, Jackson, D. V., White, D. R., Spurr, C. L., Zekan, P. J., Cruz, J. M., and Craig, J. B.,** Sequential high-dose ara-C and asparaginase in the therapy of previously treated and untreated patients with acute leukemia, *Sem. Oncol.,* 12, (Suppl. 13), 105, 1985.
27. **Haupt, H. M., Hutchins, G. M., and Moore, G. W.,** Ara-C lung: noncardiogenic pulmonary edema complicating cytosine arabinoside therapy of leukemia, *Am. J. Med.,* 70, 256, 1981.
28. **Qureshi, M. M.,** Interstitial lung disease caused by chronic nitrofurantoin reaction: case report, *Wis. Med. J.,* 83, 20, 1984.
29. **Jayasundera, N. S., Johnson, R. D., and Nicholson, D. P.,** Chronic pulmonary reaction to nitrofurantoin, *JAMA,* 243, 769, 1980.
30. **Shettar, S. P., Chattopadhyay, C., Wolstenholme, R. J., and Swinson, D. R.,** Diffuse alveolitis on a small dose of Penicillamine, *Br. J. Rheum.,* 23, 220, 1984.
31. **Morera, J., Vidal, R., Morell, F., Ruiz, J., Bernado, L. L., and Laporte, J. R.,** Amiodarone and pulmonary fibrosis, *Eur. J. Clin. Pharmacol.,* 24, 591, 1983.
32. **Sobol, S. M. and Rakita, L.,** Pneumonitis and pulmonary fibrosis associated with amiodarone treatment: a possible complication of a new antiarrhythmic drug, *Circulation,* 65, 819, 1982.
33. **Harris, L., McKenna, W. J., Rowland, E., Hold, D. W., Storey, G. C. A., and Krikler, D. M.,** Side effects of long-term amiodarone therapy, *Circulation,* 67, 45, 1983.
34. **Akoun, G. M., Gauthier-Rahman, S., Milleron, B. J., Perrot, J. Y., and Mayaud, C. M.,** Amiodarone-induced hypersensitivity pneumonitis. Evidence of an immunological cell-mediated mechanism, *Chest,* 85, 133, 1984.
35. **Dreis, D. F., Winterbauer, R. H., Van Norman, G. A., Sullivan, S. L., and Hammar, S. P.,** Cephalosporin-induced interstitial pneumonitis, *Chest,* 86, 138, 1984.
36. **de Swert, L. F., Ceuppens, J. L., Teuwen, D., Wijndaele, L., Casaer, P., and Casteels-van Daele, M.,** Acute interstitial pneumonitis and carbamazepine therapy, *Acta Paediatr. Scand.,* 73, 285, 1984.
37. **Sigvaldason, A. and Sorenson, S.,** Interstitial pneumonia due to sulfasalazine, *Eur. J. Respir. Dis.,* 64, 229, 1983.
38. **Perlow, G. M., Jain, B. P., Pauker, S. G., Zarren, H. S., Wistran, D. C., and Epstein, R. L.,** Tocainide-associated interstitial pneumonitis, *Ann. Intern. Med.,* 94, 489, 1981.
39. **Taal, B. G., Spierings, E. L. H., and Hilvering, C.,** Pleuropulmonary fibrosis associated with chronic and excessive intake of ergotamine, *Thorax,* 38, 396, 1983.
40. **Nickels, J., van Assendelft, A. H. W., and Tukiainen, P.,** Diffuse pulmonary injury associated with gold treatment, *Acta Pathol. Microbiol. Immunol. Scand.,* 91, 265, 1983.
41. **Heyd, J. and Simmeran, A.,** Gold-induced lung disease, *Postgrad. Med. J.,* 59, 368, 1983.

Chapter 32

GASTROESOPHAGEAL REFLUX AND INTERSTITIAL PNEUMONIA

Daniel V. Schidlow

TABLE OF CONTENTS

I. INTRODUCTION

Gastroesophageal reflux (GER) is defined as the retrograde passage of stomach contents into the esophagus. This condition can be asymptomatic or associated with regurgitation, recurrent vomiting, esophagitis, failure to thrive, and anemia. Aspiration of gastric juice and food particles into the respiratory tree can cause complications ranging from mild, recurrent bronchospasm, to severe necrotizing pneumonias, lung fibrosis, apnea, and death.

Decreased lower esophageal sphincter (LES) pressure is frequently due to physiologic immaturity of this area, hence, symptomatic GER tends to be more frequent and severe in younger infants. This condition, however, is seen in older children and adults as well. Severe central nervous system and neuromuscular disorders predispose to GER because of dysfunction of the swallowing mechanism, frequently present in these patients. Gastroesophageal reflux and aspiration can be particularly frequent and severe in children after repair of esophageal atresia and tracheoesophageal fistula and in children with severe neuromuscular defects. These individuals frequently exhibit marked esophageal dysmotility and LES relaxation.

Theophylline, caffeine, chocolate, and a variety of other substances decrease LES pressure and predispose to GER. Laryngospasm due to direct contact of gastric acid with the larynx has been implicated in the pathogenesis of apneic episodes associated with GER.

II. LUNG DISEASE AND GER

The association of GER and interstitial lung disease has been sufficiently documented in the literature, but a cause-effect relationship between these two conditions cannot always be proven. Repeated episodes of pneumonia, in the presence of clinical and laboratory evidence of GER, particularly when the respiratory symptoms are temporally related to episodes of regurgitation and vomiting, are suggestive of a direct relationship. Massive aspiration of gastric fluid produces diffuse alveolar damage, hemorrhage, and necrotizing bronchiolitis. Interstitial reaction follows very rapidly with acute inflammatory polymorphonuclear cell infiltration in the interalveolar septae. Bronchiolitis obliterans and fibrosis can eventually supervene. The clinical picture resembles that of the adult respiratory distress syndrome. Inhalation of milk per se can cause severe inflammatory reaction and hemorrhage in the lung, polymorphonuclear infiltration, macrophage migration into the alveoli, and interstitial fibrosis. Repeated aspiration of smaller amounts of gastric acid can also lead to pneumonia, bronchitis, and bronchiectasis, as well as fibrosis of the pulmonary interstitium.

We have uncovered a direct relationship between GER, aspiration, and bronchiolitis obliterans with interstitial pneumonia in 5 patients out of a series of 18 children with obliterative bronchiolitis followed in our Center. In three infants, the bronchiolar changes were detected in the post-mortem examination, after they succumbed to acute respiratory failure. The case of one infant with necrotizing bronchiolitis and pneumonia secondary to GER is illustrated in Figures 1 and 2.

III. CLINICAL PICTURE

The clinical picture of GER can be quite variable and depends on the frequency and severity of the reflux episodes. Gastrointestinal symptoms include dysphagia, rumination, easy regurgitation, and vomiting, especially in the supine position. In older children and adolescents, heartburn, acid-bitter taste, abdominal pain, or retrosternal pain can be present. Infants may become very irritable and exhibit poor sleeping patterns. Severe esophagitis can lead to hypochromic, microcytic anemia due to repeated bleeding. Chronic respiratory symptoms include cough, wheezing, and choking episodes which in their most severe form can

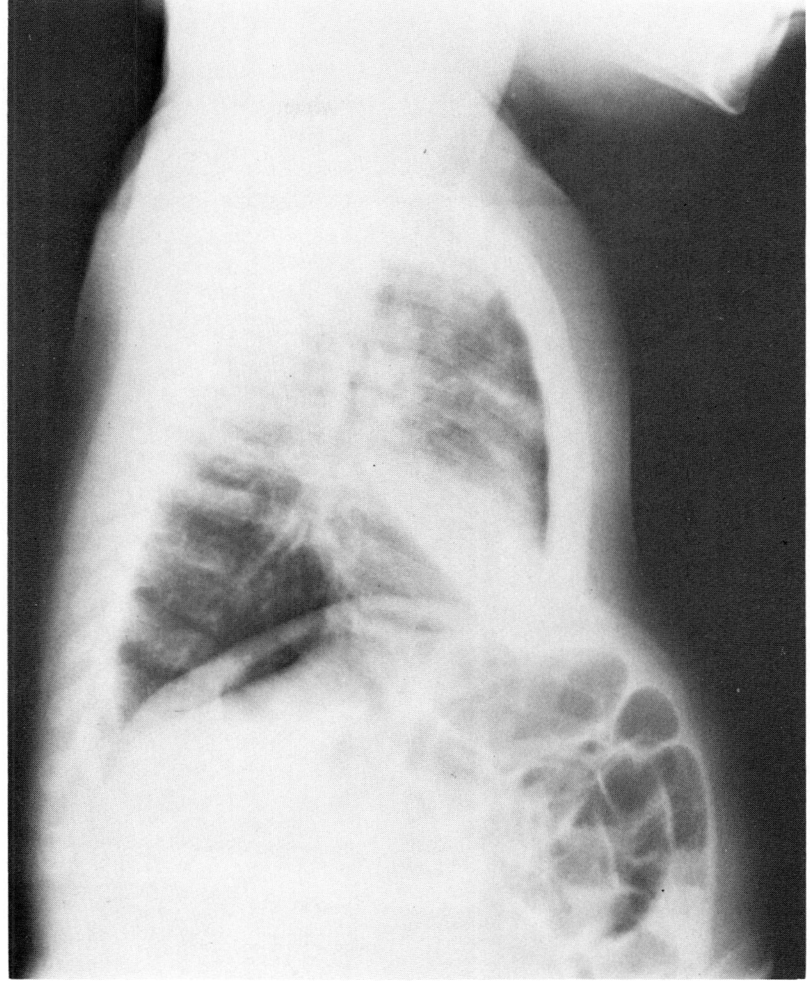

A

FIGURE 1.   Chest radiograph of an 8-month-old boy with GER showing diffuse bilateral interstitial and alveolar densities as well as right middle lobe infiltration. (A) Anteroposterior view. (B) Lateral view.

result in apneic spells (''near miss'' sudden infant death syndrome). Any one of the above can be the only manifestation of the condition.

IV. DIAGNOSIS

The radiographic appearance of the chest can vary from slight overinflation to a pattern of diffuse interstitial and alveolar densities (Figure 1). Barium esophagram and fluoroscopy allows the evaluation of esophageal motility and the detection of esophagitis. This technique is not very sensitive in that it only reflects one point in time, at which GER may or may not be present; hence, while a barium esophagram showing reflux is diagnostic, a negative study does not rule it out.

Radionuclide studies (''milk scan'') permits the observation of esophageal function for 1 hr after the administration of a bolus of milk or juice containing a radioactive tracer.

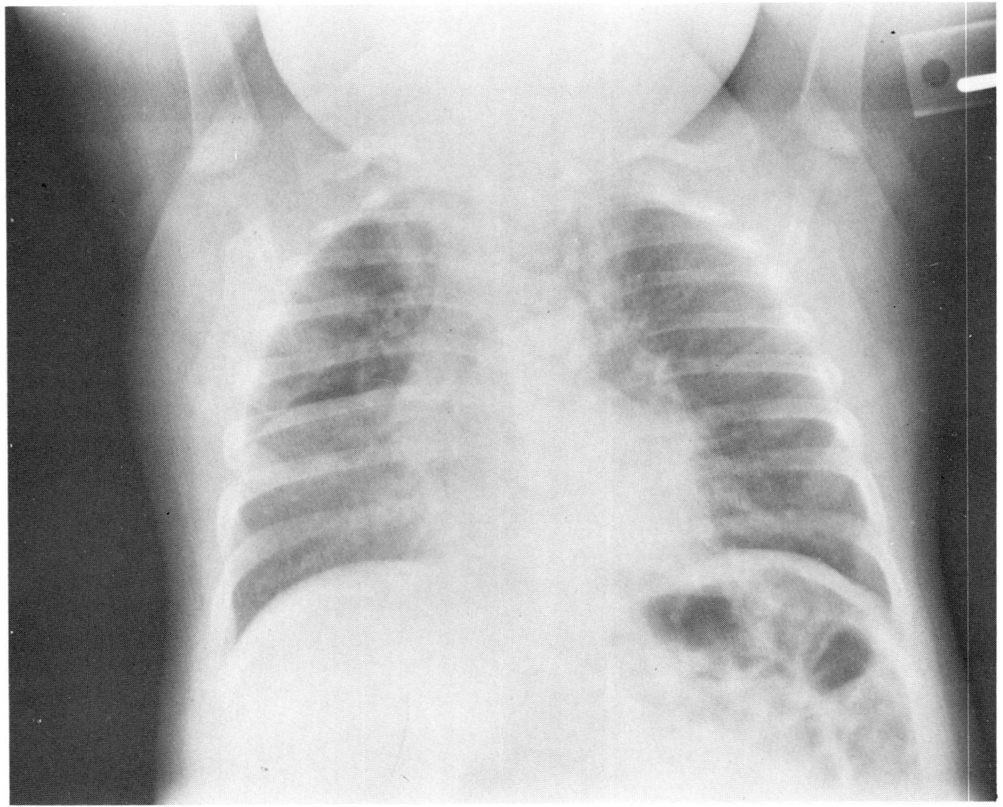

FIGURE 1B

Frequency and severity of reflux, as well as esophageal and gastric dysmotility (i.e., delayed emptying) can be detected. If aspiration occurs, the radionuclide can occasionally be detected in the lung fields.

Esophageal motility and intraluminal pressures, especially at the level of the LES, can be studied by means of manometry; pH measurement is probably the most useful test in that it allows long-term monitoring of acid reflux (up to 24 hr) by detecting the frequency, duration, and intensity of falls in intraesophageal pH. This test is the most helpful in correlating the presence of GER episodes with clinical events. Esophagoscopy is indicated to assess the extent of mucosal inflammation by direct visualization and to obtain biopsy specimens.

The examination of tracheal and bronchoalveolar fluid for lipid-laden macrophages has been suggested as a potentially useful test in the diagnosis of aspiration secondary to GER. Lipid-laden macrophages are encountered more often, in higher numbers, and contain more fat in patients who aspirate than in patients whose lung disease is not due to aspiration.

V. TREATMENT

The treatment of GER is directed to the prevention of the sliding of stomach contents into the esophagus and decreasing the risk of esophagitis and aspiration. Medical therapy includes positioning the infant upright or preferably prone at a 30° angle, with or without

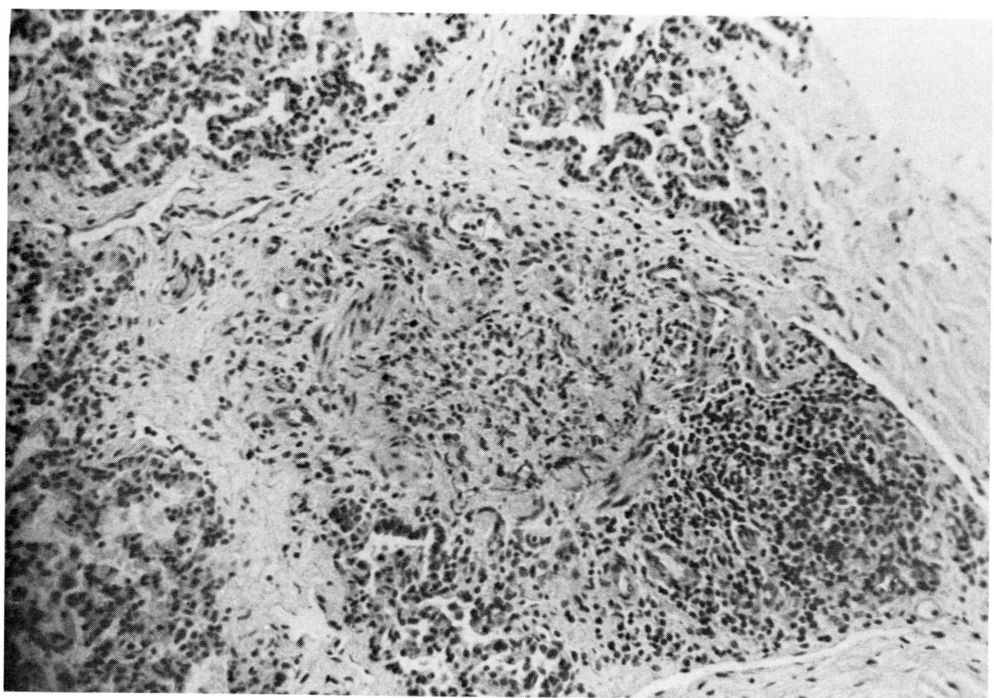

FIGURE 2.   Lung biopsy specimen of the same patient shows necrotizing bronchiolitis and interstitial inflammation. In the center of the photograph is a bronchiole; the lumen is filled with inflammatory infiltration and there is loss of the normal bronchiolar epithelial lining. The architecture of the surrounding alveoli is basically preserved but there is thickening and inflammatory infiltration of the interalveolar septae. (Picture courtesy of Nazere Zaeri, M.D., Department of Pathology, St. Christopher's Hospital for Children, Philadelphia, PA.)

the use of a harness, and thickening of feedings. Bronchodilators may be given to those children with bronchospasm who seem to respond to these drugs. We prefer the use of beta-2 agonist drugs to theophylline because of the latter's effect in decreasing LES pressure. Antacid preparations, cimetidine, and other inhibitors of H2 gastric receptors, can be used to decrease acid production or neutralize its effects. Bethanecol increases the LES pressure, however, its use in children with bronchospasm is restricted because of its broncho-constricting effect. Metoclopramide (Reglan®) can be used before meals to improve LES function and gastric emptying. Anti-reflux surgery is indicated after failure of medical therapy, in life threatening situations or in children with severe esophageal dysmotility in whom recovery is not foreseen.

VI. SUMMARY

In summary, GER in its more severe form can lead to lung damage, particularly interstitial fibrosis, and bronchiectasis. In the vast majority of children, however, this condition has a milder clinico-pathologic picture which improves with time or appropriate therapy.

REFERENCES

1. **Berquist, W. E., Rachelefsky, G. S., Kadden, M., Siegel, S. C., Katz, R. M., Fonkalsrud, E. W., and Ament, M. E.**, Gastroesophageal reflux-associated recurrent pneumonia and chronic asthma in children, *Pediatrics,* 68, 29, 1981.
2. **Christie, D. L., O'Grady, L. R., and Mack, D. V.**, Incompetent lower esophageal sphincter and gastroesophageal reflux in recurrent acute pulmonary disease of infancy and childhood, *J. Pediatr.,* 93, 23, 1978.
3. **Herbst, J. J.**, Gastroesophageal reflux, *J. Pediatr.,* 98, 59, 1981.
4. **Katzenstein, A. L. and Askin, F. B.**, Surgical pathology of non-neoplastic lung disease, in *Major Problems in Pathology,* Vol. 13, W.B. Saunders, Philadelphia, 1984, p. 356.
5. **Kennedy, J. H.**, "Silent" gastroesophageal reflux, an important but little known cause of pulmonary complications, *Dis. Chest.,* 42, 42, 1962.
6. **Krantman, H. J., Rachelefsky, G. S., Lipson, M., and Fonkalsrud, E. A.**, Recurrent pulmonary infiltrates, digital clubbing, and failure to thrive in a 4-year-old boy, *J. Allergy Clin. Immunol.,* 61, 403, 1978.
7. **Mays, E. E., Dubois, J. J., and Hamilton, G. B.**, Pulmonary fibrosis associated with tracheobronchial aspiration, *Chest,* 69, 512, 1976.
8. **Pearson, J. E. G. and Wilson, R. S. E.**, Diffuse pulmonary fibrosis and hiatus hernia, *Thorax,* 26, 300, 1971.
9. **Spencer, H.**, *Pathology of the Lung,* Vol. 1, Pergamon Press, Elmsford, N.Y., 468.
10. **Hardy, K., Schidlow, D., Zaeri, N., et al.**, Obliterative bronchitis in children, in press.
11. **Nussbaum, E., Maggi, J. C., Mathis, R., and Galant, S. P.**, Association of lipid-laden macrophages and gastroesophageal reflux in children, *J. Pediatr.,* 110, 190, 1987.
12. **Corwin, R. W. and Irwin, R. S.**, The lipid-laden alveolar macrophage as a marker of aspiration in parenchymal lung disease, *Am. Rev. Respir. Dis.,* 132, 576, 1985.

Chapter 33

METABOLIC, DEGENERATIVE, AND UNCLASSIFIED CONDITIONS ASSOCIATED WITH INTERSTITIAL LUNG DISEASE

Lourdes R. Laraya-Cuasay

TABLE OF CONTENTS

I. STORAGE DISORDER

A. Hermansky-Pudlak Syndrome

1. Introduction

Originally described in 1959 by Hermansky and Pudlak in two Czechoslovakian patients,[1] this rare congenital disorder is now known to be transmitted on an autosomal recessive basis and has multisystem involvement. The syndrome is the triad of partial oculocutaneous albinism, qualitative platelet defect, and ceroid accumulation in the reticuloendothelial system. About 200 cases have been reported in the world literature with predominance of patients from Southern Holland and the Arecibo region of Puerto Rico. Most reported cases in North America have been in Puerto Ricans. The youngest reported patients were 11 and 12 years of age, both Puerto Rican females who presented nystagmus and easy bleeding, and whose pulmonary function tests were normal.[2] The third case reported by Garay and colleagues was a 20-year-old Puerto Rican female who bled during dental extraction, and who had mild exertional dyspnea, reticulonodular densities radiographically, and a restrictive pulmonary defect.[3] Her siblings had albinism and colitis. Pulmonary interstitial fibrosis is the result of ceroid accumulation in alveolar macrophages. Davies and Tuddenham, studying a group of patients with previously diagnosed platelet function defect and another group of unrelated albinos, found a possible relationship between platelet function defect and pulmonary fibrosis.[4]

Schinella and associates reported ultrastructural studies that seem to indicate that Hermansky-Pudlak syndrome (HPS) was a disorder of lysosomal function similar to other lysosomal storage diseases. Ceroid pigment accumulates in single membrane-bound cytoplasmic organelles. Larger accumulations cause a "ballooned" appearance of macrophages with cell damage from release of lysosomal enzymes.[2] A deficiency of the lysosomal enzyme Phospholipase A has been demonstrated in the platelets of one patient.[5] Phospholipase deficiency affects prostaglandin metabolism and leads to platelet storage pool defects.[5]

2. Clinical Manifestations

The patients are albinos who usually come from the Arecibo region of Puerto Rico. They often have blond or reddish brownish hair, fair skin, and marked freckling on sun-exposure. The pigment disorder in HPS has variable phenotype expression depending on racial background.[3] Puerto Ricans who present with red or reddish brown hair and who may have some skin and eye pigmentation would look very much like Caucasians. Their regional origin may be the only important clue to the diagnosis. Rotary, horizontal or vertical nystagmus may be present. Any young Puerto Rican patient who has extreme freckling in sun-exposed areas of the skin or who has actinic keratosis should be worked up for the syndrome.

Menorrhagia, bleeding from dental extractions, easy bruisability, and occasional transient and mild hemoptyses during acute infections are frequent.

Insidious development of dyspnea on effort, digital clubbing, and basal inspiratory crackles are usual when chest roentgenograms show diffuse pulmonary infiltrates. These signs and symptoms are common in late adolescence to young adulthood.

3. Laboratory Features

Slit lamp examination and iris transillumination help diagnose tyrosine-positive albinism.[2] Patients have prolonged bleeding time, increased prothrombin consumption index, and qualitative platelet defects. Platelets fail to develop irreversible aggregation, a typical finding in platelet storage pool deficiency.

When viewed with ultraviolet light, the urine shows cytoplasmic granules with intense orange red fluorescence. Buccal scrapings may show similar findings. Chromosomal studies do not show any chromosomal breakage.[2]

Pulmonary function tests show a restrictive pattern with mild to moderate reduction in expiratory flow rates at all lung volumes without evidence of dysfunction at low lung volumes.[3] Arterial hypoxemia at rest is found in more severe cases. Diffusion capacity is reduced.

Chest roentgenograms may show diffuse interstitial infiltrates, either streaky or reticulonodular, later progressing to cystic or honeycomb lung appearance.[2-4]

4. Pathologic Features

Lung biopsy specimens show diffuse interstitial fibrosis in the alveolar septae and peribronchial fibrosis. Ceroid-like material fill alveolar macrophages. Collagen and elastic fibers are seen within the fibrous tissue that almost completely replace the parenchyma. There is no evidence of increased macrophage number in the interstitium. The ceroid-like material stain positively with periodic acid-Schiff stain and weakly-positive with Ziehl-Neilsen acid-fast stain. Fontana's stain for melanin is positive. Intense orange fluorescence of the finely divided brown pigment within the alveolar macrophages is appreciated with ultraviolet illumination. Electron microscopy shows the macrophages to contain a mixture of amorphous particulate debris (ceroid-like material) and lipid-filled vacuoles of varying sizes. No membrane enclose the pigment. Fine vacuolization is often observed in the pigment and is most prominent in bone marrow, liver, spleen, lung, and oral epithelium, with the gut and kidney showing less vacuolization. Pulmonary fibrosis is common and usually severe.

The pigment accumulations in the kidney is heaviest in the renal tubular epithelium, within macrophages. In granulomatous colitis, large numbers of pigment-filled macrophages distend the sinusoids of mesenteric lymph nodes.

Hairbulb and skin show ultrastructurally decreased melanosomes in both keratinocytes and melanocytes. Melanosomes, both premelanosome and incomplete melanosome (pheomelanosome) are considerably more in the hairbulb than in the unexposed skin.

The meninges have ceroid pigment. The substantia nigra and locus ceruleus are normally pigmented.

5. Management

The use of acetylsalicylic acid or prostaglandin blockers potentiate the hemostatic defect and *must* be avoided. Patients are cautioned against excessive sun exposure. Use of cryoprecipitate for necessary surgery is recommended.

Patients who have pulmonary fibrosis must be carefully monitored for the occurrence of viral, bacterial, or mycoplasmal infections and aggressively treated accordingly. Rapid deterioration in pulmonary function can follow acute infections especially in those with severe pulmonary fibrosis. Genetic counseling has to be given as 25% recurrence risk is present.

6. Prognosis

Decreased longevity results from severe pulmonary fibrosis, massive uncontrollable bleeding, and inflammatory bowel disease.

B. Pulmonary Lipidosis

Pulmonary lipidosis is a condition characterized by the intracellular deposition of a variety of lipid substances in the fixed and mobile macrophage cells, and in certain specialized cells, particularly the central nervous system (CNS). Gaucher disease and Niemann-Pick disease affect the lungs most commonly so that discussion will be confined to these two rare disorders.

1. Gaucher Disease

a. Introduction

Gaucher disease (GD)[6,7] is a glucosylceramide lipidosis caused by the deficiency of glycosyluramidase. An infantile form is characterized by early onset, marked hepatosplenomegaly and severe neurological progression to early death. A juvenile form with milder neurological involvement exists. The adult form of the disease may be the most commonly encountered lysosomal storage disease.

GD is often familial. The stored lipid is a cerebroside known as kerasin.

b. Clinical Features

All forms of GD have an autosomal recessive genetic basis. The disorder is about 30 times more frequent in Ashkenazi Jews. Manifestations include hepatosplenomegaly, hypersplenism, bleeding diathesis, bone pain, pathological fractures, and pulmonary involvement with associated pneumonia.

Clinical course is variable. Pulmonary involvement may lead to early death, but in many patients, life span is not shortened by the disease. Recurrent aspiration and chronic bronchopneumonia may lead to death usually at 6 to 18 months of age. Both infant and adult forms can lead to cor pulmonale. Bleeding is secondary to thrombocytopenia and this frequently responds to splenectomy with considerable benefit. Renal involvement with severe proteinuric nephropathy occurs.

c. Pathologic, Laboratory, and Radiographic Features

The Gaucher cell is a large round or polyhedral phagocyte, 20 to 100 μm in diameter containing one or more small eccentrically placed nuclei and a pale striated cytoplasm resembling tissue paper or crumpled silk. Electronmicroscopic findings show the fibrillary network consisting of numerous dilated sac-like structures resembling lysosomes containing tubules similar to twisted bilayers characteristic of glucocerebroside deposits. Periodic acid Schiff stain is strongly positive. This distinctive storage cell occurs in the bone marrow in all forms of GD.

Serum acid phosphatase is characteristically elevated. Enzyme assay of activity of glucosylceramide-B-D-glucosidase in leukocytes or cultured fibroblasts is used to diagnose relatives even if still asymptomatic, as well as confirm the disease. Enzyme assay should be performed because the Gaucher cell may also be found in patients with granulocytic leukemia and myeloma.

Glucosylceramide is increased two- to threefold in plasma and greater than 200 times in spleen and liver. Prenatal diagnosis is possible using cultured amniotic cells.

Diffuse pulmonary infiltration with direct involvement of alveoli, pleura and interstitium leads to dyspnea and cor pulmonale.[8]

d. Management

Intravenous injections of purified placental B-glucosidase in a few patients show promising results in non-neuropathic GD. Partial splenectomy to preserve splenic tissue as potential reservoir for glucosylceramide and to relieve mechanical pressure is useful. Bone marrow transplantation may have beneficial results.

e. Prognosis

Longevity in the infantile neuronopathic type varies from 2 to 3 years. Patients with the subacute type may live to their third decade. The frequency of the disease and the lack of neurological involvement in the adult form of GD is particularly worthy of research efforts to develop enzyme replacement therapy.

2. Niemann-Pick Disease
a. Introduction

Niemann-Pick disease (ND)[7-9] is a sphingomyelin lipidosis. The lipid material has been identified as the phospholipid sphingomyelin and five main clinical subvarieties of the disorder are recognized. It is often a familial condition which becomes manifest in early infancy and leads to death of the child before puberty.

b. Clinical Features

In clinical types A and B, there is a clear deficiency of sphingomyelinase, an enzyme that hydrolyzes sphingomyelin to yield ceramide and phosphorylcholine. The most common disorder is type A, the infantile neuronopathic disorder which begins shortly after birth with hepatosplenomegaly, failure to thrive, and neurological impairment. Retinal cherry spots occur, but seizures and hypersplenism are rare. Ashkenazi Jews usually have type A.

Type B is a relatively benign disorder with hepatosplenomegaly, sphingomyelinase deficiency, and sometimes pulmonary infiltrates, but there is *no* neurological involvement. These patients are most susceptible to pneumonia. Diffuse pulmonary infiltrates are found in chest radiographs.

Type C disease is characterized by sphingomyelin lipidosis, progressive neurological deterioration in childhood, and substantial or normal sphingomyelinase activity.

Type D resembles type C but is separated primarily on the basis of occurrence in a Nova Scotian population and usual occurrence in Catholics.

Type E describes a group of adult patients with visceral sphingomyelin lipidosis without neurological involvement and without sphingomyelinase deficiency.

The biochemical basis for ND types C, D, and E is not understood. Many patients described with the seablue histiocyte syndrome may have sphingomyelinase deficiency.

c. Pathologic, Radiologic Features, and Laboratory

The diagnosis can be made with considerable confidence by recognition of the distinctive Niemann-Pick cell in the bone marrow, but this should be confirmed by enzyme assay.

Tissues most frequently involved include the CNS, liver, spleen, lymph glands, adrenals, and lungs, although almost all organs contain the typical lipid-filled phagocytes. The lungs are airless, pale, and rubbery. Microscopically, lipid-laden macrophages are found both in interstitial tissues and lying free in the alveoli. Alveolar walls, peribronchial and perivascular areas, subpleural and interlobular connective tissue contain the interstitial collections of lipid-laden cells. The cells vary in size from 20 to 90 μm with very small nuclei with thick nuclear membrane containing up to four nucleoli. The nuclei are found anywhere within the cell, sometimes displaced towards the outer wall, and in others occupying a central position. The Touton cells are giant cell forms of the cells containing up to 20 nuclei often arranged around a central, more deeply staining eosinophilic and homogeneous mass. Special staining characteristics of the intracellular contents have been found with varying color response to various lipid stains. Electron-microscopic examination of the sphingomyelin deposits in alveolar macrophages shows membrane-bound cytoplasmic bodies with vacuolated structure. At high magnification, a lamellar structure with alternating osmiophilic and osmiophobic layers and at a periodicity of 5 μm are seen. This measurement of periodicity distinguishes sphingomyelin from other forms of lipid storage disease.

These foam cells should be differentiated from the foam cells in fucosidosis, mannosidosis, GM_1 gangliosidosis, Sandhoff's disease, Wolman's disease, and I-cell disease. These foam cells are frequently present in alveoli, lymphatic vessels, and branches of the pulmonary arteries, but are rarely found in sputum.

A defect in intracellular protein synthesis resulting in formation of protein with an abnormal affinity for lipids is probably the cause of the accumulation of the abnormal lipid.[8]

Diffuse reticular or finely nodular infiltrates are seen in chest radiographs. These findings ultimately lead to honeycomb lung. (See Figure 8, Chapter 6.)

Detection of carriers of type A and B by use of leukocytes and a chromogenic analogue of sphingomyelin has been reported.[7] Antenatal diagnosis is possible.[7]

d. Management

Partial splenectomy has been tried when there is bleeding or when mechanical pressure on other abdominal organs need to be alleviated. Bone marrow transplantation in those without CNS involvement is being tried. No known therapy is available.

e. Prognosis

Early death occurs with type A patients. Survival to first or early into the second decade of life is possible with type B. Type C patients experience slower deterioration and may appear normal until 2 years of age. These children die in the first decade of life. Type D patients may live up to their late second decade.

II. TRANSPORT DISORDER

A. Interstitial Lung Disease Associated with Cystic Fibrosis

1. Introduction

Although predominantly an obstructive airway disease, cystic fibrosis (CF) is discussed in this section because it manifests primarily as a transport disorder and appears to be an inborn error of metabolism involving all exocrine glands and, most likely, other tissues and organs. It also may be associated with other disorders,[10] some autoimmune, which may present with interstitial lung densities. CF as the primary disease must be ruled out and/or its association with other interstitial lung disorders[11-13] should be recognized in order to manage the person with CF comprehensively and correctly.

CF is an autosomal recessive disease that ranks as the number one killer of Caucasian children among inherited disorders. It is characterized by generalized involvement of eccrine and mucus-secreting exocrine glands. Anatomically normal eccrine sweat glands exhibit a defect in tubular reabsorption of electrolytes and/or water in the coil of the sweat duct, resulting in sweat that contains abnormally high concentrations of sodium, potassium, and chloride.[10,14,15] This abnormality forms the diagnostic basis of the confirmatory sweat test using quantitative pilocarpine iontophoresis method.[14,15] Protean manifestations of cystic fibrosis cannot be explained by a single hypothesis.[10,14,15]

Incidence of the disease is approximately 1 per 1600 to 2000 live Caucasian births. It is less frequent in other racial and ethnic groups. Carrier rate is 1 in every 20 to 25 Caucasians. CF has a heterogeneous expression so that the disease may be present in asymptomatic persons as well as in severely involved individuals.[16] The clinical course, characteristics, and severity of the disease are similar in any race.

Diagnosis can be confirmed using the quantitative pilocarpine iontophoresis tests done in duplicate. Very careful collection of uncontaminated sweat induced by pilocarpine iontophoresis or by direct thermal stimulation and subsequent titration of at least 100 mg of sweat or more should result in sweat chloride values of 70 meq/ℓ and above for the test to be considered diagnostic of CF. Borderline values of 50 to 60 meq/ℓ ought to be repeated.[10,14,15] Extreme care must be exercised in interpretation of sweat test results taking into consideration the method used and the experience in sweat testing of the laboratory from where the report originated.[17]

The reader is referred to recent books[18,19] and reviews[10,14,15] on CF for more details about the disease.

2. Anatomic and Physiologic Considerations

Mucous glands produce very thick and viscid mucus which obstructs the ducts of organs where they are located. This increased viscosity has been attributed to abnormal organic constituents such as mucous glycoproteins, alterations of electrolyte and calcium concentrations, and a relative lack of water.

The cilia in the tracheobronchial tree are unable to move the thick mucus normally, so that mucus accumulates in the smaller bronchi and bronchioles leading to obstruction with further impairment of mucociliary clearance. Stagnation of secretions favor bacterial infection which initially is with Staphylococcus aureus later with Hemophilus influenza and Pseudomonas aeruginosa usually of mucoid strain. Bronchitis and bronchiolitis result, causing hypertrophy and hypersecretion of the mucus-secreting bronchial glands further leading to more airway obstruction. Alveolar hypoplasia could result from chronic overdistention. Mononuclear cells are found in the interstitial pneumonic infiltrate which caused Esterly and Oppenheimer to raise the possibility of viral illness contributing to the progression of pulmonary disease in cystic fibrosis.[20,21] Interstitial fibrosis in alveolar septae occur. Bands of fibrous tissue separate large cavities which later form cysts and bullae.[22] Mucosal and submucosal edema contribute to more obstruction. With complete obstruction, atelectasis of a lobe or segment occurs. Air-trapping of various degrees is present with partial obstruction in different areas of the lungs. Further accumulation of viscid secretions cause impairment of mucociliary clearance especially if attempts to remove secretions are ineffective. As respiratory secretions become more purulent, DNA content of sputum becomes higher and exceeds that seen in other diseases. This increased DNA appears to come from decomposed leukocytes and contributes to increased viscosity.[23] Other substances present in respiratory secretions are I_gE antibodies, various inflammatory mediators as histamine, bradykinin, prostaglandins and leukotrienes.[24-27] The contribution of these factors to persistent infection or colonization or whether such changes secondary to the infection is not definitely known. As inflammation progresses, peribronchial thickening continues and with time leads to bronchiectasis with purulent secretions pooled in the cavities. Direct activation of the alternate complement pathway by microbial antigens and by host proteolytic activity is also possible. As more obstructive phenomenon persist, severe hyperinflation occurs with bullae or cystic formation which could rupture and cause pneumothorax. Abscess formation, hemoptysis, respiratory insufficiency, and cor pulmonale can eventually develop which ultimately leads to death.

Moss[28] presented the hypothesis that the basic defect of pulmonary fibrosis produced in CF could be abnormal glycosylation of glycoproteins which alters the lining of the respiratory tract as to permit binding and proliferation of microbes in the normally sterile bronchial tree. Two possible mechanisms for binding could be (1) alteration in the functional ability of secretory I_gA and (2) changes in the surface-binding properties of respiratory epithelial cells, e.g., deficiency in fibronectin. Colonization of the respiratory tract by potential pathogens precedes gross changes in the respiratory secretions affecting viscosity and purulence.

Once colonized, various influences, primary and secondary, mutually aggravate or accelerate each other. After colonization, several mechanisms may be involved in potentiating an I_gG antibody response, including stimulation of early reaginic (I_gE) response which allow entry of large amounts of antigen below the mucosa. Virulence factors of the colonizing agents may play a role in facilitating penetration of the submucosal line of immune defenses. As a result of the abnormal penetration, an early massive and continuing stimulation of the I_gG antibody response occurs. Two complicating factors may occur at this point. One is the dysfunction in the ability of I_gG antibodies reaching the airway to effectively opsonize the microorganisms for alveolar macrophage phagocytosis, and second, the presence of an increasingly destructive immune complex hypersensitivity reaction which would by direct complement activation and perhaps by alveolar macrophage activation also release potent chemotactic factors triggering a massive influx of neutrophiles. This neutrophile recruitment will lead to release of leukocyte proteolytic enzymes and oxidative metabolites leading to lung damage. A selection process possibly based on antiphagocytic capacity for mucoid strains of Pseudomonas aeruginosa occurs. Bronchiolitis, bronchiolectasis leading to bronchiectasis and pulmonary fibrosis follows.

Other respiratory manifestations of cystic fibrosis include sinusitis, and nasal polyps. Although nasal polyps are found in allergic individuals, sweat testing should be done when nasal polyps are found in children. Pancreatic involvement occurs in about 85% of individuals with cystic fibrosis.

3. Clinical Presentations Associated with Interstitial Lung Disease

Certain persons with cystic fibrosis may present with mild pulmonary involvement characterized radiographically by mild interstitial pattern unrelated to the presence of respiratory infection. No study is available specifically correlating these interstitial patterns in CF since pulmonary tissue has not been available in vivo from them. In this author's clinical experience, interstitial pattern may be found in some patients with or without radiographic findings of hyperinflation. This pattern persists with the addition of cystic changes on the peribronchial thickening with development of atelectasis and bronchiectasis later.

Clinicians who are presented with a child with failure to thrive in whom the chest roentgenogram shows interstitial lung disease should still consider CF in the differential diagnosis. The coexistence of superimposed viral, bacterial, and mycoplasmal infections should be remembered.[13]

Holsclaw[29] described a mixed interstitial pattern in 45 of 55 postadolescent persons with CF who had mild (7), moderate (30), and advanced (18) disease. Mixed interstitial pattern was found either alone or associated with cystic or honeycomb areas, transient nodular pattern and/or hyperinflation. Eighty two percent had mixed interstitial pattern with the frequency highest in the moderate group (26 to 30) and occurring in 7 of 18 advanced cases. Interstitial pneumonia with mononuclear cells is common in postmortem studies of lungs from persons with CF. Viral illnesses may contribute to progressive pulmonary disease in CF.[13,23]

4. Bronchial Hyperreactivity

Atopy and bronchial hyperreactivity have been reported in older patients with CF.[30] The prevalence of allergic rhinitis, atopic dermatitis, and allergic asthma in CF is probably equal to that of the normal population. Eosinophilia in nasal secretions was found in 11 to 15 allergic CF subjects but only 2 to 48 nonallergic CF individuals. Total blood eosinophil count was found higher in CF than in the control population, but this difference was not statistically significant. At least 70% of CF patients have identifiable I_gE to at least one antigen which most authors attribute to damaged respiratory epithelium. At least 40% of CF patients have bronchial hyperreactivity as defined by response to aerosolized methacholine or histamine.[31] Davis et al.[32] has recently reviewed the adrenergic and cholinergic regulation in CF and conclude that there was something abnormal in all three arms of the autonomic nervous system in CF: alpha-adrenergic, beta-adrenergic, and cholinergic at or beyond the receptor. However, the presence of this diverse array of abnormal autonomic response is not sufficient to produce either the phenotype of CF or the syndrome of asthma, since the autonomic abnormalities are present in asymptomatic nonatopic heterozygotes for CF. At this time, there is no convincing evidence linking the effect of CF gene or genes to that for allergic disease. Classic allergic disease can be developed by the person with CF in the same likelihood as anyone in the general population.

A high prevalence of skin test sensitivity for A. fumigatus[32-35] in sicker patients with CF is present. Pitcher-Wilmott et al.[36] performed a very comprehensive study of the clinical significance of positive skin test in CF in relation to clinical data, radiographs, and pulmonary function. The effect of allergy was not significant using analysis of variance. The factor found was the presence of Pseudomonas aeruginosa (PA) in the respiratory flora. The presence of PA, particularly the mucoid strain, and Aspergillus fumigatus (AF) in the airway damaged by frequent bouts of bronchitis may overwhelm the I_gE. The presence of these antibodies could mean that the atopic person could begin production with smaller antigen load or that the presence of the antibodies reflected is simply a marker for quantifying respiratory epithelial damage.

5. Allergic Bronchopulmonary Aspergillosis (ABPA)

AF may cause allergic disease in some but not all of persons with CF with skin test sensitivity to the allergen. Pepys[37] has proposed that patients who develop ABPA both have the Gell and Coombs type I and type III reaction to fungal antigen held in the airway in a sputum plug matrix. The type I reaction results in increased permeability of the mucosa with entry of complement and I_gG against AF into the airway. This permits an intense complement-mediated inflammatory reaction at the site of the sputum plug. The basic underlying pathologic process is a hypersensitivity reaction to the presence of fungus in the bronchial tree (see Chapter 41).

Long-standing involvement of the bronchial tree with these immunologic processes leads to the chronic sequelae of ABPA: pulmonary fibrosis, bronchiectasis, decreased lung size, and lobar shrinkage.[33] Primary criteria for the diagnosis of ABPA include

1. Episodic bronchial obstruction
2. Peripheral blood eosinophilia
3. Immediate skin reactivity to Aspergillus antigens
4. Precipitating antibodies against Aspergillus antigens
5. Elevated serum I_gE
6. History of infiltrates
7. Central bronchiectasis

The secondary criteria include

1. Aspergillus in sputum
2. History of mucus plug expectoration
3. Late skin (Arthus) reactivity to Aspergillus antigens

Nelson and associates[34] reviewed 46 patients and found that 4 of these met the criteria for ABPA. Positive sputum cultures for Aspergillus were found in 57% of their group. Immediate skin test reactivity to Aspergillus antigen was present in 39%; 33% had elevated precipitins, 46% had bronchospasm, and 22% had elevated serum I_gE levels. The incidence of ABPA in CF in their population was 11%. The authors cautioned about the use of steroids in patients with CF and ABPA as these patients are at increased risk of developing Pseudomonas pneumonia. Corticosteroid therapy is the treatment of choice in ABPA.[38] Resolution of infiltrates and improvement of symptoms have been associated with their use.

6. Allergic Bronchopulmonary Nonaspergillus Pneumonia

Candida albicans, helminthosporium species, and curvularia species have been reported to produce productive cough, recurrent asthmatic symptoms and hemoptysis in cystic fibrosis patients.[39-44]

7. Hypersensitivity to Airway Flora

The presence of Pseudomonas aeruginosa in the airways and sputum plugs expectorated in CF might induce allergic antibody formation. Studies[27,45,46] have been conducted that demonstrate specific I_gE as markedly increased in CF patients. PA antigen produces a basophil histamine release in CF patients by complement dependent pathways.[47] Lewiston[48] has considered that PA antigen held in the sputum matrix may possibly produce an ABPA-like disease. Such occurrence has been reported in a 2-year-old noncystic fibrosis patient who demonstrated skin-sensitizing antibody and precipitating antibody to PA and who had a disease characterized by bronchospasm, productive cough, pulmonary infiltrates, and eosinophilia, and from whom mucoid Pseudomonas was cultured from sputum, bronchoscopic washings, and tissue obtained by pulmonary biopsy. Sweat test was normal.[49]

Staphylococcus aureus which is also commonly found in CF appears not to produce hypersensitivity reaction as was found in one study showing that only 4 of 53 patients demonstrated I_gE specific for Staphylococcus.[50] Patients with CF were found to have elevated RAST scores to H. influenza but not to Staphylococcus aureus or Streptococcus pneumoniae.[51]

What viral illness does from the hypersensitivity standpoint in CF awaits further studies, but recent studies[52-54] showing specific anti-viral reactions may aid in pursuing this aspect. It is known, however, that viral and mycoplasmal infections of themselves lead to interstitial infiltrates and cause pulmonary deterioration in a stable patient with cystic fibrosis.

8. Drugs Used in the Therapy of CF

Pancreatic enzyme replacement therapy for those with malabsorption exposes hypersensitive individuals to trypsin, a protein antigen. Use of pancreatin dispensed as microspheres soluble only in the neutral pH of the duodenum should reduce to a minimum the incidence of this hypersensitivity reaction. Wheezing, sneezing, and tongue edema have been reported.[55]

Antimicrobial drugs are very commonly used in the therapy of moderate and advanced patients with CF. Penicillin hypersensitivity is present in 1 to 10% of the general population. Drug-induced lung disease includes pulmonary infiltrates but such report is lacking in CF literature. Most descriptions of penicillin sensitivity are mainly dermatologic and occur during carbenicillin therapy.[56] Ticarcillin or piperacillin may be used safely in patients who have cutaneous reactions to carbenicillin. Because penicillin-containing drugs are very useful in CF, skin testing for definite penicillin sensitivity must be done before abandoning the use of these drugs. Desensitization protocols have been used successfully.[57,58] With the advent of more frequent aerosolized use of aminoglycosides and semi-synthetic penicillins,[59] only future observations could document a higher or lower incidence of sensitivity.

9. Immune Complex (IC) Disease in CF

Using immunofluorescent staining techniques, McFarlane and his group[60] found mainly I_gG and I_gM with small amounts of I_gA and I_gE and complement (C1q, C3 and C4) in the respiratory and gastrointestinal tracts of four patients with CF at post-mortem examination. The thymus and lymphoreticular system showed some staining also. The findings were present in the submucosal areas of the gut wall, and along the walls of air spaces and bronchial submucosa. No staining was found in the lungs of a 10-year-old who was an accident victim. A biopsy of the gut of a 6-month-old child with CF showed immunoglobulin deposits in the submucosa. Staphylococcus aureus alpha-hemolysin involvement was demonstrated when the antigenic specificities of the complexed antibody in serum and sputum were examined. These complexes were of intermediate size on analytical ultracentrifugation with sedimentation coefficients between 7 and 11. In the last 8 years, a very high incidence of soluble circulating IC have been found in CF serum and respiratory tract secretions.[50,60-70] Immune complexes were found in serum, sputum sol phase, bronchial fluid, and skin biopsies using various techniques of detection of soluble circulating IC. Circulating soluble IC is an easily reproducible immunopathologic finding in CF. Immune complexes have been shown to be composed of antigens from colonizing microbes in the respiratory tract and specific I_gG or I_gM complement-fixing antibodies. Evidence of endotoxin-like activity in the complexes was shown by Berdischewsky and colleagues.[65] Moss and Hsu[64] showed that antibody was present in isolated serum IC specific for colonizing microbes. Isolated and dissociated complexes showed microbial antigens in these complexes by inhibition assays.[71] Pseudomonas antigen was isolated from dissociated complexes by Pitcher-Wilmott and his group.

There is a recognized association between the appearance of circulating IC and exacerbations of pulmonary disease.[50,66-68,70,71] Moss and Lewiston[72] reported a longitudinal study in 96 patients over a 2 year period where the incidence of pulmonary exacerbations and levels of Clq correlated very well. A dramatic return to baseline of serum Clq following hospitalization and intensive treatment of pulmonary exacerbation was recorded.

Circulating immune complexes are known to be biologically active. The pattern of bronchial proteolytic activity suggests immune-complex-mediated phagocytic cell activation as its major source.[73] Human platelets exposed to Pseudomonas antigen-antibody complexes are stimulated to release ^{3}H serotonin.[74]

A subpopulation of CF patients[75-77] have been identified who have systemic IC disease characterized by the appearance of signs and symptoms of serum sickness-like illness such as arthritis or arthralgias without evidence of rheumatoid arthritis, hypertrophic osteoarthropathy, hyperuricemia, or other known causes of rheumatic disease. Decreases in serum hemolytic complement activity and plasma complement activation along with Clq were found.[78] Higher complement activating ability or lower reticuloendothelial clearance in these patients may be speculated.

Renal involvement has been revealed in electronmicroscopic studies demonstrating subendothelial and mesangial deposition of glomerular immune deposits and positive immunofluorescence findings in 18 of 34 patients with CF showing I_gM and C3 in glomeruli and cortical arterioles. Antipseudomonas antibody activity was found in renal eluates in 2 to 3 specimens examined.[79]

Clinically apparent systemic IC disease and invitro circulating IC respond to systemic corticosteroid therapy manifested as relief in systemic symptoms, decrease in Clq accompanied by physiologic improvement.[80] The use of nonsteroidal anti-inflammatory agents awaits future trials.[81,82] The value of Pseudomonas lipopolysaccharide vaccine is unclear. However, a study in guinea pigs infected with Pseudomonas and with lung disease similar to CF lung accompanied by immunologic abnormalities: hypergammaglobulinemia, high levels of specific antibody and circulating immune complexes, use of active systemic immunization with Pseudomonas vaccine only further boosted the Pseudomonas-specific antibody levels affording no protection to the animals, exacerbating instead histologic, and seroimmunologic pathology.[83] Furthermore, Pseudomonas vaccine when available for use is best indicated in patients *prior* to Pseudomonas colonization or infection.

III. DEGENERATIVE DISORDER

A. Pulmonary Alveolar Microlithiasis (PAM)

This rare and unusual disease of unknown etiology derives its name from the characteristic expectoration of sandy material and the sandstorm appearance of the lungs on radiographic examination. PAM may show a familial tendency and is more commonly diagnosed in young adults. First described by Harbitz in 1918 and given its name "microlithiasis alveolaris pulmonum" by Puhr in 1933,[8] PAM is world-wide in distribution. Only less than 200 cases have been reported. Orientals and Caucasians predominate.[84]

Majority of cases have been in adults between 20 to 40 years old but premature infants and children have been reported. Also, it is occasionally a congenital lesion. Ravines reported nine cases occurring in three related families.[8,85] Almost always siblings were involved. No sex predilection has been observed. Insidious in onset PAM has a variable course. Lesions may gradually spread over 25 years or terminate in death within a year.[8] Associated conditions reported with PAM are chronic mitral stenosis and pulmonary fibrosis.

1. Clinical and Radiologic Features

Clinical features in children vary from no symptoms to complaints of cough and even hemoptysis.[86] Whereas expectoration of sandy material has been reported in adults, no documented report in children has been found. Tachypnea, digital clubbing, and cyanosis can occur.

The radiographic features may be the first clue to the diagnosis in a patient complaining of chest pain and shortness of breath. Dense miliary mottling or confluent shadows mainly confined in the lower two thirds of the lung fields with occasional involvement of the apices are found. Sandstorm appearance best describes these changes. Pleural abnormalities may occur. In a long-standing disease, blebs may be seen.

2. Pathology

Pathologically, the lungs feel hard and heavy. The shape is well-maintained and the lower lobes appear pale and stony-hard. The lungs are difficult to cut and may need to be sawn. Fixed lung tissue looks like sandpaper. Microscopic examination shows alveoli and bronchioles filled with psammona-like bodies called calcospherites. Electron-microscopy of these calcospherites demonstrate bodies composed of hydroxyapatite crystals. They are laminated and look like "onion skin" granules. Numerous calcifying extracellular matrix vesicles occur between the cells surrounding the mineral deposits, and these resemble the ectopic mineralization which occurs in other diseases. Less damaged parts of the lung show that the calcospherites are deposited in relation to finer blood vessels and vary in diameter from 0.1 to 0.3 mm to as large as about 1 mm. Chemical analysis reveals calcium, phosphorus, mainly phosphates, small amount of iron, and traces of magnesium. Sudanophilic and doubly refractile fatty material have appeared in frozen sections. The calcospherites have to be differentiated from corpora amylacea which occur commonly in conditions with heart failure, chronic bronchitis, and pulmonary infarction. Extrapulmonary changes include findings compatible with cor pulmonale. Hypoxemia studies demonstrate reduced vital capacity which progressively declines as the condition becomes prolonged. Arterial oxygen desaturation occurs late in the disease when more alveoli are involved. Hyperpnea is seen in the later stages at a time when lung compliance changes are more pronounced.[87]

3. Diagnosis, Treatment, and Prognosis

Expectoration of sandy material and typical radiographic features make the diagnosis of PAM. Open pulmonary biopsy is not always necessary to confirm it. Diagnosis of asymptomatic siblings is made early through radiographic examination of the chest. Since the disease may be familial, empathetic support of family members is necessary. No specific treatment is available. Supportive treatment is the rule. Bronchopulmonary lavage has been unsuccessful.[88]

As a rule the course of PAM is variable. The course is progressive in children. Death occurs in young adulthood if not earlier.

IV. UNCLASSIFIED ETIOLOGY

A. Pulmonary Alveolar Proteinosis (PAP)

Almost three decades have passed since its original description in man by Rosen and associates,[89] yet PAP remains a rare intrinsic lung disease of unknown etiology. Although still relatively uncommon, it has recently been reported in early infancy[90] and has been found at birth.[91] Indeed, with increasing clinical recognition, PAP is no longer just a pathologic curiosity.

The hallmark of PAP is the alveolar and terminal bronchiolar deposition of a periodic acid-Schiff (PAS)-staining floccular and granular type material predominantly phospholipid in nature, with dipalmitoyl lecithin forming the major component. The more proper name for the disease should therefore really be "lipoproteinosis." The mechanism by which this lipid-rich material accumulates in the terminal air spaces is ill defined. Ultrastructurally, the alveolar material is partly granular and partly fibrillar but, in addition, has lamellated structures that have been termed myeloid bodies because of their resemblance to myelin figures.[92]

In the first report of this interesting disorder in 1958,[89] a young child was also described, and since then some 50 cases of PAP in children have been well documented.[89-91,93-106] In one review of 23 cases in children,[99] thymic alymphoplasia was observed in 30%, supporting speculation about immunologic incompetence particularly in children in the first year of life as having a role in the etiopathogenesis of this disease. Indeed, adult PAP has been observed in association with hematologic malignancy and lymphoma.[107] However, it has also been observed in pulmonary infections,[108] tuberculosis,[109-111] cytomegalic inclusion virus,[108,112] busulphan treatment for leukemia,[113] and in experimental animals, exposure to dusts[114,115] and 100% oxygen.[92] This broad spectrum of associations suggests that PAP may represent one mechanism of pulmonary response to various noxious stimuli in the form of hypersecretion of a surfactant-like material. PAP in man is not an agent-specific disease but represents one of the responses of alveolar injury which may be produced by a wide variety of agents and/or disease. An identifiable primary etiologic agent has yet to be demonstrated.

PAP in one review[90] was described in five well-documented siblings and in four siblings in a family in whom PAP developed during infancy. The familial aspect of the disease is only fleetingly discussed.[116] On analysis, some cases of PAP may have a genetic basis, with possible autosomal-recessive inheritance. Consanguinity has been reported.[91] Also prominent is the presence of both affected and unaffected children of both sexes in some families.

1. Clinical Features

At the time of diagnosis, most patients are between 20 and 50 years of age. The disorder is two to three times more common in males. Whereas most adults have respiratory signs and symptoms, only 50% of children have such symptoms. A variable course is the rule, so the disease may either be abrupt or insidious in onset. Diarrhea and vomiting are frequent in children. Failure to thrive, dyspnea, and cyanosis may also be presenting symptoms. Perhaps, routine and diligent investigation of the family history may yet define the actual role, if any, of autosomal-recessive inheritance in this disorder.

2. Radiologic Considerations

As a rule, the radiologic abnormalities are more severe than the clinical findings. In children, chest roentgenograms often show a diffuse "interstitial" pattern or a miliary type pattern rather than the "pulmonary edema pattern" or consolidation found in adults.[106] Miliary pattern when noted may coalesce to larger nodular densities or small areas of consolidation. The deposition in the terminal air spaces of PAS-positive material explains small areas of atelectasis. Without superimposed infection, there is no effusion or adenopathy (refer to Chapter 6, Figure 22).

Osborne and Effman have been credited with the observation that it is the gradual increase in acinar size that occurs from birth to maturity which explains why miliary type nodules and a reticulonodular pattern are more often seen in contrast to a pulmonary edema or consolidation pattern present in adults with much larger acini.[106]

3. Pathology and Diagnosis

Macroscopically evident is the greyish white consolidation of affected lobes while the normal intervening tissue is dark red, collapsed, and soften in consistency.[117] Characteristic microscopically is the alveolar and bronchiolar proteinaceous material. Endobronchial instillation of trypsin solution or saline at pH 7.4 results in the expectoration of the distinctive PAS-staining intraalveolar contents which are subsequently histologically identified.

Diagnosis is established by light microscopic and electron microscopic examination of sputum or bronchial washings, but lung biopsy is generally regarded as the most reliable method of diagnostic confirmation. Moderate polymorphonuclear leucocytosis is frequent. Slight reduction in vital capacity, pulmonary compliance and arterial oxygen saturation at rest have been observed.[118]

4. Treatment and Prognosis

PAP is uninfluenced by steroid or antibiotic therapy. Adult PAP invariably resolves with various forms of supportive airway and expectorant therapy, including aerosolized tryspin,[119] and whole lung lavage.[120-122] Spontaneous resolution even sometimes occurs. However, in as many as one third of the patients, there is insidious progression to severe dyspnea, hypoxemia, and death. The course in adults is distinctly different from the course of PAP in children.[106] Although bronchopulmonary lavage is remarkably variable in the degree of effectiveness as therapy of PAP in adults, the results are generally satisfactory. They are not as salutary in children. Still, bronchopulmonary lavage remains the mainstay of treatment.[98,101,103,105,106]

In a review of 23 pediatric cases of PAP by Colon and others,[99] there was a 100% mortality rate at the end of 2 years as opposed to a 30% mortality in adults. Use of smaller double-lumen Carlen's tubes for bronchopulmonary lavage and extracorporeal circulation[100,101,120,122] have yet to show dramatic reversal of the inexorable progress of the disease in children. For the present, PAP remains a uniformly fatal childhood disease.

REFERENCES

1. **Hermansky, F. and Pudlak, P.,** Albinism associated with hemorrhagic diathesis and unusual pigmented reticular cells in the bone marrow. Report two cases with histochemical studies, *Blood,* 14, 162, 1959.
2. **Schinella, R. A., Greco, M. A., Garay, S. M., Lackner, H., Wolman, S. R., and Fazzini, E. P.,** Hermansky-Pudlak syndrome: a clinicopathologic study, *Human Pathol.,* 16, 366, 1985.
3. **Garay, S. M., Gardella, J. E., Fazzini, E. P., and Goldring, R. M.,** Hermansky-Pudlak syndrome, pulmonary manifestations of a ceroid storage disorder, *Am. J. Med.,* 66, 737, 1979.
4. **Davies, B. H. and Tuddenham, E. G. D.,** Familial pulmonary fibrosis associated with oculocutaneous albinism and platelet function defect, a new syndrome, *Q. J. Med.,* XLV, 178, 219, 1976.

5. **Rendu, F., Breton-Gorius, J., Trugman, G., Castro-Malaspina, H., Andrieu, J. M., Bereziat, G., Lebret, M., and Caen, J. P.,** Studies on a new variant of the Hermansky-Pudlak syndrome: qualitative ultrastructural and functional abnormalities of the platelet dense bodies associated with a phospholipase A defect, *Am. J. Hematol.,* 4, 387, 1978.
6. **Brady, R. O., Barranger, J. A.,** Glucosylceramide lipidosis: Gaucher's Disease, in *Metabolic Basis of Inherited Disease,* 5th ed., Stanbury, J. B., Wyngaarden, J. B., Frederickson, D. S., Goldstein, J. L., and Brown, M. S., Eds., McGraw-Hill, New York, 1983, 842.
7. **Swaiman, K. F.,** Niemann-Pick, Krabbe, and Gaucher disease, in *The Practice of Pediatric Neurology,* 2nd ed., Swaiman, K. F. and Wright, F. S., Eds., C.V. Mosby, St. Louis, 1982, 530.
8. **Spencer, H.,** Degenerative and metabolic disorders of the lungs, in *Pathology of the Lung,* Pergamon Press, Oxford, 1985, 750.
9. **Brady, R. O. and Berninger, R.,** Sphingomyelin lipidosis, Niemann-Pick disease, in *Metabolic Basis of Inherited Disease,* 5th ed., Stanbury, J. B., Wyngaarden, J. D., Frederickson, D. S., Goldstein, J. L., and Brown, M. S., Eds., McGraw-Hill, New York, 1983, 831.
10. **Talamo, R. C., Rosenstein, B. J., and Berninger, R. W.,** Cystic fibrosis, in *Metabolic Basis of Inherited Disease,* 5th ed., Stanbury, J. B., Wyngaarden, J. B., Frederickson, D. S., Goldstein, J. L., and Brown, M. S., Eds., McGraw-Hill, New York, 1983, 1889.
11. **Laraya-Cuasay, L. R. and Barabas, G.,** Association of cystic fibrosis and neurofibromatosis, *Cystic Fibrosis Club Abstr.,* 7, 155, 1986.
12. **Batten, J. C.,** Allergic aspergillosis in cystic fibrosis, *Mod. Probl. Pediat.,* 10, 227, 1967.
13. **Petersen, N. T., Hoiby, N., and Mordhorst, C. H.,** Respiratory infections in cystic fibrosis patients caused by virus, chlamydia and mycoplasma-possible synergism with Pseudomonas aeruginosa, *Acta Paediatr. Scand.,* 70, 623, 1981.
14. **diSant/Agnese, P. A. and Davis, P. B.,** Research in cystic fibrosis, *N. Engl. J. Med.,* 295, 481, 1976.
15. **Wood, R. E., Boat, T. F., and Doershuk, C. F.,** Cystic fibrosis, *Am. Rev. Resp. Dis.,* 113, 833, 1976.
16. **Stern, R. C., Boat, T. F., and Doershuk, C. F.,** Cystic fibrosis diagnosed after age 13: twenty five teenage and adult patients including three asymptomatic men, *Ann. Intern. Med.,* 87, 188, 1977.
17. **Denning, C. R., Huang, N. N., Cuasay, L. R., Schwachman, H., Tocci, P., Warwick, W., and Gibson, L.,** Cooperative study comparing three methods of performing sweat tests to diagnose cystic fibrosis, *Pediatrics,* 66, 752, 1980.
18. **Taussig, L. M.,** *Cystic Fibrosis,* Thieme-Stratton, Inc., New York, 1984.
19. **Lloyd-Still, J. D.,** *Textbook of Cystic Fibrosis,* John Wright PSG Inc., Massachusetts, 1983.
20. **Esterly, J. R. and Oppenheimer, E. H.,** Cystic fibrosis of the pancreas. Structural changes in peripheral airways, *Thorax,* 23, 670, 1968.
21. **Esterly, J. R. and Oppenheimer, E. H.,** Observations in cystic fibrosis of the pancreas. III. Pulmonary lesions, *John Hopkins Med. J.,* 122, 94, 1968.
22. **Oppenheimer, E. H. and Esterly, J. R., II.,** Pathology of Cystic fibrosis. Review of the Literature and comparison with 146 autopsied cases, in *Perspectives in Pediatric Pathology,* Rosenberg, H. and Bolande, P., Eds., Year Book Medical Publisher, Chicago, 1975, 241.
23. **Barton, A. D., Ryder, K., Lourenco, R. V., Dralle, W., and Weiss, S. G.,** Inflammatory reaction and airway damage in cystic fibrosis, *J. Lab. Clin. Med.,* 88, 423, 1976.
24. **Spock, A.,** State of the art of lung lavage in patients with cystic fibrosis, in *1000 Years of Cystic Fibrosis Collected Papers,* Warwick, W. J., Ed., University of Minnesota, 1981, 113.
25. **McFarlane, H., Allan, J. D., and Van der Zeil, P.,** Passive cutaneous anaphylaxis (PCA) and specific I$_g$E in cystic fibrosis and their heterozygotes, *Clin. Allergy,* 7, 279, 1977.
26. **Lopez-Vidriero, M. T. and Reid, L.,** Chemical constituents of sol and gel phases of sputum from atopic and nonatopic cystic fibrosis, in *Perspectives in Cystic Fibrosis,* Sturgess, J. M., Ed., Imperial Press, Toronto, 1980, 26a.
27. **Cromwell, O., Walport, M. J., Morris, H. R., Taylor, G. W., Hodson, M. E., Batten, J., and Kay, A. B.,** Identification of leukotrienes D and B in sputum from cystic fibrosis patients, *Lancet,* 2, 165, 1981.
28. **Moss, R. B.,** Immunology of cystic fibrosis: immunity, immunodeficiency, and hypersensitivity, in *A Textbook of Cystic Fibrosis,* Lloyd-Still, J., Ed., John Wright PSG Publishing, Massachusetts, 109, 1983.
29. **Holsclaw, D. S.,** Cystic fibrosis: overview and pulmonary aspects in young adults, *Clin. Chest Med.,* 1, 407, 1980.
30. **Tobin, M. J., Maguire, O., Reen, D., Tempany, E., and Fitzgerald, M. X.,** Atopy and bronchial reactivity in older patients with cystic fibrosis, *Thorax,* 35, 807, 1980.
31. **Rothstein, R. J., Penney, M. A., Buckley, J. M., and Cotton, E. K.,** Evaluation of reactive airway disease in atopic cystic fibrosis patients, *J. Allergy Clin. Immunol.,* 53, 100, 1974.
32. **Davis, P., Shelhamer, J., and Kaliner, M.,** Abnormal adrenergic and cholinergic sensitivity in cystic fibrosis, *N. Engl. J. Med.,* 302, 1453, 1980.
33. **McCarthy, D. and Pepys, J.,** Allergic bronchopulmonary aspergillosis, *Clin. Allergy,* 1, 261, 1971.

34. **Nelson, L. A., Callerame, M. L. C., and Schwartz, R. H.,** Aspergillosis and atopy in cystic fibrosis, *Am. Rev. Resp. Dis.,* 120, 863, 1979.

35. **Mearns, M., Longbottom, J., and Batten, J.,** Precipitating antibodies to Aspergillus fumigatus in cystic fibrosis, *Lancet,* 1, 538, 1967.

36. **Pitcher-Wilmott, R. W., Levinsky, R. J., Gordon, I., Turner, M. W., and Matthew, D. J.,** Pseudomonas infection, allergy, and cystic fibrosis, *Arch. Dis. Child.,* 57, 582, 1982.

37. **Pepys, J.,** Pulmonary aspergillosis, farmer's lung and related diseases in *Immunological Diseases,* 3rd ed., Samter, M., Ed., Little, Brown, Boston, 1978.

38. **Wang, J. and Patterson, R.,** The management of allergic bronchopulmonary aspergillosis, *Am. Rev. Resp. Dis.,* 120, 87, 1978.

39. **Galant, S. P., Rucker, R. W., Goruncy, C. E., Wells, I. D., and Novey, H. S.,** Incidence of serum antibodies to several Aspergillus species and to Candida albicans in cystic fibrosis, *Am. Rev. Resp. Dis.,* 114, 325, 1976.

40. **Warren, C. P. W., Tai, E., Batten, J. C., Hutchcroft, B. H., and Pepys, J.,** Cystic fibrosis-immunological reactions to A. Fumigatus and common allergens, *Clin. Allergy,* 5, 1, 1975.

41. **Allan, J. D., Moss, A. D., Wallwork, J. C., and McFarlane, H.,** Immediate hypersensitivity in patients with cystic fibrosis, *Clin. Allergy,* 5, 255, 1975.

42. **Dolan, C., Weed, L., and Dines, D.,** Bronchopulmonary helminthosporiosis, *Am. J. Clin. Pathol.,* 53, 235, 1970.

43. **Matthieson, A.,** Allergic bronchopulmonary disease caused by fungi other than Aspergillus, *Thorax,* 36, 719, 1971.

44. **Hendrick, D., Ellithorpe, D., Lyon, F., Hattier, P., and Salvaggio, M.,** Allergic bronchopulmonary helminthosporiosis, *Am. Rev. Resp. Dis.,* 126, 935, 1982.

45. **Shen, J., Brackett, R., Fisher, T., Holder, A., Kellog, F., and Michael, J. G.,** Specific Pseudomonas immunoglobulin E. antibodies in serum of patients with cystic fibrosis, *Infect. Immun.,* 32, 967, 1981.

46. **Hoiby, N. and Wilik, A.,** Antibacterial precipitins and autoantibodies in serum of patients with cystic fibrosis, *Scand. J. Resp. Dis.,* 56, 38, 1975.

47. **Skov, P. S., Norn, S., Schiotz, P. O., Permin, H., and Hoiby, N.,** Pseudomonas aeruginosa allergy in cystic fibrosis, Involvement of histamine release in the pathogenesis of lung tissue damage, *Allergy,* 35, 25, 1980.

48. **Lewiston, N.,** Circulating immune complexes in lung disease, *Chest,* 80, 389, 1981.

49. **Gordon, D., Hunter, R., O'Reilly, R., and Conway, B.,** Pseudomonas aeruginosa allergy and humoral antibody-mediated hypersensitivity pneumonia, *Am. Rev. Resp. Dis.,* 108, 127, 1973.

50. **Moss, R. B., Hsu, Y. P., and Lewiston, N.,** 125 I-Clq binding and specific antibodies as indicators of pulmonary disease activity in cystic fibrosis, *J. Pediatr.,* 99, 215, 1981.

51. **Tee, R. and Pepys J.,** Specific serum antibodies to bacterial antigens in allergic lung disease, *Clin. Allergy,* 12, 439, 1978.

52. **Strunk, R. C., Sieber, O. F., Taussig, L. M., and Gall, E. P.,** Serum complement depression during viral lower respiratory tract illness in cystic fibrosis, *Arch. Dis. Child.,* 52, 687, 1977.

53. **Conover, J. H., Conod, E. J., and Hirschhorn, K.,** Complement components in cystic fibrosis, *Lancet,* 2, 1501, 1973.

54. **McIntosh, K. and Fishaut, J. M.,** Immunopathologic mechanisms in lower respiratory tract disease of infants due to respiratory syncytial virus, *Prog. Med. Virol.,* 26, 94, 1980.

55. **Bergner, A. and Bergner, R. K.,** Pulmonary hypersensitivity associated with pancreatic powder exposure, *Pediatrics,* 55, 814, 1975.

56. **Møller, N., Ahlstedt, S., Skov, P., and Norm, S.,** Allergological exam of cystic fibrosis patients with skin reactions during carbenicillin treatment, *Allergy,* 35, 135, 1980.

57. **Brown, L., Goldberg, N., and Shearer, W.,** Long-term ticarcillin desensitization by the continuous oral administration of penicillin, *J. Allergy Clin. Immunol.,* 69, 51, 1982.

58. **Sullivan, T., Yecies, L., Shatz, G., Parker, C., and Wedner, H.,** Desensitization of patients allergic to penicillin using orally administered B-lactam antibiotics, *J. Allergy Clin. Immunol.,* 69, 275, 1982.

59. **Hodson, M., Penketh, A., and Batten, J.,** Aerosol carbenicillin and gentamicin treatment of Pseudomonas aeruginosa, *Lancet,* 2, 1137, 1981.

60. **McFarlane, H., Holzel, A., Brenchley, P., Allan, J. A., Wallwork, J. C., Singer, B. E., and Worsley, B.,** Immune complexes in cystic fibrosis, *Br. Med. J.,* 1, 423, 1975.

61. **Schiotz, P. O., Hoiby, N., Juhl, F., Permin, H., Nielsen, H., and Svehag, S. E.,** Immune complexes in cystic fibrosis, *Acta Pathol. Microbiol. Scand. Sect. C,* 85, 57, 1977.

62. **Schiotz, P. O., Nielsen, H., Hoiby, N., Glickmann, G., and Svehag, S. E.,** Immune complexes in the sputum of patients with cystic fibrosis suffering from chronic Pseudomonas aeruginosa lung infection, *Acta Pathol. Microbiol. Scand. Sect. C,* 86, 37, 1978.

63. **Moss, R. B. and Lewiston, N. J.,** Immune complexes and humoral response to Pseudomonas aeruginosa in cystic fibrosis, *Am. Rev. Respir. Dis.,* 121, 23, 1980.

64. **Moss, R. B. and Hsu, Y. P.**, Isolation and characterization of circulating immune complexes in cystic fibrosis, *Clin. Exp. Immunol.*, 47, 301, 1982.
65. **Berdischewsky, M., Pollack, M., Young, L. S., Chia, D., Osher, A. B., and Barnett, E. V.**, Circulating immune complexes in cystic fibrosis, *Pediatr. Res.*, 14, 830, 1980.
66. **Church, J. A., Jordan, S. C., Keens, T. G., and Wang, C. I.**, Circulating immune complexes in patients with cystic fibrosis, *Chest*, 80, 405, 1981.
67. **Beldon, I., Hodson, M. E., and Batten, J. C.**, Circulating immune complexes in the sera of patients with cystic fibrosis, in *Perspectives in Cystic Fibrosis*, Sturgess, M. M., Ed., Imperial Press, Toronto, 1980, 3a.
68. **Dasgupta, M. K., Harley, F. L., Jones, R. L., Reichert, A., and Dossetor, J. B.**, Circulating immune complexes in cystic fibrosis, *Cystic Fibrosis Club Abstr.*, 22, 109, 1981.
69. **Manthei, U., Taussig, L. M., Beckerman, R. C., and Strunk, R. C.**, Circulating immune complexes in cystic fibrosis, *Am. Rev. Respir. Dis.*, 126, 253, 1982.
70. **Pitcher-Wilmott, R. W., Levinsky, R. J., and Matthew, D. J.**, Circulating soluble immune complexes containing Pseudomonas antigens in cystic fibrosis, *Arch. Dis. Child.*, 57, 577, 1982.
71. **Moss, R. B. and Hsu, Y. P.**, Pulmonary origin of immune complexes in cystic fibrosis, *Am. Rev. Respir. Dis.*, 125, 59, 1982.
72. **Moss, R. B. and Lewiston, N. J.**, Immunopathology of cystic fibrosis, in *Immunological aspects of cystic fibrosis*, Shapira, E. and Wilson, G. B., Eds., CRC Press, Boca Raton, Florida, 1984, 5.
73. **Schiotz, P. O.**, Local humoral immunity and immune reactions in the lungs of patients with cystic fibrosis, *Acta Pathol. Microbiol. Scand. Sect. C*, Suppl. 276, 1981.
74. **Permin, H., Skov, P. S., Norn, S., Holby, N., and Schiotz, P. O.**, Platelet ^{3}H-serotonin releasing immune complexes induced by Pseudomonas aeruginosa in cystic fibrosis, *Allergy*, 37, 93, 1982.
75. **Newman, A. J. and Ansell, B. M.**, Episodic arthritis in children with cystic fibrosis, *J. Pediatr.*, 94, 594, 1979.
76. **Soter, N. A., Mihm, M. C., and Colten, H. R.**, Cutaneous necrotizing venulitis in patients with cystic fibrosis, *J. Pediatr.*, 95, 197, 1979.
77. **Goldsmith, D., Schidlow, D., Palmer, J., Cotler, M., and Huang, N.**, Rheumatic manifestations of cystic fibrosis, in *Perspectives in Cystic Fibrosis*, Sturgess, J. M., Ed., Imperial Press, Toronto, 1980, 17a.
78. **Fick, R. B., Hen, J., and Dolan, T. F.**, Acute monoarticular arthropathies in cystic fibrosis, *Cystic Fibrosis Club Abstr.*, 22, 112, 1981.
79. **Abramowsky, C. R. and Swinchart, B. A.**, The nephropathy of cystic fibrosis, *Hum. Pathol.*, 13, 934, 1982.
80. **Lewiston, N. J. and Moss, R. B.**, Circulating immune complexes decrease during corticosteroid therapy in cystic fibrosis, *Pediatr. Res.*, 16, 354, 1982.
81. **Lewis, R. A. and Austen, K. F.**, Mediation of local homeostasis and inflammation by leukotrienes and other mast cell-dependent compounds, *Nature (London)*, 293, 103, 1981.
82. **Isekutz, A. C. and Bhimji, V.**, The effect of non-steroidal anti-inflammatory agents on immune complex and chemotactic factor-induced inflammation, *Immunopharmacology*, 4, 253, 1982.
83. **Pennington, J. E., Hickey, W. F., Blackwood, L. L., and Arnaut, M. A.**, Active immunization with lipopolysaccharide Pseudomonas antigen for chronic Pseudomonas bronchopneumonia in guinea pigs, *J. Clin. Invest.*, 68, 1140, 1981.
84. **Kendig, E. L.**, Idiopathic Pulmonary Alveolar Microlithiasis, in *Disorders of the Respiratory Tract in Children*, 4th ed., W.B. Saunders, Philadelphia, 1983.
85. **Mikhailov, V.**, Pulmolithiasis endalveolaris et interstitialis diffusa, *Klin. Med. (Moskow)*, 32, 321, 1954.
86. **Thind, G. S. and Bhatia, J. L.**, Pulmonary alveolar microlithiasis, *Br. J. Dis. Chest*, 72, 151, 1978.
87. **Fulcihan, F. J. D., Abboud, R. T., Balikian, J. P., and Nucho, C. K. N.**, Pulmonary alveolar microlithiasis: lung function in five cases, *Thorax*, 24, 84, 1969.
88. **Palombini, B. C., daSilva Porto, N., Wallau, C. U., and Camargo, J. J.**, Bronchopulmonary lavage in alveolar microlithiasis, *Chest*, 80, 242, 1981.
89. **Rosen, S. H., Castleman, B., and Liebow, A. A.**, Pulmonary alveolar proteinosis, *N. Engl. J. Med.*, 258, 1123, 1958.
90. **Teja, K., Cooper, P. H., Squires, J. E., and Schnatterly, P. T.**, Pulmonary alveolar proteinosis in four siblings, *N. Engl. J. Med.*, 305, 1390, 1981.
91. **Haworth, J. C., Hoogstraten, J., Taylor, H.**, Thymic alymphoplasia, *Arch. Dis. Child.*, 42, 40, 1967.
92. **Shober, R., Bensch, K. G., and Kosek, J. C.**, On the origin of the membranous intraalveolar material in pulmonary alveolar proteinosis, *Exp. Med. Pathol.*, 21, 246, 1974.
93. **Larson, R. K. and Gordimer, R.**, Pulmonary alveolar proteinosis: report of six cases, review of the literature and formulation of a new theory, *Ann. Intern. Med.*, 62, 292, 1965.
94. **Laplane, R., Bonnet-Gajos, M., Gallet, J. P., and Dore, P.**, Pulmonary alveolar proteinosis in childhood, *Presse Med.*, 76, 1857, 1968.

95. **Wilkinson, R. H., Blanc, W. A., and Hagstrom, J. W. C.,** Pulmonary alveolar proteinosis in three infants, *Pediatrics,* 41, 510, 1968.
96. **Danigelis, J. A. and Markarian, B.,** Pulmonary alveolar proteinosis: including pulmonary electron microscopy, *Am. J. Dis. Child,* 118, 871, 1969.
97. **Preger, L.,** Pulmonary alveolar proteinosis, *Radiology,* 92, 1291, 1969.
98. **Symchuck, P. S. and Flynn, D. M.,** Pulmonary alveolar proteinosis in an infant, *Arch. Dis. Child.,* 44, 769, 1969.
99. **Colon, A. R., Lawrence, R. D., Mills, S. D., and O'Connel, E. J.,** Childhood pulmonary alveolar proteinosis (PAP), *Am. J. Dis. Child.,* 121, 481, 1971.
100. **Ramirez-Rivera, J.,** Alveolar proteinosis: importance of pulmonary lavage, *Am. Rev. Respir. Dis.,* 103, 666, 1971.
101. **Sunderland, W. A., Campbell, R. A., and Edwards, M. J.,** Pulmonary alveolar proteinosis and pulmonary cryptococcosis in an adolescent boy, *J. Pediatr.,* 80, 450, 1972.
102. **Mazyek, E. M., Bonner, J. T., Herd, H. M., and Symbas, P. N.,** Pulmonary lavage for childhood pulmonary alveolar proteinosis, *J. Pediatr.,* 80, 839, 1972.
103. **Gray, E. S.,** Autoimmunity in childhood pulmonary alveolar proteinosis, *Br. Med. J.,* 3, 296, 1973.
104. **Luppmann, M., Mok, M. S., and Wasserman, K.,** Anesthetic management for children with alveolar proteinosis using extracorporeal circulation, *Br. J. Anaesth.,* 49, 173, 1977.
105. **Coleman, M., Denner, L. P., Sibley, R. K., Burke, B. A., L'Herveux, P. R., and Thompson, T. R.,** Pulmonary alveolar proteinosis: an uncommon cause of chronic neonatal respiratory distress, *Am. Rev. Respir. Dis.,* 121, 583, 1980.
106. **McCook, T. A., Kirks, D. R., Merten, D. F., Osborne, R. F., Spock, A., and Pratt, P. C.,** Pulmonary alveolar proteinosis in children, *Am. J. Roentgenol.,* 137, 1023, 1981.
107. **Carmovale, R., Zornoza, J., Goldman, A. M., and Luma, M.,** Pulmonary alveolar proteinosis: its association with hematologic malignancy and lymphoma, *Radiology,* 122, 303, 1977.
108. **Rubin, E., Weisbrod, G. L., and Sanders, D. E.,** Pulmonary alveolar proteinosis: relationship to silicosis and pulmonary infections, *Radiology,* 135, 35, 1980.
109. **Reyes, J. M. and Putong, P. B.,** Association of pulmonary alveolar proteinosis with mycobacterial infection, *Am. J. Clin. Pathol.,* 74, 478, 1980.
110. **Payseur, C. R., Konwaler, B. E., and Hyde, L.,** Pulmonary alveolar proteinosis, *Am. Rev. Tuberculosis,* 79, 906, 1958.
111. **Ramirez-Rivera, J.,** Pulmonary alveolar proteinosis, *Arch. Intern Med.,* 19, 147, 1968.
112. **Ranchod, M. and Bissell, M.,** Pulmonary alveolar proteinosis and cytomegalovirus infection, *Arch. Pathol. Lab. Med.,* 103, 139, 1979.
113. **Doyle, A. P., Balcerzak, S. P., Wells, C. L., and Crittenden, J. O.,** Pulmonary alveolar proteinosis with hematologic disorders, *Arch. Int. Med.,* 112, 940, 1963.
114. **Davidson, J. M. and Macleod, W. M.,** Pulmonary alveolar proteinosis, *Br. J. Dis. Chest,* 63, 13, 1969.
115. **Heppleston, A. G. and Young, A. E.,** Alveolar lipoproteinosis an ultrastructural comparison of the experimental and human forms, *J. Pathol.,* 107, 1972.
116. **Webster, J. R., Battista, H., Furey, C., Harrison, R. A., and Shapiro, B.,** Pulmonary alveolar proteinosis in two siblings with decreased immunoglobulin A, *Am. J. Med.,* 69, 786, 1980.
117. **Spencer, H.,** Pulmonary edema and its complications and the effects of some toxic gases and substances on the lung, in *Pathology of the Lung,* Pergamon Press, Elmsford, N.Y.,1985.
118. **Slutzker, B., Knoll, H. C., Ellis, F. E., and Silverstone, I. A.,** Pulmonary alveolar proteinosis, *Arch. Int. Med.,* 107, 264, 1961.
119. **Jay, S. J.,** Pulmonary alveolar proteinosis successful treatment with aerosolized trypsin, *Am. J. Med.,* 66, 348, 1979.
120. **Hiratzka, L. E., Swan, D. M., Rose, E. F., and Ahrens, R. C.,** Bilateral simultaneous lung lavage utilizing membrane oxygenator for pulmonary alveolar proteinosis in an 8-month old infant, *Ann. Thorac. Surg.,* 36, 313, 1983.
121. **Selecky, P. A., Waggermann, K., Benheld, J. R., and Lippman, M.,** The clinical and physiological effect of whale lung lavage in pulmonary alveolar proteinosis, a ten-year experience, *Ann. Thorac. Surg.,* 24, 451, 1977.
122. **Lippmann, M. and Wassermann, K.,** Anesthetic management for children with alveolar proteinosis using extracorporeal circulation, *Br. J. Anesth.,* 49, 193, 1977.

Chapter 34

NEUROCUTANEOUS SYNDROMES WITH INTERSTITIAL LUNG DISEASE

Lourdes R. Laraya-Cuasay

TABLE OF CONTENTS

I. INTRODUCTION

Tuberous sclerosis and neurofibromatosis are two familial disorders with cutaneous, nervous system, and visceral manifestations. The peripheral nervous system is involved in neurofibromatosis while the central nervous system is affected in tuberous sclerosis. Interstitial fibrosis has been described in both disorders and manifests as spontaneous pneumothorax in a young adult.[1,2] Although not manifesting with dominant pulmonary symptoms in childhood, signs and symptoms which characterize the disorders occur in infancy and childhood, and recognition of these manifestations should alert the physician in anticipating the pulmonary complications, and serve as a guide in genetic counseling and prognosis.

II. TUBEROUS SCLEROSIS

Tuberous sclerosis is a relatively uncommon disorder inherited in an autosomal dominant pattern. The incidence of occurrence is about 7 per 100,000 individuals with 50 to 70% arising from new mutations. The brain, eyes, skin, heart, kidneys, lungs, and bones may be affected. The triad of seizures, mental deficiency, and cutaneous manifestations characterize the full entity. The pathognomonic skin lesions include adenoma sebaceum, shagreen patches, periungual and gingival fibromas, and hypopigmented macules. Cafe au lait spots may occur in about 26% of tuberous sclerosis. They are not considered a diagnostic sign of the disorder.[3]

A. Clinical Characteristics
1. Cutaneous Manifestations
Adenoma sebaceum occurs in 80 to 90% of cases and is the most common skin manifestation. Because these lesions histologically are found to be angiofibromas, hamartomas composed of fibrous and vascular tissue, the term adenoma becomes a misnomer. The lesions usually appear as 1 to 4 mm. dome-shaped nodules with smooth surface, and range from pink to red in color, and often accompanied by fine telangiectasia. These lesions are usually bilaterally symmetrical in distribution and located in the nasolabial folds, cheeks, chin, and sometimes in the forehead and scalp. They are rarely found in the upper lip except in the central area immediately below the nose. These lesions are rarely found at birth, may often develop between the second to fifth year, and often not seen until puberty. Only 13% of children develop the facial lesions during the first year of life; hence, this is not the best earliest marker of the disease in children. The periungual and gingival fibromas are seen in about 50% of patients and appear at puberty as firm, flesh-colored growths around and under the nails of fingers and toes. Like adenoma sebaceum, these fibromas cannot be used as an early marker of the disease.[3]

Shagreen patches develop early in childhood, from the second to the fifth postnatal year and are seen in 21 to 83% of cases. They appear as flesh-colored to yellowish or yellowish-orange slightly elevated plaques of dermal connective tissue generally found in the truncal area and most frequently in the lumbosacral region. The descriptive term comes from the shagreen leather-like appearance of the lesions which may be single or multiple, measuring 2 to 10 cm or more in diameter. An orange peel resemblance is also described.

The earliest skin lesions are the white macules[4] which are seen in 70 to 90% of cases and appear at birth or shortly thereafter. These macules enlarge as the infant grows but the shape does not change and they persist throughout life. The etiologies of hypopigmentation or hyperpigmentation are unknown. Since melanocytes are derived from the neural crest and in many ways function like nerve cells, the simultaneous finding of white macules and central nervous system involvement in this disease is not surprising. Only 18% of the white spots in tuberous sclerosis are truly ash-leaf in appearance.[5] Their sizes range from 0.4 to

7 cm or more with the majority measuring 1 to 3 cm in diameter. They are oval or semi-oval with highly irregular margins. They are to be differentiated from vitiligo but these lesions are unrelated to the latter. These lesions are a dull-white incomplete depigmentation as compared to the ivory whiteness of vitiligo. The leukoderma of tuberous sclerosis is usually present at birth, located over the abdomen, back, and anterior and lateral surfaces of the arms and legs. The lesions in vitiligo may appear on any part of the body. They are frequently bilateral and symmetrical in distribution on the skin of the face and neck, the backs of hands and forearms, over bony prominences, and in body folds and periorificial areas. They often change in size and shape, frequently spread, and may show partial to complete repigmentation.[3] By electron microscopy, the partially depigmented macules of tuberous sclerosis show normal number of melanocytes, with a decrease in the size, synthesis and melanization of melanosomes, whereas the completely depigmented lesions of vitiligo reveal an absence or a decrease in the number of melanocytes.

The presence of one or more tufts of white hair in an infant with seizures is suggestive of a diagnosis of tuberous sclerosis.[6] There seems to be an increased incidence of tuberous sclerosis in partial albinism.[7] A peculiar form of speckled leukoderma is the so-called white freckles. Characterized as multiple 1 to 3 mm hypopigmented lesions arranged in a confetti-like pattern on the pretibial area in some patients with tuberous sclerosis, it can also serve as a helpful marker of the disease. These lesions may very occasionally be found in normal individuals.[3]

In individuals with light pigmentation, recognition of the white macules can be aided by illuminating the skin with a Wood's light in a darkened room as these spots will contrast poorly against the surrounding normal skin.

Tooth pits have been recently recognized as another marker for tuberous sclerosis. Seen as punctate, round or oval 1 to 2 mm randomly arranged enamel defects particularly in permanent teeth when seen in numbers of five or more, these pits may prove to be pathognomonic of the disorder.[8]

2. Systemic Manifestations

Central nervous system involvement (62% of patients) may lead to convulsions and mild or severe mental retardation.[9,10] Sclerotic calcification in the brain is visible as "tubers" by X-ray in approximately 50 to 75% of cases. These tubers are scattered throughout the cortical gray matter. They consist of astrocytes and bizarre giant cells which stain like neurons. Multiple tumor nodules are distributed in the periventricular areas and are composed of fibrous glia, giant cells, and blood vessels. Though present at birth, these lesions enlarge and could form tumors which bulge into the lateral ventricles. Unilateral or bilateral hydrocephalus can result. Calcium is deposited in these tubers and may be visible radiographically at 1 year of age. Occasional malignant transformation to malignant astrocytoma or glioblastoma occurs. Convulsions are the commonest sign of brain involvement. Over 90% of patients affected will have seizures. Myoclonic seizures occur before 1 year of age. Grand mal and psychomotor types predominate later.[9] In infants whose skull X-rays do not show calcifications, computer assisted tomography of the skull shows calcification, ventricular dilatation, or both.[10] Mental deficiency is present in 60 to 70% of cases. Behavior disorders such as hyperactivity and destructiveness are common. Focal neurologic signs such as hemiparesis or hemianopsia suggest the possibility of malignant transformation in a paraventricular tumor. Other signs of increased intracranial pressure will also be present.[11] The electroencephalogram is usually abnormal without a specific pattern. The cerebrospinal fluid is normal or may rarely show elevated total protein.

Hamartomas may be found in the liver, spleen, and kidneys.[12] Rhabdomyomas of the heart may lead to congestive heart failure, murmurs, cyanosis, and sudden death. The retina may show phakomas or gliomatous lesions. The bones, particularly those of the hands and feet, show cysts and periosteal thickenings.[9,12,13]

The earliest reference to pulmonary symptoms and pathology in tuberous sclerosis was made by Lautenbacher,[14] who described changes in the lung of a 36-year-old woman who was dyspneic during the last 2 years of her life and who finally succumbed from bilateral spontaneous pneumothorax. At postmortem, the lung contained innumerable air-filled cystic spaces which were described as the size of "nuts". Both lungs presented a sponge-like appearance. Macroscopically, much of the lung was replaced by a honeycomb of small cystic spaces which bore no particular relationship to any part of the lung lobules. Small, solid, creamy white nodules varying in size up to 1 cm in diameter were visible on the cut surface but not related to vessels or bronchi. In advanced cases, there was evidence of hypertensive thickening in the pulmonary arteries. Sudden dyspnea may be caused by rupture of subpleural cysts resulting in spontaneous pneumothorax.

Microscopically, the appearance of the lung varies from one part to another. Some parts have a normal appearance, while others show emphysematous changes. Other areas may show nodules of fibroleiomyomatous tissue covered with flattened or cuboidal alveolar epithelium which project into the alveoli in a papillary fashion. In other parts of the lung, dilated and engorged capillaries follow obstruction of small pulmonary veins by hamartomatous tissue and lead to intra-alveolar hemorrhage and collections of siderophages. Abundance of siderophages imparts a brick-red color to the gross specimen.

It is impossible to advance any logical explanation for the bizarre neoplastic nodules that appear in this condition in so many organs, including the lung. The presence of glial nodules in the central nervous system, sebaceous adenoma in the skin, tumors composed of involuntary muscle and fibrous tissue in the kidney and lung suggests that this may be a congenital disorder of tissue organization probably involving all germinal layers.

B. Management

Anticonvulsants are the mainstay of therapy for those with seizures. Hyperactivity may be controlled with methylphenidate hydrochloride (Ritalin) or dextroamphetamine. Adenoma sebaceum requires no therapy except for cosmetic reasons. Cryosurgery, electrodessication, curettage or dermabrasion are usually successful and achieve good results. Surgical excision of tumors is indicated only if symptomatic.

The parents and their skull roentgenograms have to be examined for the stigmata of the disorder to rule out retinal, cutaneous, and cerebral manifestations. When neither parent has evidence of tuberous sclerosis, new mutation can be assumed. When evidence of the disorder is present in one parent, 50% of occurrence in subsequent children is predictable. Genetic counseling even for the mildest affected individual is usually against childbearing as the offspring may be more severely affected than the patient. Since mutations do occur in 50 to 70% of cases, genetic counseling may not be totally effective in prevention of new cases. Early recognition of the disease by discovering the early markers of the diagnosis can help screen previously unrecognized or mildly affected individuals.[3]

C. Prognosis

The course is extremely variable. Life beyond 30 years of age is a rarity. Patients with mild neurological involvement may live a full productive life. Institutional care may be needed by the mentally deficient. Premature death can occur from status epilepticus, respiratory failure, brain tumor, renal failure, or cardiac failure.

III. NEUROFIBROMATOSIS

Neurofibromatosis, or von Recklinghausen's disease, is transmitted as an autosomal dominant disorder with an incidence of approximately 1 in 2500 to 3000 births. There is no sex, race or color predilection. About 50% of cases represent new mutations.[15,16]

A. Clinical Characteristics
1. Cutaneous Manifestations

The hallmark of the disease is the cafe au lait spots which are irregularly shaped areas of increased pigmentation. The presence of six or more spots measuring greater than 1.5 cm in diameter is pathognomonic of neurofibromatosis.[16,17] A few cafe au lait spots may be found in 10 to 20% of normal individuals. These spots occur anywhere on the body. They may be as large as 15 cm in diameter, but the average size is 2 to 5 cm in length. Of diagnosed cases of neurofibromatosis, 78% have six or more cafe au lait spots.[16,17] Before the appearance of cutaneous fibromas in children, the presence of five or more cafe au lait spots measuring 0.5 cm in widest diameter or greater may indicate the presence of neurofibromatosis.[18]

Axillary freckling, another form of cafe au lait pigmentation, can serve as a useful diagnostic aid in the early recognition of neurofibromatosis. Twenty percent of patients with the disease will show these spots in the axillary vault. They measure 1 to 4 mm. Since these areas are not exposed to the sun, they can be differentiated from freckles. This finding is not seen in any other condition and therefore it is pathognomonic of von Recklinghausen's disease.[19]

The cafe au lait spots in neurofibromatosis show increased pigment in the basal layer of the epidermis, giant pigment granules in the melanocytes and keratinocytes of the epidermis,[20,21] and more DOPA-positive melanocytes per square centimeter in the cafe au lait spots than in the surrounding normal skin.[22] These characteristics distinguish these spots from those normally found in 20% of individuals.

Other cutaneous pigmentary changes include minute freckles distributed in other parts of the body, areas of leukoderma, and diffuse graying or bronzing of the skin as in argyria, but these are all not diagnostic of the disorder.[15]

Dermal fibromas and dermal or subcutaneous neurofibromas develop usually in early puberty or late childhood. These are derived from peripheral nerve sheaths. There may only be a few to many hundreds of these fibromas. They increase in size as the patient grows older. Neurofibromas may be found anywhere in the body except in the palms and soles. They are tumors measuring 1 to 2 mm or several centimeters in diameter, and they are palpated as beaded, nodular, elongated masses along the course of nerves, usually the trigeminal or upper cervical nerves. They look violaceous when small but are generally flesh-colored. They become pink, blue, or pigmented as they enlarge. The small tumors are deep-seated, sessile, or dome-shaped, then become pear-shaped, pedunculated, globular, or pendulous with continued growth. A pathognomonic feature is "button-holing" where the smaller lesions can be invaginated into an underlying dermal defect.[16,17] The course of these fibromas is generally benign but malignant transformation can occur in 2 to 3% of cases.[23] Fibrosarcomatous degeneration can occur in childhood but more often this occurs after 40 years. Malignant transformation is often preceded by rapid enlargement of the tumors and pain. Metastasis is rare and recurrences occur after excision.

2. Systemic Manifestations

Neurological involvement exists in as high as 40% of affected patients. Neurofibromas in the cranial or spinal nerve roots lead to various findings neurologically. Tumors of the VIII nerve cause tinnitus, nerve deafness, loss of corneal reflex, vertigo, ataxia, and signs of increased intracranial pressure. Increased incidence of optic glioma, meningioma, and pheochromocytoma may be found. Extramedullary spinal cord tumors resulting from fibromas involving a spinal root have been reported. Exophthalmos and decreased visual acuity are presenting findings and are seen as complications of this disorder.[9] Retardation, seizure disorders, and tumors are found in more than 50% of cases. Mild learning disabilities or severe retardation occur in 10 to 20% of cases.[12]

Kyphoscoliosis occurs in over 10% of patients when the neurofibroma involves the spine. Congenital bowing and pseudoarthrosis of the tibia, cysts of long bones, overgrowth of bone, and of soft tissue, megalencephaly, and malformation of the wing of the sphenoid bone have been described. Pulsating exophthalmos is associated with the latter malformation.[9]

Endocrine disorders associated with neurofibromatosis include cretinism, acromegaly, menstrual abnormalities, delayed or incomplete sexual development, hyperthyroidism, hypothyroidism, gynecomastia, infertility, Addison's disease, hyperparathyroidism, and diabetes. Sexual precocity is common in children. Between 5 and 20% of those with pheochromocytoma have neurofibromatosis, but only 1 of every 223 patients with neurofibromatosis is found to have pheochromocytoma.[16]

Benign bronchial and intrapulmonary neurofibromas are among the rarest tumors. Spencer has seen only three cases of bronchial neurofibroma.[24] One patient had generalized neurofibromatosis, the other had solitary extrabronchial lesion connected at one point with a nerve trunk, and the third patient had a malignant neurofibroma. Of the "acceptable" cases of benign bronchial or intrapulmonary neurofibroma, age ranged from 2 1/2 to 57 years. Although the majority of the eight reported intrabronchial schwannomas occurred in women, there is no sex predilection in intrabronchial and intrapulmonary neurofibroma.[25] Symptoms depend on the presence of obstruction of the bronchus or hemorrhage. Pain may radiate to the shoulders and interscapular regions. Joint pains, stiffness, fever, and dyspnea may occur.

These tumors are related to the bronchi and seldom exceed 3 cm in diameter. They form polypoid intrabronchial tumors or attach to the outside of a bronchus with a pedicle. These tumors are well encapsulated, lobulated, greyish-brown or pale yellow, and often contain cystic areas. They may hemorrhage and undergo calcification.[26] The collection of foam cells noted microscopically in both tumors gives them the yellow color grossly. Schwannomas contain bundles of elongated fibers showing characteristic palisading of nuclei (Antoni B tissue) separated by acellular and fine fibrillary substance (Antoni A tissue). They commonly undergo cystic degeneration and hemorrhage into the tumors and hyalinized vessel walls.[24]

Pulmonary involvement in neurofibromatosis was first described by Starck in 1928 as cystic lung disease associated with the generalized form.[24] This association was further confirmed by the later reports of Davies,[27] Massaro and colleagues,[28] and Israel-Asselain.[29] Dyspnea was the symptom that prompted previous investigators to take a chest X-ray which showed reticular densities, nodular shadows, and cystic changes. Decreased blood flow usually to the upper lobes was found angiographically. Numerous bullae were found on the surface of the lung macroscopically and honeycomb lung was found on sections. A diffuse interstitial fibrosis leading to extensive alveolar destruction and compensatory dilatation of terminal bronchioles, respiratory bronchioles and alveolar ducts were found. The distal airways were lined by cuboidal columnar or multilayered squamous-like epithelium with hyperplastic mural muscle frequently found. Hyperplasia of the neurilemmal cells occurred in the intrapulmonary nerves, especially the periarterial nerve branches. Glomus-like structures were seen in the smaller branches of the pulmonary arteries.[24]

Functional derangements include oxygen desaturation during exercise, slight increase in timed vital capacity, and hyperventilation resulting in actual or incipient respiratory alkalosis and, in the later stages, pulmonary hypertension.

Patchefsky and colleagues[30] presented the clinical and pathologic findings in a 28-year-old white woman whose symptoms started in her early childhood. Her mother had von Recklinghausen's disease. Gradually increasing exertional dyspnea occurred 2 years before admission, and productive cough was present for about 1 year. Clubbing of the fingers and toes without cyanosis was found. Chest roentgenogram done 1 year before was reported as normal. The admission chest film showed mild interstitial and diffuse infiltrates suggestive of pulmonary fibrosis in both lower lobes. The right apex showed linear fibrosis but no bullae. Ultrastructural examination of lung biopsy specimen showed increased collagen in the alveolar wall, associated with hyperplasia of granular pneumocytes. Large numbers of intra-alveolar cells, morphologically suggestive of macrophages, but having tight junction similar to epithelial cells, were also present. Direct immunofluorescent examination using goat anti IgG, IgM, IgA, complement, albumin and fibrinogen failed to show specific fluorescence.

Despite certain structural similarities to other familial and idiopathic forms of interstitial pneumonia, the pathogenesis of pulmonary findings in neurofibromatosis remains poorly understood. A mesenchymal defect which results in the primary deposition of collagen rather than a post-inflammatory reparative reaction may be the underlying mechanism of the disease. The fibrous tissue proliferation in diverse mesenchymal tissues such as blood vessels[31,32] and bone[33] that had been described in von Recklinghausen's disease support this view.

The coexistence of neurofibromatosis and interstitial pulmonary fibrosis has been previously reviewed and reported in patients ranging in age from 34 to 70 years.[28,29] Most cases showed diffuse, bilateral interstitial infiltrates suggesting pulmonary fibrosis. Apical bullae were reported in 19 of 20 patients.[28] Over 12% of patients examined in one study showed evidence of pulmonary fibrosis and alveolitis.[28] No cases were found in Crowe's large study of 223 unselected cases of neurofibromatosis.[16]

Variations in the granular pneumocytes seen in Patchefsky's patients[30] have been similarly observed in desquamative interstitial pneumonia (DIP).[34,35] Septal collagen deposition and intra-alveolar macrophages have also been reported in ultrastructural studies of DIP.[36] A case suggestive of DIP on light microscopy was reported in France.[37]

The familial occurrence of interstitial fibrosis[38] has been discussed in Chapter 2. One case of familial pulmonary fibrosis and neurofibromatosis has been reported.[29]

B. Management

Therapy is limited to excision of the fibromas or neurofibromas. Rapidly growing masses, pain, and impairment of function require tumor removal or excision.

Genetic counseling is indicated. Parents have to be examined for signs and symptoms suggestive of the disease, and if one parent is found to have evidence of the disease, 50% of subsequent children may be affected. Mutation is assumed when the parents do not manifest the disease. Genetic counseling against childbearing in an individual with the disease is recommended as 50% of the children will inherit the disorder.[9]

C. Prognosis

Life expectancy is essentially normal. The only risks to life arise from possible sarcomatous degeneration of the brain tumors, respiratory complications such as spontaneous pneumothorax resulting from chronic interstitial fibrosis, and possible intrabronchial obstructive problems.

Although not strictly a neurocutaneous syndrome, the presence of neurological and cutaneous features justify the discussion of ataxia-telangiectasia in this chapter.

IV. ATAXIA-TELANGIECTASIA

Ataxia-telangiectasia (AT) or Louis-Bar syndrome is a primary immunodeficiency transmitted on an autosomal recessive basis. The main features of this complex disease are cutaneous and bulbar telangiectases, progressive cerebellar degeneration, repeated sinopulmonary infections, endocrine abnormalities, and increased likelihood of cancer. Deficiency of immunoglobulin A and immunoglobulin E are the most common abnormalities.[39,40] Variable deficiencies in cell-mediated and/or antibody-mediated immune system are present.[41-44] The clinical expression and progression of the disease are variable but ultimate deterioration is inevitable. The variability is attributed to immunologic attrition which may

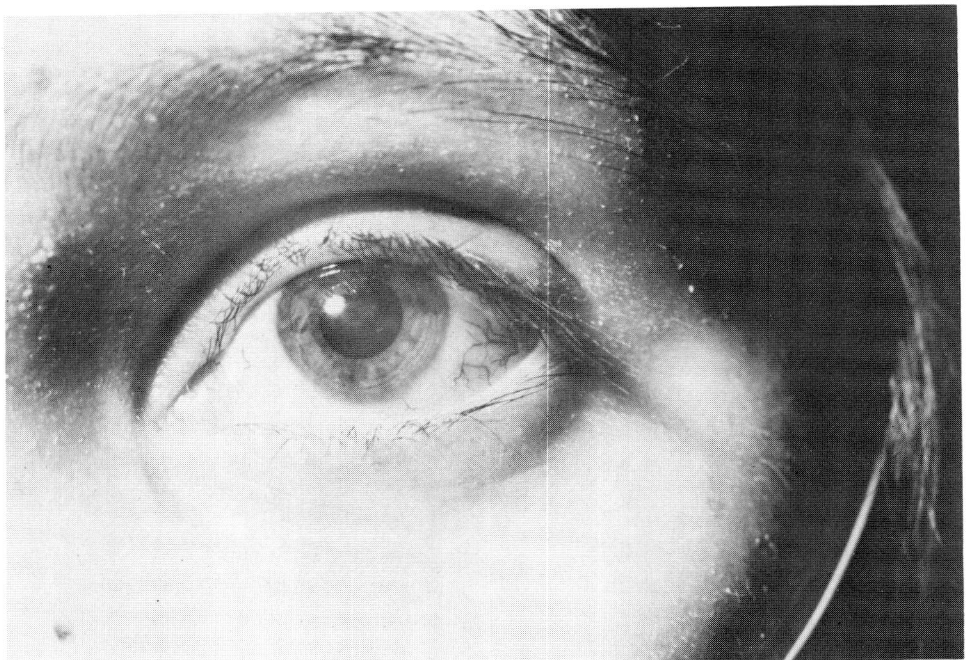

FIGURE 1.   Bulbar conjunctival telangiectasis in a patient with ataxia-telangiectasia whose lungs post-mortem showed severe pulmonary fibrosis.

be related to ''exhaustion'' of the immunologic system as a result of chronic infection or to a more basic defect. Analysis of collagen from two patients revealed deficiency of hydroxylysine suggesting a basic structural component defect.[45] This study was an attempt to support defective mesenchymal embryogenesis inasmuch as AT has thymic defect, telangiectases, and gonadal abnormalities.

A. Clinical Characteristics

1. Cutaneous Manifestations[39,46]

Telangiectases are fine, wiry, elongated vessels (see Figure 1). They may be noted in the bulbar conjunctivae as early as 1 year of age or as late as 6 years old. As the child grows older, the telangiectases become more prominent and may be found on the pinnae, butterfly area of the face, lateral aspect of the nose, the palate, neck, antecubital and popliteal areas, and dorsa of the hands and feet. Hypopigmentation and/or hyperpigmentation may be noted, as well as other skin lesions like atopic dermatitis, nummular eczema, cutaneous atrophy, skin malignancies, and excessive sweating.

2. Systemic Manifestations

Ataxia usually develops during infancy and is clinically recognized as soon as the infant is able to walk, but also, it is possible that it may not be observed until the child is 4 years of age. Although cerebellar ataxia has a variable progression and presentation, it ultimately leads to severe disability. Slurred speech gets increasingly worse with time. Tic-like movements and choreoathetosis may be present. Dysconjugate gaze, from irregular eye movements, may mimic ophthalmoplegia. Mask-like facies, strabismus, and excessive drooling have been described. Mental retardation is usually present. Muscle atrophy is secondary to muscle weakness.[47]

Diffuse cerebral atrophy and dilatation of the ventricular system may show on pneumoencephalography.[48,49] Anterior horn cell disease is suggested by fibrillation potentials demonstrated by electromyograms.[50] Loss of Purkinje and granular cell layer in the cerebellum,[49] evidence of anterior horn cell degeneration and posterior column demyelination,[47] skeletal muscle degeneration, degeneration of the acidophilic cells of the pituitary gland,[51] and rare thalamic and hypothalamic lesions have all been described.

Since 1957, recurrent sinopulmonary infections that ultimately lead to bronchiectasis have become part of the syndrome.[49] Susceptibility to recurrent infections is due to the immunologic defect. The infections may be due to bacteria, viruses, or mycoplasma. The bronchiectasis occurs often and may be diffuse. It could antedate the appearance of ataxia or telangiectasia. Pneumonia and pulmonary fibrosis are usually present.[49,51] Growth retardation is a prominent feature but the levels of thyroid, adrenal and growth hormones are normal.[52] Paucity of lymphoid tissue is noted. Lymphoid tissue is hypoplastic. The thymus may show atrophy, hypoplasia with absence of Hassall's corpuscles and corticomedullary differentiation.[53]

Patients who reach adolescence rarely demonstrate any secondary sex characteristics. Menstruation may begin in some, but menses are often irregular and may cease prematurely due to ovarian dysgenesis.[54] Testicular atrophy is common.

Increased incidence of malignancy, especially lymphomas,[55] and brain tumors, have been observed in these patients. Elevation of alpha-fetoprotein is present only in AT despite the absence of malignancy or chronic liver disease. All other immunodeficiency disorders show no elevation of alpha-fetoprotein levels.[56]

B. Management

Central nervous system degeneration proceeds at its own pace and has no known therapy. Any treatment is at best palliative except for antimicrobials given for culture-proven infections. Physical therapy and rehabilitation attempts may be frustrating. Even radiation therapy when indicated for lymphomas must be given in reduced dosage because of the unusual susceptibility of these patients to radiation effects.[57]

Frozen plasma infusions from a single family member were given to an AT patient at 3 week intervals. These resulted in good control of recurrent infections.[58] Gammaglobulin administration has been proven to be of no benefit. Immunological reconstitution has been tried but experience is limited.[59,60]

Genetic counseling must be given as there is a 25% recurrence risk in subsequently born children.

C. Prognosis

Survival to the fourth decade of life has been reported, but in general, early death from malignancy, most commonly lymphosarcomas, and the complications of repeated sinopulmonary infections, is the terminal event. Various tumors in association with AT have been reported including Hodgkin's disease, leukemia, adenocarcinoma, reticulum cell carcinoma, medulloblastoma, and dysgerminoma.

The author has managed two patients with AT. One was a 17-year-old male who developed pneumothorax and who subsequently died from chronic respiratory failure. Reticuloendotheliosis was diagnosed from a pulmonary biopsy. His sister also died from the malignant complication of AT during late adolescence. The other patient was a 14-year-old female whose major postmortem findings were acute and diffuse interstitial pneumonitis superimposed on diffuse pulmonary fibrosis with evidence of cor pulmonale. No ovaries were identifiable. Thymic tissue showed absence of Hassall's corpuscles and was very hypoplastic. Lymphoid tissue was hypoplastic.

Those who survive beyond puberty would suffer from incapacitating physical and mental disabilities and emotional problems.

REFERENCES

1. **Spencer, H.,** *Pathology of the Lung,* 4th ed., W. B. Saunders, Philadelphia, 1985, chap. 23.
2. **Petersdorf, R. G., Ed.,** *Harrison's Principles of Internal Medicine,* 10th ed., McGraw Hill, New York, 1983.
3. **Hurwitz, S.,** *Clinical Pediatric Dermatology,* W. B. Saunders, Philadelphia, 1981, 415.
4. **Hurwitz, S. and Braverman, I. M.,** White spots in tuberous sclerosis, *J. Pediatr.,* 77, 587, 1970.
5. **Fitzpatric, T. B., Szabo, G., Hori, Y., Simone, A. A., Reed, W. B., and Greenberg, M. H.,** White leaf-shaped macules; earliest visible sign of tuberous sclerosis, *Arch. Dermatol.,* 98, 1, 1968.
6. **McWilliams, R. P. and Stephensen, R. B. P.,** Depigmented hairs; the earliest sign of tuberous sclerosis, *Arch. Dis. Child.,* 53, 961, 1978.
7. **Hurwitz, S.,** Society Transactions, discussion of tuberous sclerosis, *Arch. Dermatol.,* 104, 336, 1971.
8. **Hoff, M., von Gransven, M. F., Jongeblood, W. L., and Gravenmade, E. J.,** Enamel defects associated with tuberous sclerosis, *Oral Surg. Oral Med. Oral Pathol.,* 40, 261, 1975.
9. **Behrman, R. E. and Vaughan, V. C., III,** *Nelson's Textbook of Pediatrics,* 12th ed., W. B. Saunders, Philadelphia, 1983.
10. **Martin, G. I., Kaiserman, D., Liegler, D., Amorosi, E. D., and Nadel, H.,** Computer-assisted cranial tomography in early diagnosis of tuberous sclerosis, *JAMA,* 235, 2323, 1976.
11. **Cooper, J. R.,** Brain tumors in hereditary multiple system hamartomatosis, (tuberous sclerosis), *J. Neurosurg.,* 34, 194, 1971.
12. **Callen, J. P.,** The skin, the eye, and systemic disease, *Cutis,* 24, 501, 1979.
13. **Nickel, W. R. and Reed, W. B.,** Tuberous sclerosis, *Arch. Dermatol.,* 85, 209, 1962.
14. **Lautenbacher, R.,** Dysembryomes metatypiques des reins carcinose submiliaire aigue du pomon avec emphyséme generalisé et double pneumothorax, *Ann. Med.,* 5, 435, 1918.
15. **Butterworth, T.,** Neurocutaneous syndromes — von Recklinghausen's disease, in *Clinical Genodermatology,* Williams & Wilkins, Baltimore, 1962, 101.
16. **Crowe, F. W., Schull, W. J., and Neel, J. V.,** *A Clinical, Pathologic, Genetic Study of Multiple Neurofibromatosis,* Charles C Thomas, Springfield, Ill., 1956.
17. **Crowe, F. W. and Schull, W. J.,** Diagnostic importance of the cafe au lait spot in neurofibromatosis, *Arch. Intern. Med.,* 91, 758, 1963.
18. **Whitehouse, D.,** Diagnostic value of the cafe au lait spot in children, *Arch. Dis. Child.,* 41, 316, 1966.
19. **Crowe, F. W.,** Axillary freckling as a diagnostic aid in neurofibromatosis, *Ann. Intern. Med.,* 61, 1142, 1962.
20. **Benedict, P. H., Szabo, G., and Fitzpatrick, T. B.,** Melanotic macules in Albright's syndrome and in neurofibromatosis, *JAMA,* 25, 618, 1968.
21. **Jimbo, K., Szabo, G., and Fitzpatrick, T. B.,** Ultrastructural giant pigment granules (macromelanosomes) in cutaneous pigmented macules of neurofibromatosis, *J. Invest. Dermatol.,* 61, 300, 1973.
22. **Johnson, B. L. and Charneco, D. R.,** Cafe au lait spots in neurofibromatosis and in normal individuals, *Arch. Dermatol.,* 102, 442, 1970.
23. **Braverman, I. M.,** *Skin Signs of Systemic Disease,* W. B. Saunders, Philadelphia, 1970.
24. **Spencer, H.,** *Pathology of the Lung,* 4th ed., W. B. Saunders, Philadelphia, 1985, Chap. 21.
25. **Bartley, T. D. and Arean, V. M.,** Intrapulmonary neurogenic tumors, *J. Thor. Cardiovasc. Surg.,* 50, 114, 1965.
26. **Petriat, A., Cornet, L., Leger, H., Castaing, R., and Tessier, R.,** Neurinome primitif intra-pulmonaire, *Presse Med.,* 61, 1526, 1953.
27. **Davies, P. D. B.,** Diffuse pulmonary involvement in von Recklinghausen's disease: a new syndrome, *Thorax,* 18, 198, 1963.
28. **Massaro, D., Katz, S., Matthews, M. J., and Higgins, C.,** von Recklinghausen's neurofibromatosis associated with cystic lung disease, *Am. J. Med.,* 38, 233, 1965.
29. **Israel-Asselain, R., Chebat, J., Sors, C. H., Basset, F., and LeRolland, A.,** Diffuse interstitial pulmonary fibrosis in a mother and son with von Recklinghausen's disease, *Thorax,* 20, 153, 1965.
30. **Patchefsky, A. S., Atkinson, W. G., Hoch, W. S., Gordon, G., and Lipshitz, H. I.,** Interstitial pulmonary fibrosis and von Recklinghausen's disease; an ultrastructural and immunofluorescent study, *Chest,* 64, 459, 1973.
31. **Bloor, K. and Williams, R. T.,** Neurofibromatosis and coarctation of the abdominal aorta with renal artery involvement, *Br. J. Surg.,* 50, 811, 1963.
32. **Halpern, M. and Currarino, G.,** Vascular lesions causing hypertension in neurofibromatosis, *N. Engl. J. Med.,* 273, 248, 1965.
33. **Rosenberg, R. N., Sassin, J., Zimmerman, E. A., and Carter, S.,** The interrelationship of neurofibromatosis and fibrous dysplasia, *Arch. Neurol.,* 17, 174, 1967.
34. **Farr, G. H., Harley, R. A., and Hennigar, G. R.,** Desquamative interstitial pneumonia; an electron microscopic study, *Am. J. Pathol.,* 60, 347, 1970.

35. **Shortland, J. R., Darke, C. S., and Crane, W. A. J.,** Electron microscopy of desquamative interstitial pneumonia, *Thorax,* 24, 192, 1969.
36. **Corrin, B. and Price, A. B.,** Electron microscopic studies in desquamative interstitial pneumonia associated with asbestos, *Thorax,* 27, 324, 1972.
37. **Lemenager, J., Cattan, D., Rousselot, P., and Bienard, Y.,** Pneumonie desquamative interstitielle et phacomatose pulmonaire, *J. Fr. Med. Clin. Thorac,* 25, 201, 1971.
38. **Swaye, P., Van Ordstrand, H. S., McCormack, L. J., and Wolpaw, S. E.,** Familial Hamman-Rich syndrome; report of eight cases, *Chest,* 55, 7, 1969.
39. **Louis-Bar, D.,** Sur un syndrome progressif comprenant des telangiectasies capillaires cutanées et conjunctivales symetriques, a disposition naevoide et des troubles cerebelleux, *Confin. Neurol.,* 4, 32, 1941.
40. **Tadjoedin, M. K. and Fraser, F. C.,** Heredity of ataxia-telangiectasia, (Louis-Bar syndrome), *Am. J. Dis. Child.,* 110, 64, 1965.
41. **Hanicki, Z., Hanicka, M., and Rambiesowa, E. M.,** Immunologic aspects of ataxia telangiectasia, *Int. Arch. Allerg.,* 32, 436, 1967.
42. **Gimeno, A., Liano, H., and Kreisler, M.,** Ataxia-telangiectasia with absence of IgG, *J. Neurol. Sci.,* 8, 545, 1969.
43. **Ammann, A. J., Cain, W. A., Ishizaka, K., Homg, R., and Good, R. A.,** Immunoglobulin E deficiency in ataxia-telangiectasia, *N. Eng. J. Med.,* 281, 469, 1969.
44. **Eisen, A. H., Karpati, G., Laszlo, T., Andermann, F., Robb, J. P., and Bacal, H. L.,** Immunologic deficiency in ataxia-telangiectasia, *N. Eng. J. Med.,* 272, 18, 1965.
45. **McReynolds, E. W., Dabbous, M. K., Hanissian, A. S., Deunas, D., and Kimrell, R.,** Abnormal collagen in ataxia-telangiectasia, *Am. J. Dis. Child.,* 130, 305, 1976.
46. **Reed, W. B., Epstein, W. L., Boder, E., and Sedgwick, R.,** Cutaneous manifestations of ataxia-telangiectasia, *JAMA,* 195, 746, 1966.
47. **Centerwall, S. A. and Centerwall, W. R.,** Ataxia-telangiectasia: a familial degenerative disease leading to mental retardation, *Am. J. Ment. Defic.,* 71, 185, 1966.
48. **Karpati, G., Eisen, A. H., Andermann, F., Bacal, H. L., and Robb, P.,** Ataxia-telangiectasia: Further observations and report of eight cases, *Am. J. Dis. Child.,* 110, 51, 1965.
49. **Boder, E. and Sedgwick, R. P.,** Ataxia-telangiectasia: a familial syndrome of progressive cerebellar ataxia, oculocutaneous telangiectasia and frequent pulmonary infection, *Univ. S. Calif. Med. Bull.,* 9, 15, 1957.
50. **Goodman, W. N., Cooper, W. C., Kessler, G. B., Fischer, M. S., and Gardner, M. B.,** Ataxia-telangiectasia: Report of two cases in siblings presenting a picture of progressive spinal muscular atrophy, *Bull. Los Angeles Neurol. Soc.,* 34, 1, 1969.
51. **Strich, S. J.,** Pathologic findings in three cases of ataxia telangiectasia, *J. Neurol. Neurosurg., Psychiat.,* 29, 489, 1966.
52. **Ammann, A. J., Duquesnoy, R. J., and Good, R. A.,** Endocrinological studies in ataxia-telangiectasia and other immunological deficiency diseases, *Clin. Exp. Immunol.,* 6, 587, 1970.
53. **Peterson, R. D. A., Kelly, W. D., and Good, R. A.,** Ataxia-telangiectasia: its association with defective thymus, immunological deficiency disease and malignancy, *Lancet,* 1, 1189, 1964.
54. **Bowden, D. H., Danis, P. G., and Sommers, S. C.,** Ataxia-telangiectasia: a case with lesions of ovaries and adenohypophysis, *J. Neuropath. Exp. Neurol.,* 22, 549, 1963.
55. **Peterson, R. D. A., Cooper, M. D., and Good, R. A.,** Lymphoid tissue abnormalities associated with ataxia-telangiectasia, *Am. J. Med.,* 41, 342, 1966.
56. **Waldmann, T. A. and McIntire, K. R.,** Serum alpha-fetoprotein levels in patients with ataxia-telangiectasia, *Lancet,* 2, 1112, 1972.
57. **Paterson, M. C., Smith, R. P., Lohman, P. H. M., Anderson, A. K., and Fishman, L.,** Defective excision of x-ray damaged DNA in human (ataxia-telangiectasia) fibroblasts, *Nature (London),* 260, 444, 1976.
58. **Ammann, A. J., Good, R. A., Bier, D., and Fudenberg, H. H.,** Long-term plasma infusions in a patient with ataxia-telangiectasia and deficient IgA and IgE, *Pediatrics,* 44, 672, 1969c.
59. **Ammann, A. J., Wara, D. W., Doyle, N. E., and Golbus, M. S.,** Thymus transplantation in patients with thymic hypoplasia and abnormal immunoglobulin synthesis, *Transplantation,* 20, 457, 1975.
60. **Lopukhin, Y., Morozov, Y., and Petrov, R.,** Transplantation of neonate thymus sternum complex in ataxia telangiectasia, *Trans. Proc.,* 5, 823, 1973.

Chapter 35

SARCOIDOSIS

Rosalind S. Abernathy

TABLE OF CONTENTS

I. INTRODUCTION

Sarcoidosis, a systemic granulomatous disease of unknown etiology, was originally described as a dermatologic curiosity by Hutchinson and Besnier. In 1899, Boeck, a Norwegian dermatologist, described granulomatous skin changes, which he thought resembled sarcoma. He called this sarcoid and hence the term sarcoidosis. The systemic nature of the disease was described by Schaumann in 1916, when he noted involvement of the lungs, lymph nodes, bone, liver, and spleen. It was necessary for the incidence of tuberculosis to decline before the frequency of this granulomatous disease could be fully recognized, as it has been since the first international sarcoidosis conference in 1934.[1]

II. INCIDENCE AND EPIDEMIOLOGY

The incidence of sarcoidosis varies widely with race, age, and geographic location. Caucasian subjects in northern Europe were originally described with the disease but blacks have been found to be predominantly affected in the U.S. It is most commonly seen in young adults, between 20 and 40 years of age, with an increased incidence in women, and is rare in children, 15 years or younger. McGovern and Merritt found 104 cases in childhood described in the literature in their survey published in 1956.[2] Since 1964, 9 series of 7 to 33 patients each have added 173 cases of childhood sarcoidosis to the literature. The states of Virginia, North Carolina, South Carolina, and Arkansas account for 76% of these cases, suggesting that the southeast and southcentral states are an endemic area for childhood sarcoidosis.[3-11]

Most series of childhood sarcoidosis report the majority of the cases in the 13 to 15 year age range and with an equal sex ratio. The Arkansas patients were somewhat younger, with a median age of 11 years and 60% were male. The percentage of black children in the series reported from the endemic areas ranged from 72 to 97%.[4,8-11]

III. ETIOLOGY, PATHOGENESIS, AND PATHOLOGY

Although the etiology of sarcoidosis is unknown, it appears to be an immunologic response to an unknown antigenic stimulus, which gains access to the body by the lungs. The initial response to the antigen is an alveolitis, characterized by infiltration of the alveolar septae by increased numbers of mononuclear cells, T-lymphocytes and macrophages.[12] Most of the T-lymphocytes are of the helper variety with proportionally fewer suppressor T-cells. A significant percentage of these helper T-cells are releasing mediators to attract mononuclear phagocytes to the lung with monocyte chemotactic factor, to immobilize them there with migration inhibitory factor and to provide polyclonal activation of B-cells.[13] The peripheral blood, meanwhile, shows a lower proportion of T-helper cells compared to the numbers present in normal controls.[14] The polyclonal activation of the B-cells accounts for the frequently observed hyperglobulinemia and increased levels of immunoglobulins noted in patients with sarcoidosis. The decrease in the numbers of T-helper cells in peripheral blood is a partial explanation of the parodoxical finding of a depressed response to delayed hypersensitivity skin tests to tuberculin and other antigens, another characteristic of sarcoidosis.

The mononuclear cells attracted to the lung by the activated T-lymphocytes are the precursors of the epithelioid cells and giant cells of the noncaseous granuloma, which is the characteristic pathological lesion in sarcoidosis. Granulomata are found in tissues throughout the body. They may resolve eventually spontaneously or under the influence of corticosteroid therapy, leaving no residua or they may progress to fibrosis.

The diagnosis of sarcoidosis rest on (1) compatible clinical and/or roentgenographic findings, (2) histological evidence of noncaseating granulata, and (3) proof by means of special

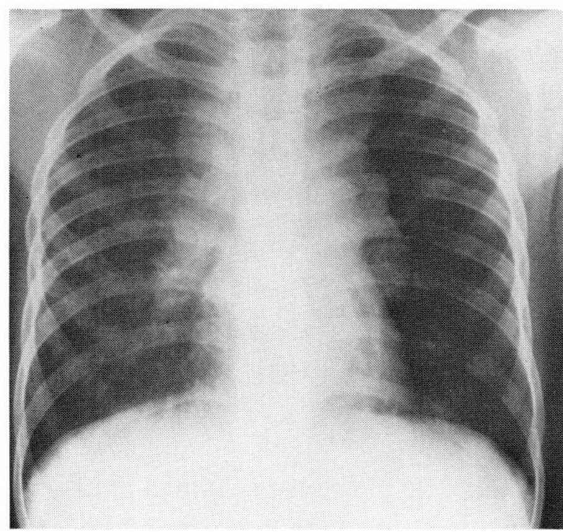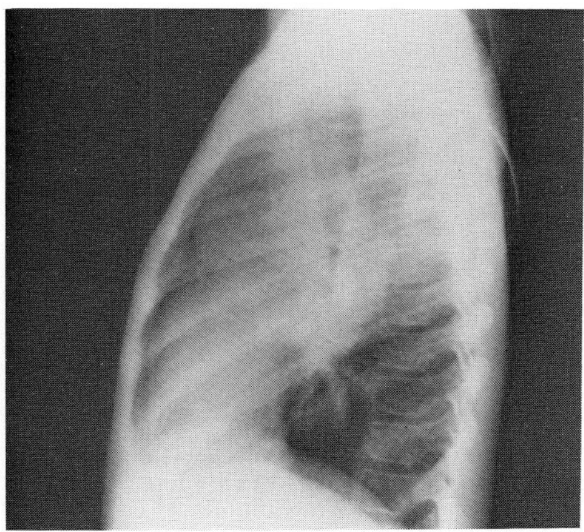

FIGURE 1.   A 12-year-old black male presented (1978) with large cervical lymph nodes, skin rash, follicular conjunctivits and mild iritis. Both skin and conjunctivitis biopsies were positive. This shows large hilar and paratracheal lymph nodes and typical reticulonodular infiltrate of Stage II.

stains and cultures that these lesions are not due to fungi, mycobacteria, or other organisms which can cause similar pathological findings.

IV. CLINICAL MANIFESTATIONS

Sarcoidosis may be asymptomatic, detected by its characteristic chest roentgenographic findings discovered on routine films. Up to 45% of adult patients may be initially diagnosed this way.[15] Since children rarely have routine roentgenograms, sarcoidosis as recognized in children is more likely to be symptomatic. Symptoms are of two varieties. Generalized constitutional symptoms, which include weight loss, fatigue or lethargy, malaise, and occasionally fever, may be present in from 42 to 68% of children.[4,10,11] Other symptoms are due to the infiltration of granulomas into various organ systems. The most commonly affected is the lung. Dyspnea, cough and to a lesser extent, chest pain were the complaints in 38 to 48% of children in the endemic area.[4,8-11] Other complaints include enlargement of peripheral lymph nodes in 15 to 30%[4,8,9,11] and ophthalmologic symptoms such as red or painful eyes and decreased visual acuity in 12 to 35%.[4,8-11]

V. ORGAN SYSTEM INVOLVEMENT INCLUDING RADIOGRAPHY

As in adults, the pulmonary system is almost universally involved in children with sarcoidosis. Physical findings of the chest are usually absent except for tachypnea in the very severely affected. Abnormalities are detected in the chest roentgenogram and by pulmonary function testing. By convention since the 1950s, the roentgenographic appearance had been classified into three categories: Stage I showing bilateral hilar and paratracheal adenopathy with normal appearing lung parenchyma, Stage II with both bilateral adenopathy and parenchymal abnormalities, and Stage III with parenchymal disease without any hilar adenopathy. A normal roentogenogram can be designated Stage O. Figure 1 shows a Stage II film with prominent adenopathy. Parenchymal abnormalities may include a diffuse reticulonodular or, less commonly, acinar pattern which may coalesce into areas of consolidation. Findings of linear strands extending out from the hilum or asymmetrical bullae are suggestive of pulmonary fibrosis. Observations by early students of the disease over many years demonstrated sequential evolution from Stage I to Stage III. Parenchymal infiltrates often appear as hilar adenopathy is diminishing. After hilar nodes disappear, they never reappear. The prognosis for remission decreases as the Stage increases.[16,17]

This classification is strictly on the basis of the appearance of the standard roentgenogram. Alveolitis and/or granulomas may be demonstrated on lung biopsy in patients with Stage I films. Despite this, as long as the roentgenographic classification remains Stage I, the prognosis is good.[16]

Pulmonary function abnormalities also correlate roughly with the roentgenographic stage. Stage I findings are associated with a normal vital capacity in 80% and normal diffusing capacity (DLCO) in 70% of patients. In the presence of parenchymal disease (Stage II and III), the vital capacity and DLCO are normal only 35% of the time. Restrictive abnormality with a decreased forced vital capacity (FVC) is the classical pulmonary function finding in sarcoidosis. Changes in the diffusion capacity usually mirror the FVC. No pulmonary function test is of any prognostic value in sarcoidosis but following changes in individual patients is an important part of ongoing evaluation.[18] Nearly all children with sarcoidosis are at least 6 years of age and capable of performing pulmonary function tests.

Granulomatous infiltration of peripheral lymph nodes is the second most common manifestation of sarcoidosis in children, occurring in 60 to 70%. The nodes are nontender, rubbery in nature, freely moveable and may be large enough to see from a distance. The table shows the incidence of organ system involvement in the three largest series of childhood sarcoidosis compared with a worldwide adult group.[4,8,11,15]

Ocular involvement is the most significant manifestation, after the lungs, with the potential for serious residua. Granulomatous uveitis, which may be asymptomatic, is very characteristic of sarcoidosis. A complete ophthalmological examination including evaluation with the slit lamp is mandatory in any patient suspected of having sarcoidosis. The presence of characteristic findings can help make the diagnosis and the patient can be offered the meticulous ophthalmologic care required to help insure that his vision is preserved. Nodules can be found on the conjunctiva; lacrimal glands can be infiltrated. Cataracts and/or glaucoma may complicate uveitis both as part of the disease and as complications of topical steroid treatment. Loss of vision is the most severe complication.[1]

A moderate degree of splenomegaly is a characteristic finding but massive enlargement can occasionally be seen. Complications of this include the possibility of traumatic rupture and hypersplenism. Hepatomegaly may be present. Although liver nearly always contains granulomas at post-mortem, liver function abnormality is rarely noted. A syndrome of febrile hepatic granulomatosis, characterized by a very large liver and high fever, has been described as a form of sarcoidosis and was present in two children and two 19-year-old patients seen at the University of Arkansas.[19]

Erythema nodosum has been seen as part of Löfgren syndrome, with other manifestations of fever, fatigue, polyarthralgia and a Stage I chest film. Spontaneous resolution without therapy occurs within 6 months in 80% of cases. This is most commonly seen in young adult white women and is rare in children and black patients.[1]

Children do have cutaneous lesions which show noncaseating granulomas on biopsy. The most characteristic forms are small flat-topped papules on the face and 2 to 3 cm round pigmented plaques on the trunk. Subcutaneous nodules may also be seen. Skin lesions often appear first with a systemic exacerbation of the disease.[11]

Parotid gland enlargement may be seen, either as an initial finding or developing during the course of the illness (Table 1).

Arthralgias without physical findings occur in some patients. Arthritis with nonpainful effusions and boggy synovial thickening in the large joints is characteristic of a small group of pediatric sarcoidosis patients in whom the disease has its onset at 4 years of age or less. Other characteristic findings in this group are diffuse dermatitis and granulomatous uveitis. These children do not have pulmonary involvement and only 2 of the 28 cases so far reported have been black.[20,21]

Table 1
ORGAN SYSTEM INVOLVEMENT IN SARCOIDOSIS

| Location (Reference) no. cases | Children 15 years and under | | | | | | Adults world-wide[15] 1,609 |
| | North Carolina[4] 25 | | Virginia[8] 33 | | Arkansas[11] 30 | | |
	No.	(%)	No.	(%)	No.	(%)	(%)
Chest roentgenogram abnormality	25	100	33	100	30	100	88
Peripheral lyphadenopathy	18	72	23	70	19	63	28
Splenomegaly	10	40	9	27	12	40	10
Hepatomegaly	14	56	11	33	9	30	—
Eyes	12	48	8	24	12	40	22
Uveitis	12	48	7	21	8	26	—
Skin	8	32	9	27	9	30	18
Parotid	6	24	4	12	7	23	6
7th nerve palsy	2	—			2		—

Involvement of the bones is nearly always asymptomatic and detectable only on roentgenograms. The characteristic finding is small, round lytic lesions in the small bones of the hands or feet. These may remain unchanged for years. Larger, irregular lytic lesions in the long bones are occasionally seen. These may heal without therapy.[11]

Renal disease in children is primarily the result of hypercalciuria, which causes the development of kidney stones and sometimes ureteral obstruction and secondary infection. Increased gastrointestinal absorption of calcium is due to elevated 1,25 dihydroxyvitamin D levels in the blood. It has been demonstrated that this material is synthesized in the sarcoid granulomas.[22,23]

The most common neurological complication of sarcoidosis in children is facial (7th) nerve palsy, always transient in nature.[24]

VI. LABORATORY STUDIES

Hyperglobulinemia, present in two thirds of the cases, is the most common laboratory abnormality in sarcoidosis.[4,11] Often there is hyperimmunoglobulinemia. This is most often seen in black patients and in children, most of whom are black. A white count less than 5000 and a modest degree of eosinophilia are both common findings, but by no means diagnostic of sarcoidosis. Hypercalcemia, with serum calcium levels greater than 11 mg% is present in about one third of childhood cases.[4,8,11] Hypercalciuria, much more common than hypercalcemia but difficult to document, can be detected by measuring creatinine and calcium in a single voided specimen. A calcium/creatinine ratio of greater than 0.20 is indicative of hypercalciuria.[25] This technique has not been widely used in evaluating pediatric sarcoidosis patients but should be studied.

Delayed hypersensitivity skin testing with PPD, candida and tetanus help to complete the evaluation. A negative PPD is less of an indicator of sarcoidosis than a reassurance that the granulomatous disease is not tuberculosis. The combination of elevated immunoglobulins with negative skin tests to candida and tetanus would certain be supportive of the diagnosis of sarcoidosis.

VII. DIAGNOSTIC BIOPSIES

The diagnosis of sarcoidosis rests on finding noncaseating granuloma in a biopsy specimen and proving that this is not due to a known granuloma producing infection. Less invasive biopsies should be done whenever possible. Biopsies of skin lesions and subcutaneous nodules are nearly always positive. Specimens from less obviously diseased tissue such as from the lower lip for minor salivary glands often have a significant yield.[26] The conjunctival biopsy is nearly always positive if a small millet-seed nodule can be biopsied, but even in the absence of this, granulomas can be obtained 70% of the time if bilateral biopsies are taken.[27] All of these can be performed on an ambulatory basis. The most frequently biopsied site in children has been a peripheral lymph node, including the scalene fat pad biopsy. This a low risk procedure but usually requires anesthesia and admission to the hospital or ambulatory surgery. Other biopsy sites in children have been liver, lung parenchyma, parotid gland, bone, striated muscle and testes.[4,8,11] Figure 2 shows the microscopic features of sarcoidosis.

Transbronchial biopsy with the flexible bronchoscope has become the procedure of choice for adults because it is simple, safe and may be performed without anesthesia. Roethe has shown that multiple specimens are needed, five for Stage II and ten for Stage I disease, to ensure a positive biopsy.[28] Mediastinoscopy provides a very high yield in any patient with hilar adenopathy. It is safe but requires anesthesia.[29] Either of these procedures could be done in a cooperative teen-age patient.

Three new diagnostic techniques described in the past 10 years were promoted as being much more sensitive measures of the inflammatory response in sarcoidosis, which would allow more accurate diagnosis and prognosis than with traditional means of evaluation. Bronchoalveolar lavage has been the tool by which much of the pathophysiology of pulmonary sarcoidosis has been worked out,[31] but it is too invasive to use in children. Gallium 67 scanning of the lungs appears to reflect the presence of granulomas accurately,[12] but because of its generalized radiation exposure, should not be used in children. Determination of the serum angiotensin-converting enzyme (ACE) level can be done in children. Normal values for children, higher than for adults, were established and it was demonstrated that children with sarcoidosis had significantly higher values than did normal children.[31] Unfortunately, false negative serum ACE tests are found in both Stage I and Stage III patients. Regrettably, none of these new tests are specific for sarcoidosis and they offer less diagnostic aid than originally expected. They also have failed to predict the long-term prognosis in pulmonary sarcoidosis or to differentiate those who will develop pulmonary fibrosis.[32]

The major diseases for differentiation from pulmonary sarcoidosis are tuberculosis, systemic fungal diseases, Hodgkins disease, and lymphomas. The tuberculin skin test, serologic tests for the fungal antigens and cultures should help differentiate the first of these and the diagnostic biopsy should rule out lymphomas.

VIII. TREATMENT

The indications for treatment of pulmonary sarcoidosis vary with the radiologic appearance at diagnosis. About 70% of patients with Stage I disease will have a spontaneous remission and should be followed until this occurs or they progress to Stage II. Spontaneous remission rates with Stage II and Stage III chest roentgenograms are 50% and 30% respectively. Patients with parenchymal disease (Stage II or III) should be treated if they are symptomatic or abnormalities appear to be progressing. The response will be good if granulomatous inflammation is present but fibrosis will not respond. Since there is no way to determine if fibrosis is present, all patients should have the benefit of a trial of treatment. Some authorities feel that early treatment with corticosteroids may suppress inflammation and decrease the

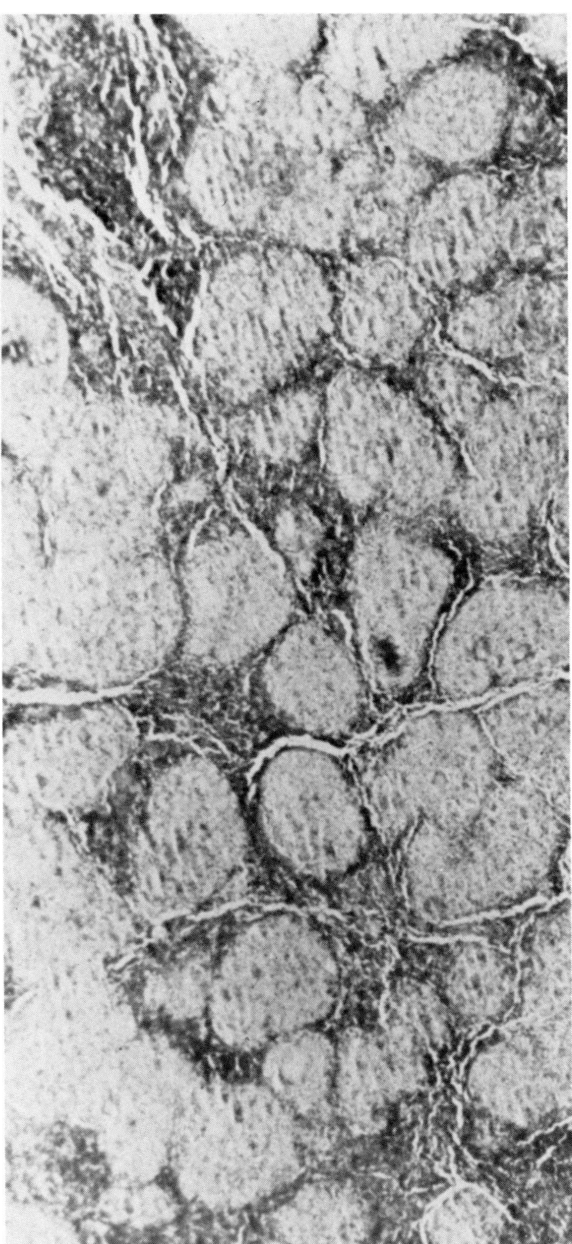

A

FIGURE 2.   (A) Lymph node showing extensive infiltration with non-caseating granulomata (H & E × 100). (B) Multinucleated giant cell, epithelioid cells and lymphocytes in lung tissue (× 750). (C) Skin with a large giant cell containing two astroid bodies, characteristic but not diagnostic inclusions sometimes seen in sarcoidosis (× 1000).

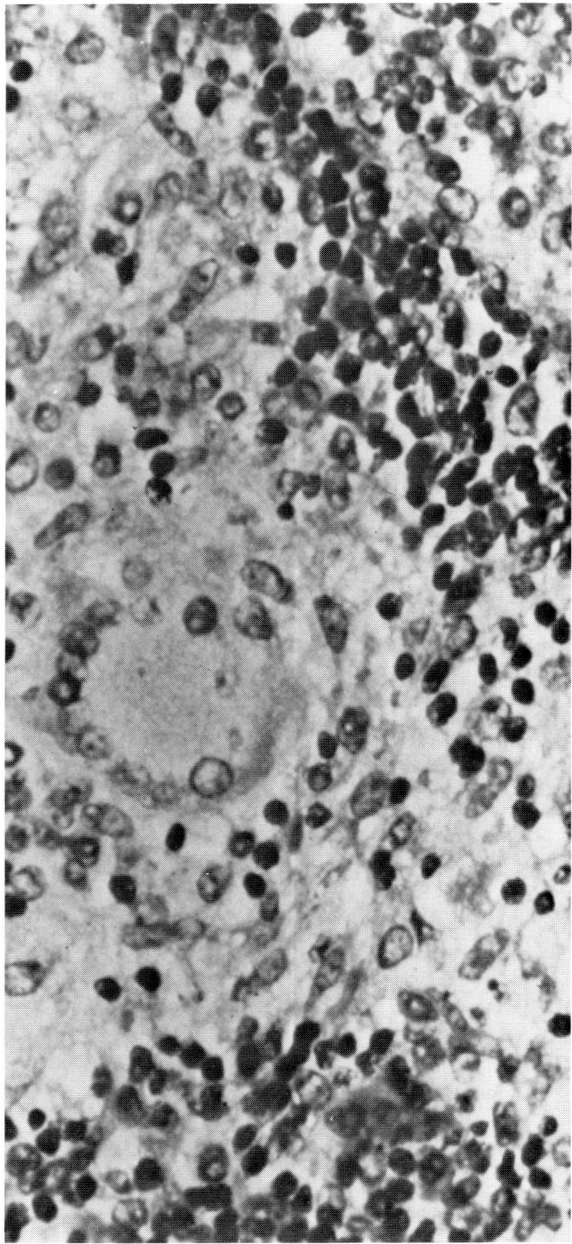

FIGURE 2B

possibility of progression to fibrosis.[33] Extrapulmonary sarcoidosis is often the indication for treatment. These indications include persistent hypercalcemia and hypercalciuria, massive splenomegaly with hypersplenism, infiltration into vital structures such as the myocardium and the central nervous system, uveitis uncontrolled by topical steroids, disfiguring skin disease, severe hepatic involvement and progressive constitutional symptoms such as fever and weight loss.

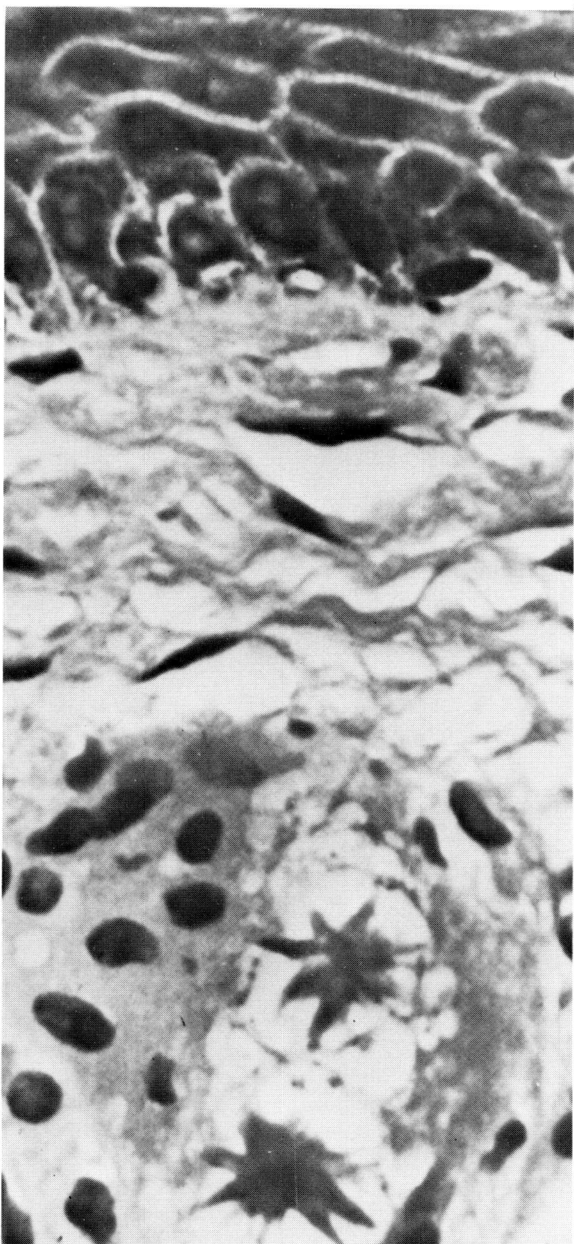

FIGURE 2C

When treatment is indicated, oral prednisone is the drug of choice, beginning with 1 mg/ kg daily and changing to an alternative day schedule once improvement has occurred. The duration of therapy depends upon the rapidity of clearing of signs and symptoms but usually is many months and often years.

Children with generalized sarcoidosis may have a 50% incidence of systemic exacerbation after initial improvement either spontaneously or induced by prednisone treatment. This is usually heralded by weight loss. Other manifestations are the appearance of skin lesions, the onset or recurrence of hypercalcemia or hypercalciuria, splenomegaly or parotid swelling. Granulomatous uveitis may progress or abnormality of the chest roentgenogram or pulmonary functions may worsen. Exacerbations are usually equally responsive to prednisone treatment.[11]

The overall prognosis of children is similar to that of adults, and is less favorable for blacks and those with generalized disease. Most children fall into both of these categories. World-wide statistics show a mortality of 5% in London and New York but only 1.8% in Paris where 84% of the patients were white.[15] Katuria reported a death rate of 5.5% in black patients but only 1.4% in white patients.[34] Pediatric reports include 1 death in 43 cases,[35] 1 in 25,[4] 1 in 18,[9] and 2 in 30.[11] Four of these were pulmonary deaths. This is a death rate of 5/116 or 4.3%, comparable to reports in adults from largely black populations.

IX. SUMMARY

Sarcoidosis, a generalized granulomatous disease of unknown etiology occurs most commonly in black people in the USA. Children, who are uncommonly affected except in the southeast and southcentral areas of the county, show a similar clinical picture to adults. Pulmonary involvement is almost universal. The most characteristic finding on chest roentgenogram is large hilar lymph nodes bilaterally. Many also have parenchymal disease and abnormalities of pulmonary function. Peripheral lymph nodes, eyes, skin, spleen, and liver can also affected. Treatment, if necessary, is with prednisone. The death rate, over time, is about 5%, usually as a result of respiratory failure from pulmonary fibrosis. Significant visual impairment may also result.

REFERENCES

1. **Kerdel, F. A. and Moschella, S. L.,** Sarcoidosis, an updated review, *J. Am. Acad. Dermatol.,* 11, 1, 1984.
2. **McGovern, J. P. and Merritt, D. H.,** Sarcoidosis in childhood, *Adv. Pediatr.,* 8, 97, 1956.
3. **Beier, F. R. and Lahey, M. E.,** Sarcoidosis among children in Utah and Idaho, *J. Pediatr.,* 65, 350, 1964.
4. **Jasper, P. L. and Denny, F. W.,** Sarcoidosis in children with special emphasis on the natural history and treatment, *J. Pediatr.,* 73, 499, 1968.
5. **Siltzbach, L. E. and Greenberg, G. M.,** Childhood sarcoidosis — a study of eighteen patients, *N. Engl. J. Med.,* 279, 1239, 1968.
6. **Reed, W. G.,** Sarcoidosis: a review and report of eight cases in children, *J. Tenn. Med. Assoc.,* 62, 27, 1969.
7. **Schmitt, E., Appelman, H., and Threatt, B.,** Sarcoidosis in children, *Radiology,* 106, 621, 1973.
8. **Kendig, E. L., Jr.,** The clinical picture of sarcoidosis in children, *Pediatrics,* 54, 289, 1974.
9. **Schabel, S. I., Stanley, J. H., and Shelley, B. E., Jr.,** Pediatric sarcoidosis, *J. S.C. Med. Assoc.,* 76, 419, 1980.
10. **Merten, D. F., Kirks, D. R., and Grossman, H.,** Pulmonary sarcoidosis in childhood, *Am. J. Roentgenol.,* 135, 673, 1985.
11. **Abernathy, R. S.,** Childhood sarcoidosis in Arkansas, *South Med. J.,* 78, 435, 1985.
12. **Abe, S., Munakata, M., Nishimura, M., et al.,** Gallium-67 scintigraphy, bronchoalvelar lavage, and pathologic changes in patients with pulmonary sarcoidosis, *Chest,* 85, 650, 1984.
13. **Keogh, B. A., Hunninghake, G. W., Line, B. R., et al.,** The alveolitis of pulmonary sarcoidosis, *Am. Rev. Respir. Dis.,* 128, 256, 1983.
14. **Ceuppens, J. L., Lacquet, L. M., Mariën, G., et al.,** Alveolar T-cell subsets in pulmonary sarcoidosis, *Am. Rev. Respir. Dis.,* 129, 563, 1984.
15. **Sitzbach, L. E., James, D. G., Neville, E., et al.,** Course and prognosis of sarcoidosis around the world, *Am. J. Med.,* 57, 847, 1974.

16. **DeRemee, R. A.,** The roentgenographic staging of sarcoidosis. Historic and contemporary perspectives, *Chest,* 83, 128, 1983.
17. **Paré, J.A.P. and Fraser, R. G.,** *Synopsis of Diseases of the Chest,* W. B. Saunders, Philadelphia, 1983, chap. 14.
18. **Winterbauer, R. H. and Hutchinson, J. F.,** Clinical significance of pulmonary function tests. Use of pulmonary function tests in the management of sarcoidosis, *Chest,* 78, 640, 1980.
19. **Israel, H. L., Margolis, M. L., and Rose, L. J.,** Hepatic granulomatosis and sarcoidosis, *Dig. Dis. Sci.,* 29, 353, 1984.
20. **North, A. F., Fink, C. W., Gibson, W. M., et al.,** Sarcoid arthritis in children, *Am. J. Med.,* 48, 449, 1970.
21. **Hetherington, S.,** Sarcoidosis in young children, *Am. J. Dis. Child.,* 136, 13, 1982.
22. **Chesney, R. W., Hamstra, A. J., DeLuca, H. F., et al.,** Elevated serum 1,25-dihydroxyvitamin D concentration in the hypercalcemia of sarcoidosis: correction by glucocorticoid therapy, *J. Pediatr.,* 98, 919, 1981.
23. **Barbour, G. L., Coburn, J. W., Slatopolsky, E., et al.,** Hypercalcemia in an anephric patient with sarcoidosis: evidence for extrarenal generation of 1,25-dihydroxyvitamin D, *N. Engl. J. Med.,* 305, 440, 1981.
24. **Weinberg, S., Bennett, H., Weinstock, I.,** Central nervous system manifestations of sarcoidosis in children, *Clin. Pediatr.,* 22, 477, 1983.
25. **Roy, S., III, Stapleton, F. B., Noe, H. N., et al.,** Hematuria preceding renal calculus formation in children with hypercalciuria, *J. Pediatr.,* 99, 712, 1981.
26. **Nessan, V. J. and Jacoway, J. R.,** Biopsy of minor salivary glands in the diagnosis of sarcoidosis, *N. Engl. J. Med.,* 301, 922, 1979.
27. **Karcioglu, Z. A. and Brear, R.,** Conjunctival biopsy in sarcoidosis, *Am. J. Ophthalmol.,* 99, 68, 1985.
28. **Roethe, R. A., Fuller, P. B., Byrd, R. B., et al.,** Transbronchoscopic lung biopsy in sarcoidosis. Optimal number and sites for diagnosis, *Chest,* 77, 400, 1980.
29. **Munkgaard, S. and Neukirch, F.,** Comparison of biopsy procedures in intrathoracic sarcoidosis, *Acta Med. Scand.,* 205, 179, 1979.
30. **Crystal, R. C., Roberts, W. C., Hunninghake, G. W., et al.,** Pulmonary sarcoidosis: a disease characterized and perpetuated by activated lung T-lymphocytes, *Ann. Intern. Med.,* 94, 73, 1981.
31. **Rodriquez, G. E., Shin, B. C., Abernathy, R. S., et al.,** Serum angiotensin-converting enzyme activity in normal children and in those with sarcoidosis, *J. Pediatr.,* 99, 68, 1981.
32. **Rubinstein, I. and Baum, G. L.,** The persistent need to improve our approach to sarcoidosis (editoral), *Chest,* 87, 710, 1985.
33. **DeRemee, R. A.,** Sarcoidosis, current perspective on diagnosis and treatment, *Postgrad. Med.,* 76, 167, 1984.
34. **Kataria, Y. P., Shaw, R. A., and Campbell, P. B.,** Sarcoidosis: an overview II, *Clin. Notes Respir. Dis.,* 20, 3, 1982.
35. **Kendig, E. L., Jr.,** Sarcoidosis, *Am. J. Dis. Child.,* 136, 11, 1982.
36. **Lieberman, J., Ed.,** *Sarcoidosis,* Grune & Straton, Inc., New York, 1985.

Chapter 36

HYPERSENSITIVITY PNEUMONITIS

Bettina C. Hilman

TABLE OF CONTENTS

I. GENERAL CONSIDERATIONS

Hypersensitivity pneumonitis (HP) or extrinsic allergic alveolitis (EAA), is a descriptive term for a group of immunologically mediated inflammatory pulmonary diseases which result from sensitization and recurrent exposure to a variety of inhaled finely dispersed organic dusts. The size of the inhaled particles inducing HP vary but are usually in the range of 3 to 5 μ. Antigens in inhaled organic dusts include thermophilic actinomycetes, fungi, bacteria, animal proteins, arthropods, chemicals, and other agents such as Bacillus subtilis or amoebae (Table 1). Hypersensitivity pneumonitis is a diffuse inflammatory disease of the lung parenchyma (particularly the alveoli and terminal bronchioles) and interstitium; the inflammatory response, predominately mononuclear, often organizes into granulomas and may progress to fibrosis.

There is no single clinical finding or laboratory study which is diagnostic of hypersensitivity pneumonitis. The diagnosis is made by a combination of characteristic clinical, roentgenographic, and pulmonary function findings in addition to supportive immunologic studies. Clinical manifestations vary with: (1) immunologic responses of the host, (2) the characteristics of the antigen, and (3) the intensity, frequency, or consistency of exposure to the offending antigens. History is the key to the diagnosis. Suspicion of hypersensitivity pneumonitis is essential to obtaining a good history of exposure to organic dusts in patients with respiratory symptoms or a chest roentgenogram suggestive of it. Precipitating antibodies to the suspected inhaled organic dust when suitable antigens are available for immunodiffusion testing, are helpful in identifying exposure and an immune response, but are not diagnostic of disease. Inhalational challenges with the suspected antigen can be confirmatory of the suspected diagnosis of HP. Environmental challenges are usually preferred since severe immediate or delayed respiratory symptoms may occur after a laboratory challenge. Skin tests with serum proteins in pigeon-breeder's disease may be of value; both immediate (wheal and flare) and delayed (4 to 6 hr) skin reactions can occur. Skin tests with suspected thermophilic antigens are unreliable because of nonspecific irritative reactions and can result in skin necrosis. Lung biopsies help clarify the diagnosis, especially after chronic exposure to organic dusts, when the antigen is not evident or the clinical evaluation of the patient is uncertain.

Children as well as adults are at risk of developing HP from sensitizing organic dusts through contamination of forced-air heating, humidification, or air-conditioning systems in homes or as a result of contact with animal proteins from pets in home, hobby-related contacts or through the medical use of pituitary snuff. Although a variety of organic antigens have been associated with HP in adults, especially from occupational exposure, the majority of the reported cases in children have been due to exposure to avian proteins.[1-13]

II. SOURCE OF ANTIGENS IN HYPERSENSITIVITY PNEUMONITIS

The inhalation of and sensitization to antigens found in a wide variety of organic dusts originating from many different sources can result in hypersensitivity pneumonitis. The offending antigen can be bacterial (Thermophilic actinomyectes), fungal (Alternaria or Phoma species, *Aspergillus clavatus, Penicillium frequentans, caseii,* and *roqueforti, Mucor stolonifer,* and *Cryptostroma corticale*), animal proteins (dove, parakeet, parrot, pigeon, gerbil, bovine, porcine, or rat), chemicals (anhydrides, diisocyanates), other agents (amoeba, various fungi, *Bacillus subtilis*) and unknown agents in coffee dust.[14] The Thermophilic actinomycetes, bacteria less than 1 μ with the morphology of fungi, are ubiquitous in soil, grain, and compost which contaminate moldy vegetation and forced-air heating and cooling systems. Microorganisms in this group responsible for HP seen in farmer's lung, bagassosis, and ventilation pneumonitis are *Micropolyspora faeni, Thermoactinomyces sacchari,* and

Table 1
AGENTS OF HYPERSENSITIVITY PNEUMONITIS

Agent	Disease
Thermophilic actinomycetes	
Micropolyspora faeni	Farmer's Lung
Thermoactinomyces sacchari	Bagassosis
Thermoactinomyces vulgaris	Mushroom Worker's Lung
Thermoactinomyces viridis	Mushroom Worker's Lung
Thermoactinomyces candidus	Ventilation Pneumonitis
Fungi	
Alternaria species	Wood Worker's Lung
Pullularia pullulans	Sequoiosis
Aspergillus clavatus	Malt Worker's Lung
Penicillium frequentans	Suberosis
Penicillium caseii	Cheese Worker's Lung
Penicillium roqueforti	Cheese Worker's Lung
Phoma species	Shower Curtain Disease
Mucor stolonifer	Paprika Splitter's Lung
Cryptostroma corticale	Maple Bark Stripper's
Cephalosporium	Humidifier's Disease
Animal proteins	
Chicken proteins	Chicken Handler's Disease
Turkey proteins	Turkey Handler's Disease
Unknown (bat excreta) antigens	Bat Lung
Dove, parakeet, parrot	Bird-Fancier's Disease
Gerbil	Gerbil Keeper's Disease
Pig or ox	Pituitary Snuff-taker's Lung
Pigeon	Pigeon-Breeder's Disease
Rat	Rat-Handler's Disease
Vegetable products	
Unknown	Grain Measurer's Lung
Unknown	Thatched Roof Disease
Unknown (tobacco plants)	Tobacco Grower's Disease
Unknown (tea plants)	Tea Grower's Disease
Unknown (cloth wrappings of mummies)	Coptic Disease
Arthropods	
Sitophilus grainarius	Wheat Weevil
Chemicals	
Phthalic anhydride	Epoxy Resin Worker's Lung
Toluene diisocyanate	Porcelain Refinisher's Lung
Trimellitic anhydride	Plastic Worker's Lung
Other agents	
Amoeba, various fungi	Ventilation Pneumonitis
Bacillus subtilis	Enzyme Worker's Lung
Hair dust	Furrier's Lung
Coffee dust	Coffee Worker's Lung
Thatched roof dust	New Guinea Lung

Thermoactinomyces candidus respectively. Contaminated home humidifiers in forced-air heating or air-conditioning systems are another source of exposure to organic antigens from amebae and other fungi.

III. PATHOGENESIS

The precise pathogenic mechanisms in hypersensitivity pneumonitis have not been completely clarified; however, the disease is characterized by the demonstration of precipitating antibodies, circulating antigen-antibody complexes and altered immune regulatory cell function.[20-23] Immediate type IgE hypersensitivity reactions are not thought to be involved in the pathogenesis of HP. There is no evidence of specific IgE antibody in symptomatic individuals and the total serum levels of IgE are normal. The characteristic immunologic feature in hypersensitivity pneumonitis is the presence of precipitating antibodies against the offending agent which can be demonstrated in the serum by immunodiffusion testing when suitable antigens are available.[18] Precipitating antibodies in the serum are usually of the IgG class, although smaller quantities of IgM and IgA have been detected. Although the presence of precipitating antibodies suggests a role of immune complexes in the pathogenesis of HP, raises the question of the significance of these antibodies to disease.

Patients with pigeon breeder's disease and farmer's lung have been the predominant focus for studies to delineate pathogenic mechanisms of hypersensitivity pneumonitis. Serum precipitins have been found in up to 50% of asymptomatic pigeon breeders as well as in most symptomatic individuals[17] and thus reflect exposure but do not indicate the presence of disease. These precipitating antibodies are usually demonstrated by such simple tests as Ouchterlony gel diffusion; however, more sensitive tests such as countercurrent immunoelectrophoresis can be used for the detection of serum precipitins. Some patients have low titers of serum precipitins and it may be necessary to concentrate their serum to detect these antibodies.

Approximately 80% of symptomatic pigeon breeders exhibit immediate wheal and flare reactions on skin testing. Dual-phase skin test reactions may occur and include an immediate wheal and flare followed in 4 to 8 hr by a dermal and subcutaneous swelling resembling an Arthus phenomenon indicative of vasculitis due to a precipitin-antigen reaction. The latter reaction subsides after 18 to 24 hr and suggests the involvement of soluble immune complexes in the pathogenesis. Some individuals with HP up to 10% may have a two-stage reaction after inhalational exposure: an immediate asthmatic-type pulmonary function response (decreased forced vital capacity (FVC), forced expiratory flow volumes (FEV1), and expiratory flow rates) and the late 4 to 6 hr response (decreased FVC, FEV1, and expiratory flow rates). It has been suggested that such asthma-type responses may be mediated by short-term or short-latent sensitizing antibody of the IgG subclass (IgG4).[15] This IgG subclass has been reported to be elevated in bronchoalveolar lavage fluids of symptomatic pigeon-breeders but not in those without symptoms.[16] IgA and IgM antibodies have also been detected in the sera of patients exposed to organic dusts by techniques more sensitive than gel diffusion.[18]

Granulomatous pulmonary inflammatory response seen in some patients with HP suggests the role of cell-mediated immunity (CMI). Other studies suggesting involvement of CMI include: the production of migration inhibition factor by peripheral blood lymphocytes of symptomatic pigeon breeders on exposure to pigeon antigen,[19,20] antigen-induced blastogenesis by circulating sensitized T-lymphocytes of pigeon breeders,[19] significant increase in the percentage of T cells in bronchial lavage fluid of patients with chronic HP,[21] asymptomatic but similarly exposed individuals,[22] and the proliferation of T cells in bronchial lavage fluid of symptomatic pigeon breeders when stimulated with pigeon serum.[22] In vitro tests of cell-mediated immunity appear to discriminate symptomatic from asymptomatic pigeon breeders better than tests of circulating antibodies.[19,20]

Recent studies by Keller et al.[23] demonstrated functional differences in peripheral blood suppressor cell activities and significant differences in bronchial lavage (BAL) fluid suppressor cell function between asymptomatic and symptomatic pigeon breeders which suggests a discrepancy between the phenotype and function of immunoregulatory T-cell subsets in BAL lymphocytes.[23] These studies indicate the role of immunoregulation in the pathogenesis of HP, but shed no light on the initial pathogenetic mechanism(s) inducing the immune inflammation.[23]

Studies by Moore et al.[22] of in vitro stimulation of BAL lymphocytes with phytohemagglutinin and pigeon antigens in patients with pigeon breeder's disease indicate the presence of specifically activated lymphocytes in the lung parenchyma. The recent study of Costabel et al.[24] evaluated the presence of Ia plus T-cells, (another sign of T-cell activation), in patients with hypersensitivity pneumonitis. OKT4 plus helper and OKT8 plus suppressor lung cells express in part Ia antigens. These findings suggest that different T-cell subpopulations are activated in HP in contrast to sarcoidosis.

Serum complement levels are usually not lowered in symptomatic individuals after inhalation challenge with the offending antigen.[25] Although some lung biopsies have shown antigen, antibody and complement components in lung tissue, the characteristic vasculitis of immune complex injury is not usually observed in the lung parenchyma of HP patients.

The delay in obtaining lung biopsies may account for this as vasculitis may be seen early after the challenge only to disappear with time.[14] Immune complex lesions have been detected in the walls of small vessels in the skin 4 to 6 hr after antigen injection.[14]

IV. CLINICAL MANIFESTATIONS

The clinical findings of hypersensitivity pneumonitis are essentially the same regardless of the offending organic dusts. Although the time necessary for sensitization in HP varies from months to years, the onset of symptoms may be acute or insidious. The diagnosis of hypersensitivity pneumonitis should be considered in patients who present with a history of recurrent influenza-like episodes with pneumonitis or acute interstitial changes on chest roentgenogram. Acute symptoms include cough, dyspnea, chills, fever, malaise, and myalgia. Recovery is rapid and spontaneous following removal of the antigen, although easy fatigability may persist for several weeks. During an acute episode of HP include bilateral end-inspiratory rales are most prominent in the lung bases with cough and injected conjunctiva. Wheezing is uncommon, except in patients with underlying asthma.

Acute episodes recur regularly on re-exposure to the offending organic antigens. The severity of each episode varies with the degree of exposure and the sensitivity of the individual. These episodes can be confused with acute viral bronchitis or pneumonia.[26] When exposure is less intense but prolonged, chills and fever may not occur but nonproductive cough or cough productive of scanty mucopurulent sputum, exertional dyspnea, easy fatigability, anorexia, and weight loss are frequent symptoms.[14] Chest roentgenogram findings are variable in HP and related to the frequency of the acute episodes and the time interval at which the X-ray is taken following exposure to the offending organic antigens.[14,27]

In the chronic form of hypersensitivity pneumonitis, the symptoms include progressive shortness of breath which may be associated with mucopurulent sputum production, anorexia, and weight loss.[14] As exposure to offending organic dusts continues, progressive pulmonary disability occurs and, in some cases, progresses even after institution of avoidance measures.[26] With progression of the pulmonary disease, fibrosis with parenchymal contraction and honeycombing, characteristic of end-stage chest pulmonary disease, may be seen on chest roentgenograms.

V. LABORATORY FEATURES

During the acute episodes of HP, a polymorphonuclear leukocytosis with a shift to the left may be seen; with recovery, the leukocytosis resolves and the slight eosinophilia which may occur during the acute phase often persists.[14] Serum IgE is usually normal except in atopic individuals.[26] There is usually generalized elevation of other serum immunoglobulins.[14] Rheumatoid factor can be detected in moderate to high titers during periods of illness, but becomes negative after periods of prolonged exposure to the offending organic antigens.[28]

Although there are several types of abnormalities in pulmonary function in HP, the most common finding is a restrictive pattern with reduction in both forced vital capacity (FVC) and 1-sec forced vital capacity (FEV 1) with a constant ratio between these two parameters.[26,29] A bi-phasic response may occur with an acute reduction in FEV1 and FVC, followed by a plateau and return to normal, and then a late-phase reaction with a reduction in both FEV1 and FVC several hours later.[26,29] During the acute episodes, there may be a fall in diffusion capacity and hypoxemia, especially during exercise.[14] A decrease in compliance indicating lung stiffness and an increase in closing volumes may also be demonstrated during the acute episode.[14] With parenchymal damage, hypercapnia and flow and volume abnormalities may be detected during asymptomatic phases.[14] In patients with the subacute or chronic form, persistent abnormalities in pulmonary function such as restrictive impairment, diffusion defects, and hypoxemia may be demonstrated, even after cessation of exposure (CE) to the offending organic antigen.[13,29] In a series of 12 children with HP reported by Chiron et al., persistent hypoxemia after 2 months following CE was an unfavorable prognostic sign, dynamic lung compliance was normal by the 8th month CE, and diffusing capacity improved more slowly and remained significantly decreased in one case. Major abnormalities of pulmonary function persisted in the one child with no CE.[13]

VI. PATHOLOGIC FINDINGS

Pathologic features include interstitial and alveolar inflammatory responses, depending upon the state of the disease and the time the biopsy is taken. During acute episodes of HP, the lung morphology is an acute granulomatous interstitial pneumonitis with the alveolar spaces containing macrophages, foreign body giant cells, neutrophils and some eosinophiles, and the alveolar walls thickened with infiltration by neutrophils, macrophages and eosinophils.[14,28] The granulomatous lesions can involve the bronchioles as well as the parenchyma.[14] With repeated insults, the inflammation may persist in the interstitial and alveolar septa which become thickened by connective tissue deposition and residual chronic inflammatory cells.[14] Results of pulmonary biopsies in children with HP were reported by Chiron et al.[13] in one case from their series and from a review of eight others from the literature which showed interstitial infiltration of mononuclear cells in all cases, five had fibrosis, eight had alveolar exudate, two had granulomas, and two demonstrated bronchiolar lesions. In the one case of Chiron et al.[13] without CE, interstitial and peribronchial fibrosis were found on biopsy.

VII. TREATMENT

Avoidance measures are the most important aspect of management in HP with removal of the individual from the contaminated environment. During the acute episodes symptomatic treatment may include bed rest, antipyretics, and supplemental oxygen. Cromolyn sodium has been tried in preventing acute episodes, but the effect is variable.[26] Bronchodilators and antihistamines are not of value in HP. Although there is some controversy in regard to the use of corticosteroids, they may be associated with dramatic responses in patients with recurrent acute episodes with significant pulmonary and chest roentgenographic abnormalities.[26] The duration of therapy should be determined based on clinical and laboratory changes.[26] The use of corticosteroid therapy did not significantly modify respiratory function in the two children with HP treated in Chiron's series.[13] Chiron et al.[13] suggest that the prognostic value of corticosteroid therapy be evaluated in terms of the results of pulmonary biopsies performed within the first 2 months after cessation of exposure.

VIII. PROGNOSIS

The prognosis for an individual patient with hypersensitivity pneumonitis is primarily determined by the amount of reversible pulmonary impairment present at the time of diagnosis and the avoidance of exposure to the offending organic dusts. The severity of the initial symptoms does not influence the prognosis in hypersensitivity pneumonitis. The length of exposure to the offending antigens in the inhaled organic dusts after the onset of the initial symptoms may affect prognosis. Longer duration of exposure is associated with a more unfavorable prognosis.[13] The prognosis is excellent if the diagnosis of HP is recognized early and exposure to the offending organic dusts is avoided before irreversible pulmonary damage occurs.

Pulmonary function studies can be used to follow the functional course of hypersensitivity pneumonitis in children after cessation of exposure (CE) to the offending antigens in the inhaled dust. Caution should be exercised in utilizing pulmonary function data to predict prognosis in the first 2 months after CE. In the initial 2 months period following CE, hypoxemia at rest or with exercise is present and is probably related to both interstitial and bronchiolar lesions noted on lung biopsies.[13] The persistence of hypoxemia after 2 months following CE was considered an unfavorable prognostic indicator in the series of children with HP reported by Chiron et al.[13] The length of time for the functional recovery in those children appeared to be related to the degree of impairment in the initial pulmonary function studies.[13] Functional sequelae were found to persist in the midterm (2 to 8 months) and long-term (greater than 8 months) period following CE; the presence and severity of these sequelae were greater in children over 10 years of age. Lung biopsy data in the initial period after CE can also be useful in the prognostic evaluation of patients with hypersensitivity pneumonitis. The presence of fibrosis appears to be associated with an unfavorable prognosis.[13] Avoidance of inhaled organic antigens or even the use of corticosteroids may have little effect in the chronic form of hypersensitivity pneumonitis with irreversible pulmonary damage, fibrosis, and/or obstructive bronchiolitis.[14]

REFERENCES

1. **Stiehm, E. R., Reed, C. E., and Tooley, W. H.,** Pigeon breeder's lung in children, *Pediatrics*, 39, 904, 1967.
2. **Dinda, P., Chatterjee, S. S., and Riding, W. D.,** Pulmonary function studies in bird breeder's lung, *Thorax*, 24, 374, 1969.
3. **Shannon, D. C., Andrews, J. L., Recavarren, S., and Kazemi, H.,** Pigeon breeder's lung disease and interstitial pulmonary fibrosis, *Am. J. Dis. Child.*, 117, 504, 1969.
4. **Heersma, J. R., Emanuel, D. A., Wenzel, F. J., and Gray, R. L.,** Farmer's lung in a 10-year old girl, *J. Pediatr.*, 75, 704, 706, 1969.
5. **Hughes, W. F., Mattimore, J. M., and Arbesman, C. E.,** Farmer's lung in an adolescent boy, *Am. J. Dis. Child.*, 118, 777, 1969.
6. **Chandra, S. and Jones, H. E.,** Pigeon fancier's lung in children, *Arch. Dis. Child.*, 47, 716, 1972.
7. **Reiss, J. S., Weiss, N. S., Payette, K. M., and Strimas, J.,** Childhood pigeon breeder's disease, *Ann. Allergy*, 32, 208, 212, 1974.
8. **Cunningham, A. S., Fink, J. N., and Schlueter, D. P.,** Childhood hypersensitivity pneumonitis due to dove antigens, *Pediatrics*, 58, 436, 1976.
9. **Bureau, M. A., Fecteau, C., Patriquin, H., Rola-pleszczynski, M., Masse, S., and Begin, R.,** Farmer's lung in early childhood, *Am. Rev. Respir. Dis.*, 119, 671, 1979.
10. **El-Hefny, A., Ehladiosis, E., El-Sharhawy, S., El-Ghadban, H., El-Heneidy, F., and Frankland, A. W.,** Extrinsic allergic bronchiolo-alveolitis in children, *Clin. Allergy*, 10, 651, 1980.
11. **Keith, H. H., Holsclaw, D. S., and Dunsky, E. H.,** Pigeon breeder's disease in children. A family study, *Chest*, 79, 107, 1981.
12. **Barker, P. M. and Warner, J. O.,** Atypical pneumonia due to parakeet sensitivity: bird fancier's lung in a 10-year-old girl, *Br. J. Dis. Chest*, 78, 404, 1984.
13. **Chiron, C., Gaultier, CL., Boule, M., Grimfeld, A., and Girard, F.,** Lung function in children with hypersensitivity pneumonitis, *Eur. J. Respir. Dis.*, 65, 79, 1984.

14. **Fink, J. N.,** Hypersensitivity pneumonitis, *J. Allergy Clin. Immunol.,* 74, 1, 1984.
15. **Bryant, D. H., Burns, M. W., and Lazarus, I.,** New type of allergic asthma due to IgG "reaginic" antibody, *Br. Med. J.,* 4, 589, 1973.
16. **Calvanico, N. J., Ambegaonkar, S. P., Schleretter, D. P., and Fink, J. N.,** Immunoglobulin levels in bronchoalveolar lavage fluid from pigeon breeders, *J. Lab. Clin. Med.,* 96, 129, 1980.
17. **Fink, J. N., Schlueter, D. P., and Sosman, A. J.,** Clinical survey of pigeon breeder's, *Chest,* 62, 271, 1972.
18. **Patterson, R., Schatz, M., and Fink, J. N., et al.,** Pigeon breeder's disease. I. Serum immunoglobulin concentrations; IgG, IgM, IgA, and IgE antibodies against pigeon serum, *Am. J. Med.,* 60, 144, 1976.
19. **Hansen, P. J. and Penny, R.,** Pigeon breeder's disease. Study of the cell-mediated immune response to pigeon antigens by the lymphocyte culture technique, *Int. Arch. Allergy Appl. Immunol.,* 37, 498, 1974.
20. **Fink, J. N., Moore, V. L., and Barboriak, J. J.,** Cell-mediated hypersensitivity in pigeon breeders, *Int. Arch. Allergy Appl. Immunol.,* 49, 831, 1975.
21. **Reynolds, H. Y., Fulmer, J. D., Kazmierowski, J. A., Roberts, W. C., Frank, M. M., and Crystal, R. G.,** Analysis of cellular and protein content of bronchoalveolar lavage fluid from patients with idiopathic pulmonary fibrosis and chronic hypersensitivity pneumonitis, *J. Clin. Invest.,* 59, 165, 1977.
22. **Moore, V. L., Pederson, G. M., Hauser, W. C., and Fink, J. N.,** A study of lung lavage materials in patients with hypersensitivity pneumonitis. In vitro response to mitogen and antigen in pigeon breeder's disease, *J. Allergy Clin. Immunol.,* 65, 365, 1980.
23. **Keller, R. H., Swartz, S., Schlueter, D. P., Bar-Sela, S., and Fink, J. N.,** Immunoregulation in hypersensitivity pneumonitis: phenotypic and functional studies of bronchoalveolar lavage lymphocytes, *Am. Rev. Respir. Dis.,* 13, 766, 1984.
24. **Costabel, U., Bross, K. J., Ruhle, K. H., Lohr, G. W., and Matthys, H.,** Ia-like antigens on t-cells and their subpopulations in pulmonary sarcoidosis and in hypersensitivity pneumonitis, *Am. Rev. Respir. Dis.,* 131, 337, 1985.
25. **Baur, X., Dorsch, W., and Becker, T.,** Levels of complement factors in human serum during immediate and late asthmatic reactions and during acute hypersensitivity pneumonitis, *Allergy,* 35, 383, 1980.
26. **Levy, M. B. and Fink, J. N.,** Hypersensitivity pneumontis, *Ann. Allergy,* 54, 167, 1985.
27. **Unger, J. D., Fink, J. N., and Unger, G. F.,** Pigeon breeder's disease - a review of the roentgenographic pulmonary finding, *Radiology,* 90, 683, 1968.
28. **Fink, J. N., Sosman, A. J., Barboriak, J. J., Schlueter, D. P., and Holmes, R. A.,** Pigeon breeders disease, a clinical study of hypersensitivity pneumonitis, *Ann. Intern. Med.,* 68, 1205, 1968.
29. **Schlueter, D. P., Fink, J. N., and Sosman, A. J.,** Pulmonary function in pigeon breeder's disease. A hypersensitivity pneumonitis, *Ann. Intern. Med.,* 70, 457, 1969.

Chapter 37

IDIOPATHIC PULMONARY HEMOSIDEROSIS

Brad E. Alpert and Daniel V. Schidlow

TABLE OF CONTENTS

I. INTRODUCTION

Pulmonary hemosiderosis (PH) is a rare disease which primarily affects children and adolescents, and was described first by Virchow in 1864. It is characterized by acute and chronic blood loss which occurs from pulmonary capillaries and often results in the triad of hemoptysis, interstitial pulmonary infiltrates, and anemia. PH can result from conditions such as mitral stenosis, systemic lupus erythematosis, and Goodpasture's syndrome. When a thorough investigation does not reveal an underlying cause, it is then classified as idiopathic pulmonary hemosiderosis (IPH).

II. PATHOLOGY

Macroscopic examination of the lung reveals multilocular or diffuse brown induration. Light microscopy shows degeneration, desquamation and hyperplasia of alveolar epithelial cells, and alveolar capillary dilatation. Hemosiderin-laded macrophages are seen within the alveoli, bronchioles, and lung interstitium. The interalveolar septa become thickened due to interstitial fibrosis, hemosiderin deposits, capillary dilatation, and inflammatory infiltrates;[1-3] mast cell infiltrates have also been reported.[4] During acute exacerbations, alveoli may be filled with erythrocytes (see Figure 1).

Reports of electronmicroscopic findings have varied considerably among observers. Most agree that there is degeneration and desquamation of type I pneumocytes and hyperplasia of type II pneumocytes.[5] These changes are thought to be secondary to some insult or defect which has yet to be identified. Further discussion of ultrastructural abnormalities is included below in the section on pathogenesis.

III. PATHOGENESIS

The hypothesis that the primary defect in IPH is an inherent weakness of the vascular walls dates back to 1931 when Ceelen proposed a developmental abnormality of elastic fibers in pulmonary capillaries.[5,6] Hyatt et al., found a focal discontinuity in the pulmonary capillary basement membrane, and proposed that this was the etiology of IPH.[7] Gonzalez-Cruzzi et al. found two types of abnormalities: first, the basement membrane was irregularly and diffusely thickened, and second, the normal single laminar structure was replaced by discontinuous deposits which tended to form concentric layers.[8] The authors proposed that these lesions were the result of some primary defect or injury. However, none of these ultrastructural abnormalities has thus far been confirmed as the cause of IPH.[9]

An immune-mediated mechanism for the pathogenesis of IPH was first proposed in 1954 by Steiner.[10] He theorized that an autoimmune reaction was the basis for this disease; an idea supported by the fact that several of the known etiologies of PH are immunologic in nature. These include Goodpasture's Syndrome, Heiner's Syndrome, systemic lupus erythematosus, and immune complex nephritis. In addition, eosinophilia, high serum IgA, cold agglutinins, circulating immune complexes, lymphadenopathy, splenomegaly, autoimmune hemolytic anemia and thombocytopenia, and improvement after plasmapheresis have all been reported in association with IPH.[5,11-15] However, there has been no consistently detected immunologic abnormality associated with IPH.

A genetic basis for IPH has been suggested by a few reports of familial masses. One report describes it in a 26-year-old man and his 62-year-old mother,[16] while affected siblings have been described by others.[17-19] Although these cases may represent an hereditary form of IPH, common exposure to a toxic or infectious agent is also possible.[20]

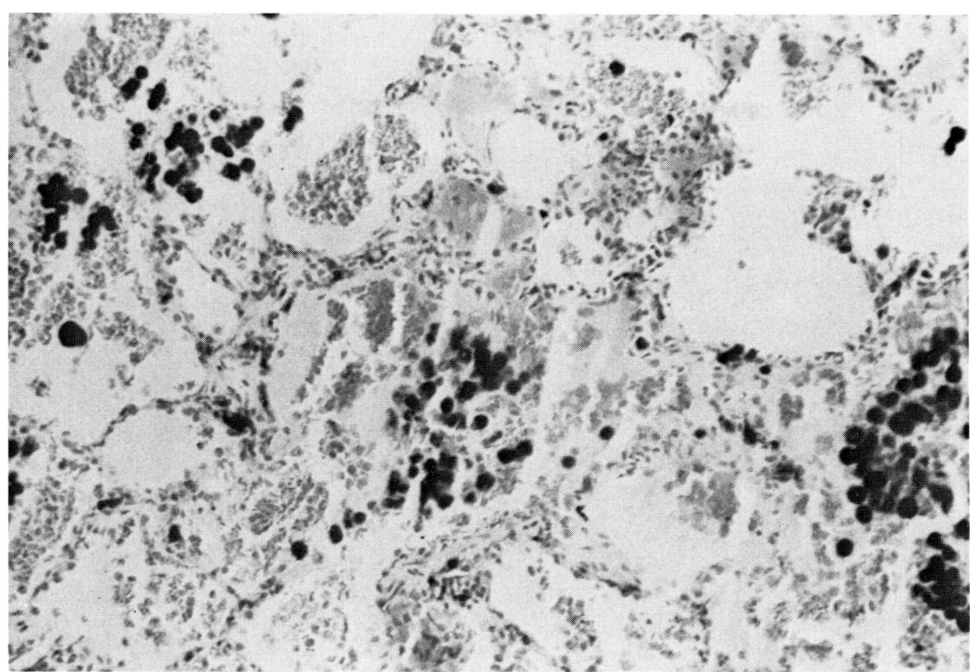

FIGURE 1.   Idiopathic pulmonary hemosiderosis. Alveoli and alveolar ducts contain large numbers of hemosiderin-laden macrophages and free particles of hemosiderin. The alveolar ephithelial cells are very prominent, and the interstitium is markedly thickened due to fibrosis, deposits of hemosiderin granules, lymphocytes and macrophages, some containing hemosiderin.

IV. EPIDEMIOLOGY

About 80% of the cases of IPH occur in children less than 16 years of age. The majority present between the ages of 1 and 7 years with a peak at 2,[1,20,21] and it has even been reported in a newborn.[22] Most adults present before age 30. The sex distribution is equal in children,[1,21] but males predominate 2 to 1 in adults.[1] The actual incidence of IPH in children is not well described, but is reported to be about 0.24 new cases per year per million children in Sweden.[23]

V. CLINICAL PRESENTATION

The presentation and clinical course of IPH are variable and depend upon the intensity, duration and frequency of the hemorrhages.[1,21,24] The intrapulmonary bleeding may be continuous and mild with intermittent acute exacerbations, or acute episodes may be separated by periods of quiescence. A chronic nonproductive cough, dyspnea on exertion, anemia, and poor weight gain frequently become manifest during periods of mild continuous bleeding. Digital clubbing, jaundice, lymphadenopathy, hepatomegaly and splenomegaly may develop, and blood-tinged sputum and occult hematochezia occasionally occur. Cor pulmonale and heart failure may eventually supervene.

Acute large hemorrhages may be accompanied by fever, hemoptysis, coughing spells, tachypnea, tightness in the chest, cyanosis, and epigastric or substernal pain. Young children are less likely to have hemoptysis, since they often swallow their sputum. Rales and dullness to percussion may occur, especially over the lower lobes. Pallor may result from severe anemia and poor perfusion due to massive blood loss, and shock, respiratory failure, and death may supervene.

VI. DIAGNOSIS

A. Hematology

Chronic and acute blood loss occurs in IPH, and since the iron contained in hemosiderin trapped within the lung is only scantily reutilized for erythropoiesis, iron deficiency anemia develops in most cases. Red cells are microcytic and hypochromic, total iron binding capacity may be elevated, and iron is decreased in the serum and absent from the bone marrow,[25,26] but paradoxically, reticulocytosis is not uncommon.[27] Indirect hyperbilirubinemia and eosinophilia sometimes occur.[1]

B. Cytology

Hemosiderin-laden macrophages can usually be recovered from gastric washings, sputum, or bronchoalveolar lavage fluid, and identified by staining with potassium ferrocyanide.[24,38] Since these cells may be found within 48 to 72 hr and persist for 2 to 4 weeks after an acute hemorrhage from the lung parenchyma or a peripheral airway, they are of more diagnostic significance when recovered during a remission.[26,28] Some consider finding these cells sufficient to make the diagnosis of PH without obtaining a lung biopsy; however, they do not distinguish idiopathic from secondary causes.

C. Histology

The gold standard for the diagnosis of IPH is microscopic examination of lung tissue. When PH is present without histologic lesions or a history suggestive of a known etiology, a presumptive diagnosis of IPH can be made.

D. Roentgenology

The radiographic appearance of the chest is highly variable. During episodes of acute bleeding, there can be unilateral or bilateral confluent alveolar consolidation due to blood filled alveoli, which resolves in 1 to 2 weeks. In chronic cases an interstitial pattern of fine reticulonodularity or miliary stippling occurs as pulmonary fibrosis develops. The apical lung fields are generally spared, and mediastinal lymphadenopathy is occasionally present.[1,24]

Pulmonary hemorrhage can be detected with nuclear scans using 59 Fe, 51 Cr or 99 m Tc-labeled red blood cells, which accumulate in areas of bleeding. 15 C-labeled carbon monoxide is retained in the lung in abnormally large amounts during episodes of pulmonary hemorrhage, because of its high affinity for the hemoglobin in extravasated blood.[29,30]

E. Pulmonary Function Tests

Pulmonary function abnormalities generally indicate restrictive lung disease;[31] however, an obstructive pattern may sometimes occur.[24] Carbon monoxide diffusion capacity is usually decreased once chronic interstitial disease develops,[32] but may be supranormal during an acute hemorrhage due to increased uptake by hemoglobin in extravasated blood.[24] Pulmonary functions improve during remissions, and may revert to normal before interstitial fibrosis supervenes.

VII. DIFFERENTIAL DIAGNOSIS

IPH should be included in the differential diagnosis of recurrent pneumonia, chronic interstitial infiltrates, or hemoptysis, especially when anemia is present. When PH is present, a thorough search for known causes must be made before IPH can be diagnosed.

Cardiovascular disease leading to pulmonary venous hypertension, especially mitral valve stenosis, can cause diffuse pulmonary hemorrhage and PH. A careful physical examination along with an electrocardiogram and echocardiogram should be performed.

Renal disease may be associated with pulmonary hemosiderosis. In Goodpasture's Syndrome autoantibodies against glomerular basement membrane (GBM) can be demonstrated in the serum, lung, or kidney. It is primarily a disease of young white males with a median age at onset of 21 years, but it does occur rarely in children. Pulmonary symptoms generally precede renal involvement, and although the clinical course is variable, the disease is often fatal despite treatment with corticosteroids, immunosuppressives and plasmapheresis. Biopsy specimens often reveal linear deposits of immunoglobulins on the basement membranes of the glomerulus or alveolus.[3,32] Another form of renal disease associated with PH was reported by Loughlin et al. who described it in association with glomerulonephritis and circulating immune complexes.[34] A urinalysis, BUN, creatinine, and serum for anti-GBM antibodies and circulating immune complexes should be obtained.

Collagen vascular diseases, especially systemic lupus erythematosus can cause pulmonary vasculitis which occasionally results in PH. These diseases and their treatment are beyond the scope of this chapter, and are discussed elsewhere. Antinuclear antibody and rheumatoid factor should be included in the work-up.[3]

Heiner et al. described an association between the ingestion of cow milk and PH.[35] These children frequently have serous or purulent otitis media, chronic rhinitis, vomiting, diarrhea, anorexia, poor weight gain, and wheezing. Hypertrophy of the tonsils and adenoids occasionally occurs, and may lead to cor pulmonale.[36] Precipitins to cow milk proteins are found in the serum, and removing milk from the diet usually results in a dramatic improvement of symptoms.[37]

VIII. TREATMENT

The treatment of PH depends on the etiology. If no cause is identified, therapy is primarily supportive and includes blood transfusion, oxygen, and mechanical ventilation when necessary. High doses of intravenous corticosteroids are probably beneficial for controlling acute bleeding, but chronic therapy with these drugs does not appear to alter the clinical course.[3,38] Azathioprine, iron chelating agents, and plasmaphoresis have been used with some reported success, but splenectomy is probably of no value.[3,15]

IX. PROGNOSIS

Although the clinical course is variable, the ultimate prognosis for pulmonary hemosiderosis when no etiology is found is usually bleak.[1,38,39] The duration of symptoms is frequently less than 3 years before death supervenes, and a massive fatal pulmonary hemorrhage can occur at any time.

Some patients, however, have a protracted course of exacerbations followed by relatively asymptomatic remissions lasting weeks to years. Severe restrictive lung disease and cor pulmonale with heart failure usually occur eventually, and almost always lead to a fatal outcome.[38]

REFERENCES

1. **Soergel, K. H. and Sommers, S. C.,** Idiopathic pulmonary hemosiderosis and related syndromes, *Am. J. Med.,* 2, 499, 1962.
2. **Soergel, K. H. and Sommers, S. C.,** The alveolar epithelial lesion of idiopathic pulmonary hemosiderosis, *Am. Rev. Respir. Dis.,* 85, 540, 1962.
3. **Bradley, J. D.,** The pulmonary hemorrhage syndromes, *Clin. Chest Med.,* 3, 593, 1982.

4. **Dolan, J., McGuire, S., Sweeney, E., Bourke, J., and Ward, O. C.,** Mast cells in pulmonary hemosiderosis, *Arch. Dis. Child.,* 59, 276, 1984.
5. **Bailey, P. and Gorden, B. M.,** Idiopathic pulmonary hemosiderosis: report of two cases and review of the literature, *Postgrad. Med. J.,* 55, 266, 1979.
6. **Ceelen, W.,** Die Kreislaufstorengen der Lungen, *Anatomie Histologie,* 3, 20, 1931.
7. **Hyatt, R. W., Adelstein, E. R., Halazun, J. F., and Lukeng, J. N.,** Ultrastructure of the lung in idiopathic pulmonary hemosiderosis, *Am. J. Med.,* 42, 822, 1972.
8. **Gonzalez-Crussi, F., Hull, M. T., and Grosfeld, J. L.,** Idiopathic pulmonary hemosiderosis: evidence of capillary basement membrane abnormality, *Am. Rev. Respir. Dis.,* 114, 689, 1976.
9. **Irwin, R. S., Cottrell, T. S., and Hsu, K. C.,** Idiopathic pulmonary hemosiderosis. An electronmicroscopic and immunofluorescent study, *Chest,* 65, 41, 1974.
10. **Steiner, B.,** Essential pulmonary hemosiderosis as an immunohematological problem, *Arch. Dis. Child.,* 29, 391, 1954.
11. **Valassi-Adam, H., Rouska, A., Karpousas, J., and Matsaniotis, N.,** Raised IgA in idiopathic pulmonary hemosiderosis, *Arch. Dis. Child.,* 50, 320, 1975.
12. **Blanco, A., Solis, P., Gomez, S., Linares, P., and Sanchez-Villares, E.,** C1q binding immune complexes and other immunological studies in children with pulmonary hemosiderosis, *Allergol. Immunopathol.,* 12, 37, 1984.
13. **Rafferty, J. R. and Cook, M. K.,** Idiopathic pulmonary hemosiderosis with autoimmune haemolytic anemia, *Br. J. Dis. Chest.,* 78, 282, 1984.
14. **Buchanan, G. R. and Moore, G. C.,** Pulmonary hemosiderosis and immune thrombocytopenia, initial manifestation of collagen-vascular disease, *JAMA,* 146, 861, 1981.
15. **Poso-Rodriguez, F., Freire-Campo, J. M., Gutierrez-Millet, V., Barbosa-Ayucar, C., Diaz De Atauri, J., and Martin-Escribano, P.,** Idiopathic pulmonary hemosiderosis treated by plasmapheresis, *Thorax,* 35, 399, 1980.
16. **Thaell, J. F., Greipp, P. R., and Stubb, S. E.,** Idiopathic pulmonary hemosiderosis: two cases in a family, *Mayo Clin. Proc.,* 53, 113, 1978.
17. **Choremis, C. B., Messaritakis, J. M., and Karpouzas, J. G.,** Idiopathic pulmonary hemosiderosis, *Lancet,* 2, 499, 1965.
18. **Beckerman, R. C., Taussig, L. M., and Pinnas, J. L.,** Familial pulmonary hemosiderosis, *Am. J. Dis. Child.,* 133, 609, 1979.
19. **Breckenridge, R. L. and Ross, J. S.,** Idiopathic pulmonary hemosiderosis, a report of familial occurrence, *Chest,* 75, 636, 1979.
20. **Cassimos, C. D., Chytssanthopoulos, M. D., and Panagiotidou, M. D.,** Epidemiologic observations in idiopathic pulmonary hemosiderosis, *J. Pediatr.,* 102, 698, 1983.
21. **Matsaniotis, N., Karpouzas, J., Apostolopoulou, E., and Messaritakis, J.,** Idiopathic pulmonary hemosiderosis in Children, *Arch. Dis. Child.,* 43, 307, 1968.
22. **Livingstone, C. S. and Baczarow, B.,** Idiopathic pulmonary hemosiderosis in a newborn, *Arch. Dis. Child.,* 42, 543, 1967.
23. **Kjellman, B., Elinder, G., Garwicz, S., and Svan, H.,** Idiopathic pulmonary hemosiderosis in Swedish children, *Acta Pediatr. Scand.,* 73, 584, 1984.
24. **Turner-Warwick, M. and Dewar, A.,** Pulmonary hemorrhage and pulmonary hemosiderosis, *Clin. Radiol.,* 33, 361, 1982.
25. **Giovanni, B., Morandi, S., Genova, R., and Ascari, E.,** Idiopathic pulmonary hemosiderosis: ferrokinetic remarks, *Haematologica,* 60, 322, 1975.
26. **Morgan, P. G. M. and Turner-Warwick, M.,** Pulmonary hemosiderosis and pulmonary hemorrhage, *Br. J. Dis. Chest.,* 75, 225, 1981.
27. **Donlan, C. J., Srodes, C. H., and Duffy, F. D.,** Idiopathic pulmonary hemosiderosis: electron microscopic, immunofluorescent, and iron kinetic studies, *Chest,* 68, 577, 1975.
28. **Boat, T. F.,** Pulmonary hemosiderosis, in *Pediatric Respiratory Disorders: Clinical Approaches,* Nussbaum, E. and Galant, S. P., Eds., Grune & Stratton, New York, 1984, chap. 7.
29. **Miller, T. and Tanaka, T.,** Nuclear scan of pulmonary hemorrhage in idiopathic pulmonary hemosiderosis, *Am. J. Roentgenol.,* 132, 120, 1979.
30. **Kurzwail, P. R., Millop, D. R., Freeman, J. E., Reinan, R. E., and Mayer, K.,** Use of sodium chromate Cr51 in diagnosing childhood idiopathic pulmonary hemosiderosis, *Am. J. Dis. Child.,* 138, 746, 1984.
31. **Allue, X., Wise, M. B., and Beaudry, P. H.,** Pulmonary function studies in idiopathic pulmonary hemosiderosis in children, *Am. Rev. Resp. Dis.,* 107, 410, 1973.
32. **Repetto, G., Lisboa, C., Esparaza, E., Ferretti, R., Naira, M., Etchart, M., and Menghello, J.,** Idiopathic pulmonary hemosiderosis. Clinical, radiological and respiratory function studies, *Pediatrics,* 40, 24, 1967.

33. **Martini, A., Binda, S., Mariani, G., Scotta, M. S., and Ruberto, G.,** Goodpasture's Syndrome in a child: natural history and effect of treatment, *Acta Pediatr. Scand.,* 70, 435, 1981.
34. **Loughlin, G. M., Taussig, L. M., Murphy, S. A., Strunk, R. C., and Kohnen, P. W.,** Immune complex mediated glomerulonephritis and pulmonary hemorrhage simulating Goodpasture's syndrome, *J. Pediatr.,* 93, 181, 1978.
35. **Heiner, D. C., Sears, J. W., and Kniker, W. T.,** Multiple precipitins to cow's milk in chronic respiratory disease. A syndrome including poor growth, gastrointestinal symptoms, evidence of allergy, iron deficiency anemia, and pulmonary hemosiderosis, *Am. J. Dis. Child.,* 103, 634, 1962.
36. **Boat, T. F., Polmar, S. H., Whitman, V., Kleinerman, J. I., Stern, R. C., and Doershuk, C. F.,** Hyperreactivity to cow milk in young children with pulmonary hemosiderosis and cor pulmonale secondary to nasopharyngeal obstruction, *J. Pediatr.,* 87, 23, 1975.
37. **Heiner, D. C.,** Respiratory disease and food allergy, *Allergy,* 53, 657, 1984.
38. **Scully, R. E., Galdabini, J. J., and McNeely, B. U.,** Weekly Clinicopathological exercises case 30-1979, *N. Engl. J. Med.,* 301, 201, 1979.
39. **Chryssanthopoulos, Ch., Cassimos, Ch., and Panagiotidou, Ch.,** Prognostic criteria in idiopathic pulmonary hemosiderosis in children, *Eur. J. Pediatr.,* 140, 123, 1983.

Chapter 38

PULMONARY INVOLVEMENT IN SYSTEMIC CANCER

Michael R. Bye and Daniel V. Schidlow

TABLE OF CONTENTS

I. INTRODUCTION

Children who are receiving chemotherapy for malignant diseases are subject to a variety of pulmonary insults, many of which result in an interstitial pattern of disease. The malignancy itself may invade the pulmonary parenchyma, as part of primary disease or metastatic disease. Many of the *chemotherapeutic agents* have been shown to have pulmonary toxicity. Lastly, due to the therapy and/or the underlying disease, these children are frequently immunosuppressed. They may therefore develop pulmonary infections which present as interstitial disease. Drug-induced interstitial lung diseases and these infections are discussed elsewhere in this text.

II. MECHANISMS OF LUNG INVOLVEMENT

Tumor cells enter the pulmonary parenchyma by direct infiltration, lymphatic, hematogenous, transpleural and/or intrabronchial spread.[1] Because the tumors involved in the latter two mechanisms are so uncommon in children, those mechanisms will not be discussed.

Direct infiltration from an adjoining solid tumor can invade the pulmonary parenchyma. Such tumor invasion will usually not cause an interstitial pattern of disease. Tumors which may invade the lung in this manner include chest wall tumors (i.e., Ewings sarcoma in a rib), Hodgkin's or other lymphomas affecting the mediastinal nodes, and neuroblastomas. Other tumors may spread to the lung by contiguous invasion (neuroblastoma) or by hematogenous spread (Wilm's tumor, osteogenic sarcoma, Ewing's sarcoma, germ cell tumors, tumors of the sex organs and rhabdomyosarcomas). However, these metastatic lesions usually produce nodular disease, not an interstitial pattern. Thus, they are not the province of this textbook.

The lung has a rich network of lymphatics which communicate with those in the neck and upper abdomen. The pulmonary lymphatics drain into the mediastinal nodes and then to the thoracic duct. Obstruction to lymph flow in the mediastinum may result in its retrograde flow with concomitant spread of tumor cells into the lung. Anastomoses between the lymphatics of the lower lobes of the lung and those of the esophagus and upper abdomen occasionally permit tumor spread into the lung.

Diffuse permeation through the pulmonary lymphatics is known as lymphangitis carcinomatosis. This entity is due to lymphatic and hematogenous spread. Because the tumors that usually cause lymphangitis carcinomatosis (carcinomas of the stomach, lung, breast, ovary, pancreas, and prostate) are very rare in childhood the entity itself is rare in the pediatric age group.

Since the lung receives the entire cardiac output and is constructed to serve as a filtering system, it should not be a surprise that tumor cells entering the bloodstream are often trapped in the lung. Most of these cells are destroyed by the normal lung defense mechanisms. Some cells may leave the blood vessels into the perivascular spaces where they may either multiply *in situ* or enter the lymphatics and spread further. Cells may also adhere to the endothelial wall and become encased in a fibrous plaque. The latter cells develop into nodular lesions, rather than interstitial infiltrates. However, either can occur, and in leukemia such infiltrates are more likely to have a diffuse interstitial pattern.

III. TUMORS

A. Leukemia

Although pulmonary involvement in children dying of leukemia is frequently seen,[2] clinical lung disease is not usually significant. Pulmonary disease is rare at initial presentation but is more commonly part of a relapse or generalized progression of disease, when it may play a more significant clinical role.[3,4] Isolated pulmonary relapse has been described, raising the possibility of the pulmonary parenchyma occasionally serving as a "sanctuary".[5]

On microscopic examination, the blood vessels in the lung contain large numbers of leukemic cells. Leukemic infiltrates are found in the perivascular and peribronchial areas, and in the alveolar walls. This represents hematogenous spread, although spread from blocked lymphatic vessels is also possible. Extravasation of leukemic cells may also play a role in the development of these lesions.

The clinical picture ranges from an incidental autopsy finding to tachypnea, dyspnea, dry cough, or crackles on auscultation. The chest roentgenogram may show interstitial disease, but it may be normal. Pulmonary function tests often show restrictive disease, decreased diffusion capacity, and hypoxemia. The clinical picture is indistinguishable from that of the drug-induced lung injuries causing diffuse alveolar damage. Only lung biopsy can definitively distinguish between the two. Figure 1 shows the radiographs of a 12-year-old patient with acute lymphoblastic leukemia with diffuse interstitial pneumonia who subsequently died of respiratory failure. Figure 2 demonstrates the markedly enlarged interalveolar septae with rounded nuclei and prominent nucleoli in the infiltrate. Mitosis is shown in multiple cells. The alveoli show thick proteinaceous exudate.

B. Lymphomas

Non-Hodgkin's Lymphoma (NHL) may be divided into T-cell and B-cell varieties.[6] The non-T-cell, non-B-cell lymphomas are not common in children. There are several subclassifications of the tumors, with at least three classifying schema.[7-9] The most common childhood T-Cell NHL is the lymphoblastic lymphoma.[10] Pulmonary involvement in this tumor is most commonly due to pleural effusion and/or invasion by mediastinal nodes although blockage of the thoracic duct may lead to lymph backflow with tumor spread. If the tumor invades the bone marrow, hematogenous spread to the lung may occur, as in leukemia.

The most common form of B-cell NHL is Burkitt's lymphoma. The non-African form, which is the form most commonly seen in the U.S., usually presents as an abdominal mass. Pulmonary involvement with this tumor is distinctly rare.

Mention should be made here of Lymphoid Interstitial Pneumonitis (LIP). This is a diffuse lung disease with interstitial infiltration of mature lymphocytes, some of which form lymphoid follicles. It is considered a prelymphomatous state and has developed into a more malignant entity in some patients.[11,12] Until recently LIP was very uncommon in childhood.[13-15] However LIP is being frequently seen in infants with the Acquired Immune Deficiency Syndrome.[16,17] This entity is described fully in Chapter 4A.

C. Hodgkin's Disease

There are four patterns of lung involvement in Hodgkin's disease.[18,19] There may be contiguous spread from the mediastinal or hilar nodes into the pulmonary parenchyma. The mediastinal and/or hilar nodes are involved in 25% of those patients with right cervical node involvement. With left cervical node involvement, mediastinal nodes are usually spared. In the pattern of peribronchovascular disease there is infiltration and spread along the lymphatic vessels from the mediastinum. The radiographic pattern is one of "radiating streaks" from the hilum, almost in a fan-like pattern. Tumor cells may invade the bronchus and cause endobronchial lesions. Subpleural spread can occur when the subpleural network is involved, which is more likely with anterior mediastinal node disease. Pleural effusion is also more commonly associated with anterior mediastinal node involvement. Finally, there may be parenchymal disease which can be either nodular or alveolar.[20] The latter is indistinguishable from other forms of interstitial pneumonitis, except by tissue diagnosis. Parenchymal disease occurs by hematogenous and/or lymphatic spread.

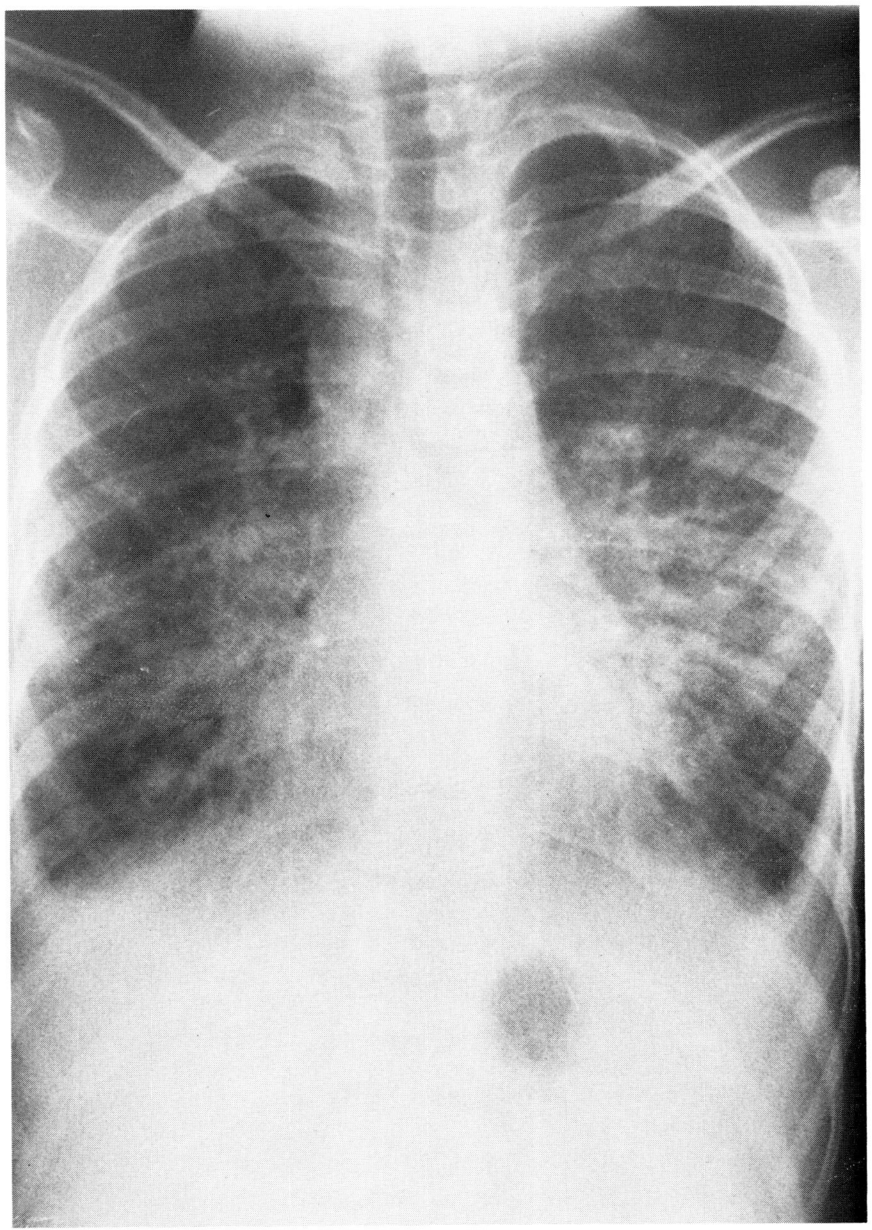

A

FIGURE 1.   Chest radiograph of a 12-year-old patient with acute lymphoblastic leukemia and diffuse interstitial pneumonia. (A) Diffuse interstitial infiltration is present bilaterally, especially in the lower halves of both lungs. (B) Close-up of the right lower lobe and the pattern of interstitial infiltration. This patient went on to die of respiratory failure. (Radiographs courtesy of the Department of Radiology, St. Christopher's Hospital for Children, Philadelphia, Pennsylvania).

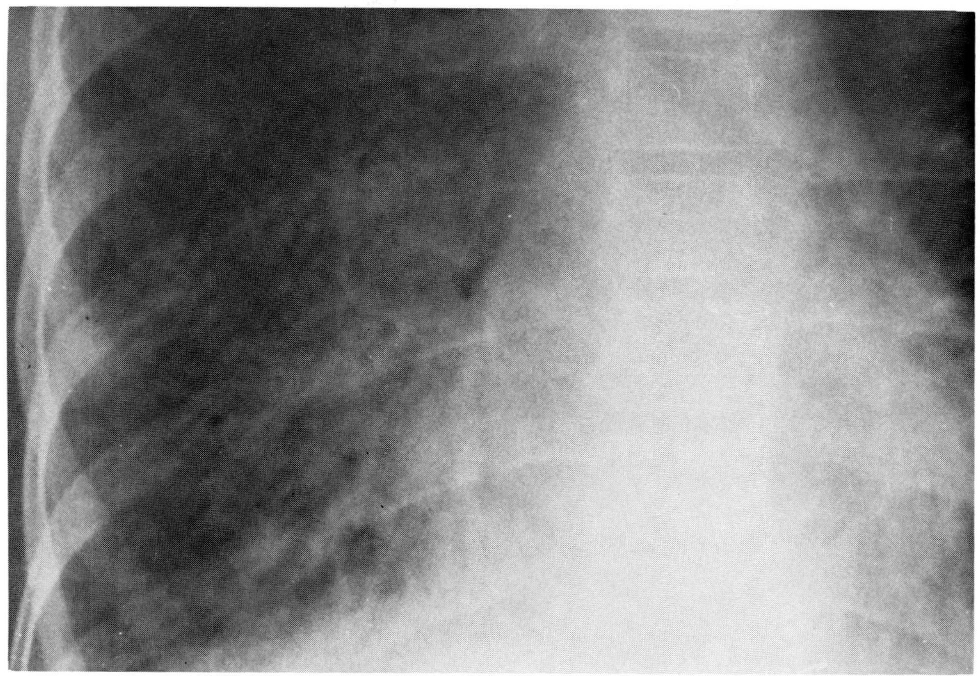

FIGURE 1B

IV. HISTIOCYTOSIS X

Histiocytosis X encompasses a spectrum of pathologic entities and is itself included among the histiocytic syndromes.[21] The pathology of histiocytosis X primarily consists of proliferation and tissue invasion by Langerhans cells.[22] Other cells may be found in conjunction with the Langerhans cells, but it is the invasion of the Langerhans cells that is believed to pathologically define the entity. In the lung these cells usually invade the interstitium with subsequent development of interstitial fibrosis. Clinical manifestations of pulmonary involvement include tachypnea, cough, crackles, dyspnea, and hypoxemia. Chest radiographs will reveal an interstitial pattern of disease, as found in 12% of 57 children with histiocytosis X[23] (see Chapter 1A, Case 1).

Letterer-Siwe Disease is an acute disseminated form of histiocytosis X occurring primarily in children under 3 years of age. Pulmonary involvement as described above plays a prominent clinical role in the patients,[24] causing significant morbidity and mortality. In addition, a cystic dilatation of bronchiolar walls can occur, possibly as a result of a weakening of those walls by Langerhans cell invasion. This may also be the etiology of the pneumothorax occasionally seen in these young children.

A less severe form of the disease, Hand-Schuller-Christian Disease typically affects slightly older children than does Letterer-Siwe. The common manifestations of Hand-Schuller-Christian Disease are in the bones but there may be a concomitant diabetes insipidus. Pulmonary involvement may be diffuse or occur as nodular invasions by Langerhans cells. Eosinophilic granuloma is the most localized and benign form of the disease. Involvement may be unifocal, or multifocal but limited to one organ or organ system. Most often the lesions are in the bones. A pulmonary syndrome may fit in this category, with the lung being the sole organ

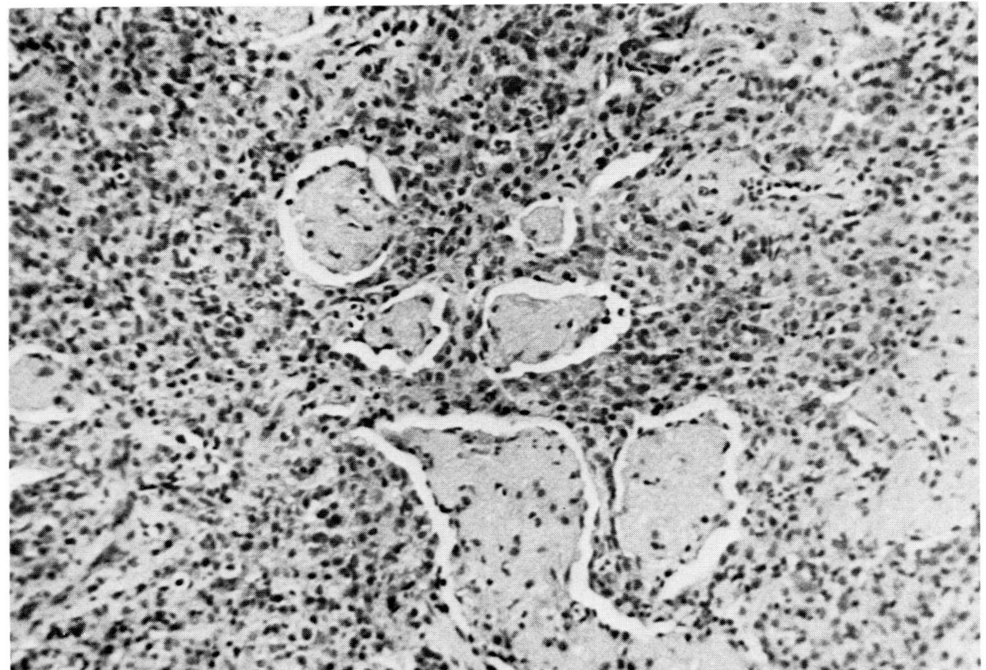

FIGURE 2.   Lung section of same patient showing markedly enlarged interalveolar septae due to diffuse interstitial infiltration. The infiltrate is comprised by cells with rounded nuclei and prominent nucleoli; multiple cells show mitosis. Thick proteinaceous exudate is present in the alveoli. (Photograph courtesy of Nayere Zaeri, M.D., Department of Pathology, St. Christopher's Hospital for Children, Philadelphia, Pennsylvania).

involved.[23] Pathologic findings in the lung may include alveolar filling by histiocytes and eosinophils; interstitial infiltration by the cells occasionally with formation of nodules 2 to 4 mm; or an endarteritis may lead to interstitial fibrosis with honeycomb lung or spontaneous pneumothorax.[25,26]

Children who survive the acute disease are susceptible to long-term pulmonary sequelae.[27,28] Such children are prone to opportunistic infections by Aspergillus, Pneumocystis carinii, nontuberculous mycobacteria, and Pseudomonas aeruginosa. Pulmonary fibrosis may give rise to long-term pulmonary dysfunction. Some of the long-term manifestations may also be due to the chemotherapeutic agents being used in the treatment of this underlying disorder.

REFERENCES

1. **Spencer, H.,** Secondary tumours in the lung, in *Pathology of the Lung,* Pergamon Press, Oxford, 1985.
2. **Bodey, G. P., Powell, R. D., Hersh, E. M., et al.,** Pulmonary complications of acute leukemia, *Cancer,* 19, 781, 1966.
3. **Wells, R. J., Weetman, R. M., Ballantine, T. V. N., Grosfeld, J. L., and Baehner, R. L.,** Pulmonary leukemia in children presenting as diffuse interstitial pneumonia, *J. Pediatr.,* 96, 262, 1980.
4. **Kelleher, J. F., Miale, T. D., and Donnelly, W. H.,** Respiratory distress secondary to pulmonary leukemia, *Am. J. Dis. Child.,* 135, 716, 1981.
5. **Georgitis, J., Eigen, H., Provisor, D., and Baehner, R. L.,** Isolated pulmonary leukemic relapse following successful bone marrow transplant in a child with acute lymphoblastic leukemia, *Pediatrics,* 64, 913, 1979.
6. **Quinn, J. J.,** The lymphoproliferative disorders, in *Malignant Diseases of Infancy and Childhood and Adolescence,* Altman, A. J. and Schwartz, A. D., Ed., W. B. Saunders, Philadelphia, 1983.

7. **Berard, C. W., Greene, M. H., Jaffe, E. S. et al.,** A multidisciplinary approach to non-Hodgkin's lymphomas, *Ann. Int. Med.,* 94, 218, 1981.
8. **Lukes, R. J. and Collins, R. D.,** New approaches to the classification of the lymphomata, *Br. J. Cancer,* 3 (Suppl.), 1, 1975.
9. **Rappaport, H., Winter, W., and Hicks, E.,** Follicular lymphoma, *Cancer,* 9, 792, 1956.
10. **Nathwani, B. N., Kim, H., and Rappaport, H.,** Malignant lymphoma, lymphoblastic, *Cancer,* 38, 964, 1976.
11. **Spencer, H.,** Pulmonary reticuloses, in *Pathology of the Lung,* Pergamon Press, Oxford, 1985.
12. **Fleetham, J. A. and Thurlbeck, W. M.,** in *Disorders of the Respiratory Tract in Children,* Kendig, E. L. and Chernick, V., W. B. Saunders, Oxford, 1983.
13. **Church, J. A., Isaaca, H., Saxon, A., Keens, T. G., and Richards, W.,** Lymphoid interstitial pneumonitis and hypogammaglobulinemia in children, *Am. Rev. Resp. Dis.,* 124, 491, 1981.
14. **O'Bradovich, H. M., Moser, M. M., and Lu, L.,** Familial lymphoid interstitial pneumonia. A long term followup, *Pediatrics,* 65, 523, 1980.
15. **Lovell, D., Lindsley, C., and Langston, C.,** Lymphoid interstitial pneumonitis in juvenile rheumatoid arthritis, *J. Pediatr.,* 105, 947, 1984.
16. **Joshi, V. V., Oleske, J. M., Minnefor, A. B., Singh, R., Bokhari, T., and Rapkin, R. H.,** Pathology of suspected acquired immune deficiency syndrome in children, *Pediatr. Pathol.,* 2, 71, 1984.
17. **Scott, G. B., Buck, B. E., Leterman, J. G., Bloom, F. L., and Parks, W. P.,** Acquired immunodeficiency syndrome in infants, *N. Eng. J. Med.,* 310, 76, 1984.
18. **Altman, A. J. and Schwartz, A. D.,** *Malignant Diseases of Infancy, Childhood and Adolescence,* W. B. Saunders, Philadelphia, 1983.
19. **Ultman, J. E. and Moran, E. M.,** Clinical course and complications in Hodgkin's disease, *Arch. Int. Med.,* 131, 332, 1973.
20. **Grossman, N. J., Luddy, R. E., and Schwartz, A. D.,** Stage IV A Hodgkin's disease of the lung, *Am. J. Ped. Hem./Onc.,* 6, 332, 1984.
21. **Lanzkowsky, P.,** *Pediatric Oncology,* McGraw-Hill, New York, 1983.
22. **Nezelof, C., Frileux-Herbert, H., and Cronier-Saibot, J.,** Disseminated histiocytosis X. Analysis of prognostic factors based on a retrospective study of fifty patients, *Cancer,* 44, 1824, 1979.
23. **Carlson, R. A., Hattery, R. R., O'Connell, E. J., and Fontana, R. S.,** Pulmonary involvement by histiocytosis X in the pediatric age group, *Mayo Clin. Proc.,* 51, 542, 1976.
24. Case records of the Massachusetts General Hospital, *N. Engl. J. Med.,* 313, 874, 1985.
25. **Smith, M., McCormack, L. J., Van Ostrand, H. S. et al.,** Primary pulmonary histiocytosis X, *Chest,* 65, 176, 1974.
26. **Nadeau, P. J., Ellis, F. H., Harrison, E. G., et al.,** Primary pulmonary histiocytosis X, *Dis. Chest.,* 37, 325, 1960.
27. **Komp, D. M.,** Long-term sequelae of histiocytosis X, *Am. J. Ped. Hem-Oncol.,* 3, 165, 1981.
28. **Sims, D. G.,** Histiocytosis X: follow-up of 43 cases, *Arch. Dis. Child.,* 52, 433, 1976.

Chapter 39

NONINFECTIOUS PULMONARY MANIFESTATIONS OF RENAL DISEASE IN CHILDREN

Stephen T. Lawless and H. Jorge Baluarte

TABLE OF CONTENTS

I. INTRODUCTION

Management of pediatric renal disease has become especially complex by the introduction of peritoneal dialysis, hemodialysis, renal transplantation, and new immunosuppressive agents. At the same time, it is becoming increasingly important therapeutically, diagnostically, and financially for the primary physician to be aware of how commonly an underlying kidney disease interacts with other organ systems. It should be noted, however, that 75% of all pulmonary infiltrates found in patients with renal diseases are of an infectious etiology and only 25% are noninfectious.

II. SPECIFIC RENAL CONDITIONS

A. Renal Failure

Pulmonary disease with renal failure includes pulmonary edema, pleural effusion, uremic pneumonia, pleuritis, pulmonary calcification, hemosiderosis, and fibrosis.

The presence of renal failure is associated with a defect in gas transfer due to decreased diffusing capacity across the alveolar capillary membrane. Even more overt respiratory symptoms or radiographic findings can occur[1] and will increase in severity as azotemia worsens. The radiographic appearance of pulmonary edema in renal failure assumes a classic "bat's wing" or "butterfly" pattern also called uremic pneumonia. It is described as bilaterally symmetric alveolar infiltrates in the inner two thirds of the lung fields with sparing of the apex and periphery. This represents a fibrinous pleuritis with protein rich edema and perihilar infiltrates.[2]

In acute renal failure, the degree of uremic pulmonary edema is related to the degree of azotemia.[3] Microscopically, one sees alveolar septal swelling, proteinacious exudate in the alveoli and hyalinization of membranes. In chronic renal failure the severity of uremic pulmonary edema is not directly associated with the degree of azotemia as one sees hyalinization of alveolar septa, casts of bronchioles, and interstitial fibrosis. The etiology of these pulmonary infiltrates in renal failure could be related to the toxic effect of uremia on the pulmonary vasculature. Most commonly, however, it is due to a combination of factors which include overhydration, hypertension, uremia, anemia, and myocardial dysfunction.

It is important to distinguish between uremic pulmonary edema and pulmonary edema secondary to congestive heart failure and fluid overload. In uremic pulmonary edema, there is a lack of hilar congestion, no pleural effusion, and a normal heart size. A complex occurs, however, when the two states can exist simultaneously. In early renal failure, for example, the heart may be of large or normal size with pericarditis. However, as the uremia progresses the pericarditis can progress to a subacute and fibrosing constrictive condition which could make the heart appear small on radiograph. Subsequently, with some overhydration and fluid overload, heart failure could present with a normal or small heart. Echocardiogram and EKG are essential in making this diagnosis.

As azotemia progresses the radiograph of the chest may also show persistent pulmonary edema-like features with punctate or patchy infiltrates in the lungs. These may represent pulmonary calcifications.[3] Over 50% of patients on chronic hemodialysis show some evidence of pulmonary calcifications. Often patients are asymptomatic when the calcifications are microscopic. The patients may also have fever and symptoms of hypoxia. The calcifications are then perivascular and rarely nodular.[2] Microscopically, the calcifications are located in the alveolar septa and at the opening of the alveolar duct. The picture can be identical to pneumonia or pulmonary edema.

This picture of metastatic calcification is related partly but not entirely to secondary hyperparathyroidism. All the etiologic factors are not completely understood as serum calcium, phosphate, the Ca $\times$ PO$_4$ solubility product, and parathyroid hormone in those patients with histologic calcification are only slightly altered.[4] The diagnosis of metastatic lung calcification can be made by Technetium 99 (Tc99) diphosphate lung scan. Technetium seeks bone and calcium, so the lungs show enhancement on bone scan if calcifications are present. The calcifications may reverse somewhat with more frequent and efficient dialysis. Surprisingly, the incidence of pulmonary embolus among patients with renal insufficiency appears less than in the general population. In one series of adult patients, the incidence of embolus on autopsy was 32%, while in those with a serum creatinine > 5 mg% the incidence was 9.5%,[5] in spite of the usually high risk factors present in adults. It is possible that there are nonspecific platelet abnormalities inherent in the uremic condition which help decrease the incidence of emboli. Pulmonary hemosiderosis with fibrosis can occur as a result of multiple blood transfusions and iron overload.

B. Nephrotic Syndrome

The definition of nephrotic syndrome remains unchanged: massive proteinuria, hypoalbuminemia, hyperlipemia, and edema. The nephrotic syndrome is the mere clinical manifestation of a large number of morphologically distinct glomerular disorders which, in 90% of the cases is secondary to systemic disease. The terminology used to describe the disorders associated with nephrotic syndrome may seem confusing. The term more commonly used is "lipoid nephrosis" which refers to uncomplicated primary nephrotic syndrome with no glomerular change by light microscopy. Other descriptive titles are "nil" disease or idiopathic primary nephrotic syndrome, but all these synonyms are now supplanted by the more descriptive term "minimal change" nephrotic syndrome.

Two additional histologic lesions often discussed are mesangial proliferation and focal glomerulosclerosis, which account for 9 to 15% of the total children with nephrotic syndrome. Children with these glomerular lesions are clinically indistinguishable at presentation from those with minimal change nephrotic syndrome but show a relative lack of response to the usual regimen of prednisone therapy. Other histologic lesions in patients with nephrotic syndrome are membranous nephropathy and membranoproliferative glomerulonephritis. The latter type is rarely confused with minimal change nephrotic syndrome either at clinical presentation or after initial diagnostic studies.

The primary pulmonary findings in the nephrotic syndrome are pulmonary edema and pleural effusion. They are the result of decreased plasma volume and decreased glomerular filtration rate (GFR) which leads to an activation of the renin/angiotensin system which in turn produces a hyperaldosterone state. The end result is sodium and water retention, which along with the already low protein state leads to interstitial space and edema.

Effusions can be unilateral or bilateral with some mediastinal widening. There may also be some pericardial fluid and evidence of pulmonary edema. As renal disease progresses, azotemia can occur and the so-called "butterfly" infiltrates may appear even without systemic evidence of edema or overhydration. Patients with nephrotic syndrome are predisposed to renal vein thrombosis and systemic thromboembolism.[6] Acquired antithrombin III deficiency, caused by excess urinary excretion of this protein, has been suggested to be the major factor in the pathogenesis of thrombosis in these patients. However, the exact nature of the hypercoagulable state in patients with the nephrotic syndrome is unclear and other factors, such as the accompanying hyperlipidemia, may also be involved.[6]

C. Peritoneal Dialysis

Peritoneal dialysis is a viable option for treatment of renal disease and is widely available in pediatrics. All the pulmonary changes of acute and chronic renal failure may be seen in the patient who is on peritoneal dialysis. However, there are a few pulmonary complications that one must be aware of which are directly related to peritoneal dialysis. Pulmonary problems during peritoneal dialysis may be the result of abdominal distention during dialysis with elevation of the diaphragm and pressure on the lower lobes of the lung.[2] This may lead to a reduction in vital capacity and decreased perfusion to the lung bases. In about one third of patients basilar atelectasis occurs. There may also be a pleural effusion due to either lymphatic connections or fenestrations through the diaphragm. These complications, except perhaps the effusion, are all reversible and can be lessened with smaller dialysate volumes.

D. Hemodialysis

This dialysis modality is also occasionally associated with respiratory symptoms. Roughly 3 to 5% of patients using cuprophane dialyzers will experience some type of mild respiratory complaints. The so-called "first use" syndrome involves complement activation triggered by the exposure to new cuprophane dialysis membranes.[7] Patients may experience chest pain, dyspnea, hypotension, urticaria, angioedema, bronchospasm, and sometimes cardiopulmonary collapse, 2 to 3 min after the beginning of dialysis. The full range of this syndrome is rare, its rate of occurrence is roughly 3.5 reactions per million dialysis treatments. If this reaction occurs it is better to switch to a polyacylnitrite or polymethylacrylate membrane, although these can also be associated with complement activation.

Besides acute anaphylactoid reaction with cuprophane membranes, other immunologic pulmonary reactions can occur during chronic maintenance hemodialysis: hypereosinophilia, "asthma-like" reactions, and pulmonary leukotaxis leading to pulmonary infiltrates[8] consisting of entrapped granulocytes and monocytes.

Nonimmunologic pulmonary changes that occur with chronic hemodialysis can result from either hypoventilation secondary to hypocarbia (as carbon dioxide is cleared) or microemboli from the dialysis material and peripheral vascular access which show as pulmonary infiltrates.

E. Renal Transplant

Despite significant advances in dialytic technology, successful renal transplantation remains the optimal form of therapy for children with end-stage renal disease. A well functioning renal transplant brings about both physiologic and rehabilitative improvement in a child's quality of life which cannot be attained with the current dialysis therapies.

The major medical complications after renal transplantation are unusual infections, steroid and cyclosporin A toxicity, hypertension, and malignant disease. Infection is the primary cause of death after renal transplantation.[9] Although common bacterial and viral infections occur in recipients of transplants, unusual infections often occur with bacteria, viruses and parasites.

Various problems associated with transplantation are potential sources of pulmonary infiltrates — infection, embolus, rejection, fluid overload, and tumor. Pulmonary disease has been said in adults to complicate the course of 20% of renal transplants and cause 50% of the fatalities. In a recent adult series, approximately 75% of the pulmonary disease that was seen in transplant recipients was due to infection, and the most common noninfectious lesion was that of pulmonary infarction.[10] The risk of embolus is low in children. The greatest risk of pulmonary infarct was in the first 2 months post-transplant. Predisposing factors in kidney disease leading to thromboembolus were the presence of A-V fistulas, an abdominal surgical procedure, vascular procedures, and prolonged bed rest. However, recent advances in surgical techniques and early post-operative mobilization have further decreased the risk. Unfortunately, the diagnosis of pulmonary embolism in pediatrics usually takes a few days before suspicion and diagnosis are made and by that time there is a high incidence of superinfection.

The timing and the acute or chronic nature of the pulmonary event in relation to the renal transplant are also important. Post-operative atelectasis secondary to hypoventilation, mechanical ventilation, analgesia, pain, and splinting is common. Acute infiltrates tend to be noninfectious with the exception of cytomegalovirus infection which usually occurs 1 to 4 months post-transplantation. Chronic infiltrates developing over days to weeks, have a higher chance of being secondary to embolism or edema. Emboli tend to be focal or multifocal with occasional consolidation while edema is usually multifocal, diffuse and peribroncho-vascular.[11] Whereas the incidence of emboli peaks at 3 weeks post-transplant, edema occurs at anytime.

Fluid overload is not uncommon post operatively. Maintenance of good fluid status keeps the new kidney well perfused, although this increases the risk of a fluid overload state and pulmonary edema. Edema is a very real possibility especially in someone who already is prone to renal pulmonary edema as a consequence of azotemia. At any time post-transplant, rejection can occur. There are some changes in the lungs with transplant rejection. They probably occur secondary to indistinct immune mechanisms which release "factors" that act at the alveolar capillary bed creating and increasing pulmonary edema. This can often occur with decreasing steroid dose.[3]

F. Drug Effects

Many different types of medications used in renal disease are associated with interstitial lung disease (see Chapter 31). Cyclophosphamide in a synthetic antineoplastic drug chemically related to nitrogen mustard, which has been used alone or in addition to steroids to treat a variety of immune mediated primary renal or systemic diseases. It causes dysplasia of type II pneumocytes that line the alveoli. The pulmonary toxicity has been reported within weeks or years after multiple courses of chemotherapy. The clinical presentation in these patients is of fever, hypoxemia, and bilateral lung infiltrates.[10]

The differential diagnosis of these infiltrates is of infection vs. underlying disease vs. drug induced change. The diagnosis is made by biopsy where the combination of alveolar cell dysplasia and interstitial inflammation in the absence of alveolar fluid, inflammation, or hyaline membrane thickening suggest a pneumonitis due to either a drug or radiation.[10]

Azathioprine, an alkylating agent used in organ transplantation has been rarely associated with pulmonary infiltrates. Bleomycin, carnistine, busulfan, methotrexate, and nitrofurantoin are all associated with interstitial lung disease. Nitrofurantoin has also been associated with the occurrence of pleural effusion and eosinophilic pneumonia. D-penicillamine rarely can cause alveolar hemorrhage and crescentric glomerulonephritis.

G. Cancer

Neoplasms of the kidneys occur at a rate of 7.8 per million children. Almost all the renal neoplasms consist of Wilm's tumor. The median age for Wilm's tumor is 3 years, with 80% presenting before age 5 years. It is unusual in the second decade but it can occur in adults. Metastasis to the lungs (80%), liver, CNS and bone marrow occur. Pulmonary metastasis are evident on roentgenograms in about 19% of patients at the time of diagnosis.[12] Renal cell carcinoma, infrequent in children; also metastasizes to the lungs.

Any subacute or chronic lung infiltrate in renal disease, especially in those who have had immunosuppression could represent a malignancy. Immunosuppression increases the risk of malignancy and the incidence about six times more frequent among organ transplant recipients.[13] In a study among transplant patients there was a 21-fold increase in cancer of the skin but pulmonary metastasis of primary squamous cell cancer was unusual.[10] The risk of lymphoma is 35 times higher in transplant recipients. The majority of the lymphomas are reticular cell sarcomas with primary metastasis to the brain. Lymphomas that metastasize to the lungs appear as infiltrates, nodules, cavitary lesions, effusions, and hilar or mediastinal nodes.

However, the risk of lymphoma is even higher when cyclosporin and prednisone is used as the primary immunosuppressive regimen as opposed to azathioprine and prednisone. Interestingly, the characteristics of the lymphoma associated with cyclosporin are also different. It appears earlier (5.6 months vs. 24 months with conventional) and rarely involves the CNS.[14] The overall incidence of lymphoma with cyclosporin is 0.7%.[15] There is a suggestion that the incidence of cyclosporin-induced lymphoma is related to dosage.

Certain malignancies that present with pulmonary findings can also cause specific renal syndromes. For example, Hodgkin's lymphoma can in 10% of cases present with nephrotic syndrome, simulating lipoid nephrosis or membranous glomerulonephritis.[16] This occurs without evidence of renal vein thrombosis, amyloidosis, or tumor invasion. Incidentally, in patients with uremia, there does not appear to be an increased incidence of cancer.[17] With the exception of immunosuppression, it appears that the effect of age is more significant than the underlying renal disease or treatment.

III. GENERAL DISEASE STATES

There are a number of syndromes and diseases that have prominent pulmonary manifestations and renal disease. One clue to these syndromes is hemoptysis. The differential diagnosis of hemoptysis and renal failure includes pulmonary edema, infection, or hemorrhage. The infiltrate that occurs in these disorders may be patchy or diffusely involve both lung fields, simulating pulmonary edema or infection. Pulmonary edema and infection usually do not decrease the hemoglobin. Alveolar hemorrhage is usually a manifestation of systemic disease. Goodpasture's syndrome, systemic lupus erythematosus (SLE), hypersensitivity angiitis, hemosiderosis, Henoch-Schonlein Purpura, mixed IgG/IgM cryoglobulinemia, renal vein thrombosis with pulmonary embolism, Wegener's granulomatosis and polyarteritis nodosa all should be considered in the differential diagnosis of pulmonary hemorrhage.

Bilateral involvement is the rule with alveolar hemorrhage, however, at times it may be asymmetric or entirely unilateral. Any segment of lung could be involved. The apex and costophrenic angles are most often spared.

These diseases can produce a wide spectrum of findings ranging from proteinuria to crescentric glomerulonephritis (rapidly progressive glomerulonephritis). Rapidly progressive glomerulonephritis is a clinically descriptive term applied to cases in which irreversible renal failure ensues relentlessly within a few weeks to several months. Histologic examination of the renal tissue may or may not reveal a proliferative glomerular lesion, but a constant feature is one of diffuse florid epithelial crescents filling Bowman's space. Crescentric glomerulonephritis can be seen in Goodpasture's syndrome, SLE, Wegener granulomatosis, and polyarteritis, subacute bacterial endocarditis, Henoch-Schonlein purpura, post-streptococcal glomerulonephritis and idiopathic glomerulonephritis.

A. Goodpasture's Syndrome

Is defined as a disorder consisting of the triad of glomerulonephritis, pulmonary hemorrhage, and antiglomerular basement membrane antibody (anti-GBM) formation. Synonyms for this disease are lung purpura with nephritis, hemorrhagic pneumonia and nephritis, pulmonary hemosiderosis with nephritis, and hemorrhagic pulmonary renal syndrome. Unfortunately, the eponym of Goodpasture's syndrome has been applied to many patients in whom no evidence was available to confirm or deny the presence of anti-GBM antibody.

The disease process consists of a cytotoxic type II autoimmune disease in which antibody is directed primarily against the glomerular basement membrane. This antibody can cross react with the alveolar basement membrane and choroid plexus. Immunoglobulin reacts against a cell surface or cell attached antigen which results in opsonization or destruction of that tissue often with complement activation.[18] However, serum complement levels are classically normal.

Evidence of anti-GBM antibody formation may be obtained in several ways. The first is by the demonstration of linear, ribbon-like deposits of IgG along the glomerular capillary walls by immunofluorescent study of renal biopsy material. These deposits are frequently (80%), but not necessarily, accompanied by C_3, usually in an irregular or interrupted linear fashion. The association of these deposits with proliferative glomerulonephritis, particularly of the crescentric variety, can confidently be assumed to represent in vivo fixation of anti-GBM antibody. Second, circulating anti-GBM antibody may be demonstrated by precipitation in-gel, indirect immunofluorescence, passive hemagglutination, or radioimmunoassay procedures.[19] Third, if sufficient renal or lung tissue is available, elution studies may be carried out to demonstrate directly the antibody nature and specificity of deposited IgG.

Approximately 90% of the patients have the anti-GBM antibodies, but such antibodies by themselves are not absolutely diagnostic of Goodpasture's syndrome as they have been found in cases of lupus, polyarteritis nodosa, diabetic nephropathy, penicillamine sensitivity, focal glomerular sclerosis, and Henoch-Schonlein purpura. These diseases, however, are not characterized by the linear ribbon-like glomerular deposits that are seen with Goodpasture's syndrome. This syndrome is more prevalent among young adult males, the usual age of onset being between 20 and 30 years. There is a male to female ratio of 3:1. The classic presentation is with pulmonary hemorrhage, although pulmonary symptoms may precede or may present coincident with the renal lesion. Clinically one will see hemoptysis, anemia, and nephritis with symptoms of dyspnea, cough, malaise, and fever. Sputum samples may have hemosiderin-laden macrophages. The radiograph of the lungs may show patchy lung infiltrates in a ''butterfly'' pattern or an acinar, reticular, or reticulonodular pattern. These radiographic findings may be transitory. Pulmonary insufficiency with recurrent hemoptysis also occurs.

Approximately 60 to 80% of patients will have both pulmonary hemorrhage and glomerulonephritis. The latent period between the first episode of hemoptysis and the discovery of the renal disease (usually in the form of abnormal urinalysis) may vary from a few weeks to several years, but averages about 3 months. Unfortunately the renal lesion progresses rapidly over time requiring some form of dialysis usually after 3 1/2 months (range <1 to 14 months). The glomerular injury is mediated by the interaction of the circulating autoantibody with intrinsic GBM glycoproteins, resulting in activation of the complement cascade and thus leading to the infiltration by inflammatory cells. Coagulation mechanisms and monocytes are seen to participate actively in the generation of crescents. Lung injury may be induced in a similar fashion; however, the lack of correlation between levels of anti-GBM antibody and pulmonary manifestations is difficult to account for. It is possible that nonantibody factors, perhaps released by the acutely damaged kidney, participate in the pulmonary injury. The triggering factor for Goodpasture's syndrome is not known, but it is perhaps a combination of genetic factors and an exposure to an environmental agent like influenza, hydrocarbon, or penicillamine that damage the alveolar walls which then release an autoantigen.[3]

Uncontrolled observations suggest that high dose parenteral (''pulse therapy'') or oral steroid treatment produces a prompt improvement in the pulmonary hemorrhagic manifestations. Unfortunately, steroids alone seem to have little demonstrable beneficial effect on the rapidly progressive glomerular disease. Similarly, cytotoxic agents, although widely employed, have not been generally associated with clear-cut benefit in well documented cases in which renal failure and extensive crescent formation were present. The role of anticoagulation in treatment is unclear, but might be expected to be exceptionally hazardous in these patients because of the unpredictable appearance of pulmonary hemorrhage. Uncontrolled studies have reported dramatic results using intensive plasma exchange (plasmapheresis).[20,21] The prompt disappearance of pulmonary bleeding and the reversal of renal function deterioration by aggressive plasma exchange therapy make it difficult to justify a controlled clinical trial.

As with other forms of rapidly progressive renal failure, early and aggressive therapy is required. Poor results can be expected in oliguric patients or in those with renal failure severe enough to need dialysis support (e.g., >8 mg/dℓ creatinine). Initial therapy with daily 3 to 4 ℓ plasma exchanges combined with 2 mg/kg/day of azathioprine or cyclophosphamide plus 1 mg/kg/day of prednisone has been recommended, at the same time monitoring the degree of renal and pulmonary function, and level of anti-GBM antibody. Although many uncertainties exist, it appears at the present time that bilateral nephrectomy should be reserved for those patients with presumptive evidence of irreversible glomerular damage who have life-threatening pulmonary hemorrhage and who have failed to respond to a brief trial of high dose corticosteroid and/or intensive plasma exchange.

B. Idiopathic Pulmonary Hemosiderosis

Idiopathic pulmonary hemosiderosis is a disease occurring most frequently in childhood and in young adults. It is characterized by dyspnea, cyanosis, fever, cough, blood-streaked sputum, and pallor, with laboratory evidence of iron-deficiency anemia. The basic pathologic process is blood extravasation in the pulmonary alveoli by repeated hemorrhages. A chest roentgenogram shows a variety of findings from bilateral perihilar patchy infiltration to diffuse pulmonary infiltration. Clearing of the pulmonary fields can occur with treatment but the lesions may progress to interstitial fibrosis.

A high incidence of specific renal lesions have been noted with hemosiderosis, even a rapidly progressive form of diffuse glomerulonephritis, which may dominate the clinical picture.[22] It is unknown whether this rapid progression of renal failure has an immune pathogenesis similar to other known acute or chronic nephridities or whether the iron deposition plays any role in the pathogenesis of the renal lesion.

C. Wegener's Granulomatosis

Wegener's granulomatosis is a rare syndrome in pediatrics that is characterized by destructive granulomatous lesions of the upper and lower respiratory tract associated with a systemic necrotizing arteritis, most prominently in the lung and kidney.[12] The disease affects patients of any age but is more common in males in their 40s and 50s.

Type I Wegener's is described as necrotizing angiitis and aseptic necrosis of the upper respiratory tract and lung with glomerulonephritis. Type II (15%) is limited to the respiratory tract. Type III is called lymphomatoid granulomatosis which is a vasculitis and granulomatoid reaction characterized by an angiotrophic and angiodestructive infiltrate of various tissues particularly the lung with atypical lymphocytoid and plasmacytoid cells. The lungs develop multiple infiltrates and nodules that cavitate. One sees involvement of the skin (45%), kidney (45%), and CNS (20%). In contrast to type I, the vasculitis is not leukocytoclastic or fibrinoid and there are rare upper airway findings. The renal picture is almost never one of a necrotizing glomerulonephritis but nodular infiltrates of renal parenchyma appear.[23] Type IV is called necrotizing sarcoid granulomatosis and does not involve the kidney.

Respiratory symptoms are prominent initial symptoms. There may be nasal stuffiness or discharge with crusted or pustular lesions in the nares. The lesions progress to involve the sinus, palate, nares, larynx, and pharynx. The kidney is affected in 85% of cases, nasopharynx 75%, paranasal sinus 90%, eyes 60%, ears 35%, heart 15%, nervous system 20%, skin 40%, and joints 50%.[23] About 90% present with nasal symptoms.[24] Cough and hemoptysis occur but frank pulmonary hemorrhage is rare. The spectrum of renal disease may range from focal segmental glomerulonephritis with minimal hematuria and little or no renal insufficiency to rapidly progressive glomerulonephritis with hematuria, pyuria, cylindruria, and frank renal failure.[12] In one series only 5% of patients presented with renal failure.[25]

Pathologically, the disease is characterized by epitheloid cell granulomas of both arteries and veins with fibrinoid necrosis, microabscesses, focal vasculitis, thrombosis, and fibrous obliteration of the vascular lumen. The underlying lesion is probably of immunologic origin.

The role of immune complexes in the pathogenesis of Wegener's is not clear. Perhaps immune complexes are partly responsible for triggering the granulomatous reactivity seen in the disease. A delayed hypersensitivity-like response to a suspected antigen itself may elicit the granulomatous response characteristic of the upper and lower airway, with immune complex formation being a secondary phenomenon. This may or may not contribute to the pathogenesis of disease in organs such as the kidney.[23] Complement levels are usually normal.

Renal biopsy may show granular deposits of Ig and C_3 along the glomerular basement membrane or mesangium or both. However, glomerular deposits containing Ig and complement may be sparse or absent or nonspecific.[26] Pulmonary radiographic findings may be diffuse. Multiple or solitary nodular densities or infiltrates can be present. The nodules can be <1 cm or >10 cm and have vague or sharply demarcated borders. They can cavitate (50%) or be transient. Atelectasis, mediastinal nodes, and pleural effusion are rare present. There is a predilection for the upper lung with wide bilateral distribution.

The dismal outlook for patients with Wegener's has been considerably altered by combined treatment with steroids and cytotoxic agents.[23] The drug of choice is cyclophosphamide with dramatic long term remissions of the pulmonary and renal lesions. Chlorambucil and azathioprine have also been used. However, it appears that once severe renal failure occurs, it cannot be reversed. The side effects of the drugs include bone marrow suppression, gonadal dysfunction, hemorrhagic cystitis, and pulmonary fibrosis.

D. Systemic Lupus Erythematosus

Systemic lupus erythematosus (SLE) is a disease of unknown etiology characterized by the presence of multiple antibodies that participate in immunologically mediated tissue damage.[27] Only the musculoskeletal, cutaneous, renal and nervous systems are commonly involved, yet the pulmonary manifestions of SLE are frequent and occasionally are the presenting symptoms. Most common signs and symptoms include butterfly rash, Raynaud's phenomenon, purpura, alopecia, arthralgias, myositis, polyserositis, hepatosplenomegaly, cardiomegaly, carditis, seizures, cerebritis, neuritis, diarrhea, abdominal pain, bowel infarction, episcleritis, iritis, retinal vascular involvement, and hypertension.

Of primary diagnostic significance in determining the presence of activity of systemic lupus erythematosus is the degree of reactivity and the pattern of the antinuclear factor (ANA), its titer, and the levels of serum complement components. The pulmonary manifestations of SLE can be grouped into two categories: disease-related (pleurisy with/without effusion, lupus pneumonitis, diffuse interstitial disease, pulmonary hypertension, diaphragmatic dysfunction, atelectasis, and pulmonary hemorrhage); and disease associated (infection, uremic pulmonary edema, pulmonary embolus, pneumothorax, pseudolymphoma, sarcoidosis).[27]

Even though the presentation of SLE with pulmonary hemorrhage and glomerulonephritis is rare, if there is renal involvement by SLE there is an increased risk of pulmonary hemorrhage. Pleuropulmonary complications occur in 50 to 60% of patients. About 10% of patients will experience hemoptysis.

With pulmonary hemorrhage biopsy of the lungs shows deposits of IgG along the alveolar capillary wall. On electron microscopy, electron dense deposits are present with some organized ''finger print'' patterns associated with DNA — anti-DNA aggregates, which can also be found in the renal deposits.[28] Signs of renal involvement include variable degrees of proteinuria (transient to >6 gm/24 hr) and hematuria (microscopic or macroscopic). Nephrotic syndrome, hypertension, and renal insufficiency are present less frequently and are usually in those patients having a more extensive renal lesion. Several types of glomerular lesions may be seen in disseminated lupus erythematosus and a specific histologic alteration may be accompanied by different symptoms. Since the outcome correlates best with the severity of the disease as judged by glomerular pathology, a renal biopsy is usually indicated in all patients with suspected renal involvement. Nephritis is characteristic. The types present include mesangial nephritis (mesangial widening with hypercellularity); focal proliferative lupus nephritis (some glomeruli and lobules affected by mesangial hypercellularity with increased matrix and polymorphonuclear infiltration); diffuse proliferative lupus nephritis (crescentric formation, obliteration of capillaries, and necrosis of glomerular lobules); membranous lupus (little cell proliferation but diffuse thickening of the basement membrane); and interstitial lupus (interstitial infiltration and glomerular changes). In all forms, glomerular sclerosis may develop.[29]

While segmental glomerulitis with or without a necrotizing glomerular lesion is common, only the so-called "wire loop" lesion is specifically characteristic of lupus nephritis. It is the result of abundant subendothelial immune complex deposition. Immune deposits may be mesangial, subendothelial, or epimembranous in location. The deposits are abundant and pleomorphic varying from fine granules to large coalescent lumps. They can be fragmentary or coarsely linear. They always contain IgG and C_3 and react to a variable degree with labeled antibody to IgA, IgM, IgE, and fibrin. Fluorescent-labeled antibody to Clq and properdin are present with severe active disease, but are absent or in trace amounts in patients with mild disease or in those patients who exhibit minimal proteinuria following therapy.

As renal disease progresses the radiologic pattern of uremic lung or "butterfly wing" appearance appears. When hemorrhage occurs the diagnosis of Goodpasture's syndrome should be entertained. The majority of pulmonary infiltrates in SLE are of infectious etiology. Both the renal and pulmonary findings are related to the disease itself or are secondary to infection, or as in the case of the lungs, secondary to renal failure. As the overall progression of disease may be slow, there may be rapid onset of pulmonary distress. A child may become rapidly ill with pneumonia, uremia, pulmonary edema (secondary to fluid retention), cardiomegaly (due to myocarditis and/or pericarditis), and mild to moderate pleuritis. This clinical complex makes radiologic distinction and diagnosis difficult.[30]

Despite extensive study there is a great deal of uncertainty regarding the optimal treatment of lupus nephritis. Corticosteroids alone can reverse many of the features of active disease such as low complement levels, elevated sedimentation rate and circulating anti-nuclear factors. However, corticosteroids have a relatively unfavorable balance of efficacy and toxicity. Cytotoxic drugs, including azathioprine and cyclophosphamide have been associated with more favorable trends in the outcome of lupus nephritis.[31,32] More recent controlled studies demonstrate that cytotoxic drug therapy is more likely than prednisone to prevent progressive, irreversible paranchymal destruction in patients with lupus nephritis.[29,33]

E. Polyarteritis Nodosa

Polyarteritis nodosa is a systemic vasculitis in which the basic disease process involves inflammation and necrosis of medium and small sized muscular arteries. Necrosis, thrombosis, or aneurysm formation may occur, and the occlusion of the affected vessels may infarct various organs. In the subsequent healing stages there is gradual resolution of inflammation, with increasing luminal obliteration and fibrosis in the aneurysms, detectable arteriographically.[34] Malaise, weight loss, abdominal pain, and fever are common. Clinical manifestations vary with organ involvement and can include arthritis, myalgias, cutaneous manifestations, ulcers, peripheral neuropathy (mononeuritis multiplex), flank pain, hematuria, hypertension, cough, pleuritis, seizures, strokes, iridocyclitis, tachycardia, congestive heart failure, myocardial infarction, carditis, orchitis, or epididymitis. Hypertension, usually related to increased levels of plasma renin, is common and may be severe, even malignant. Nonspecific laboratory data include anemia and elevated sedimentation rate. Complement levels, usually normal, may be reduced or increased. A significant number of patients (10 to 30%) may be found to be carriers of hepatitis B virus.[35] Angiographic diagnosis is made by finding aneurysmal dilatation up to 1 cm in size in medium sized renal, hepatic, or visceral arteries.

In polyarteritis only 30% of patients have pulmonary involvement. Infantile polyarteritis rarely affects the lungs. The chest shows nothing characteristic, as engorgement and nonspecific increased lung markings are common. Cardiac enlargement may also be present. Chest radiographs can show edema, pleuropericardial effusion, nodules, or patchy infiltrates.[26] The pulmonary infiltrates tend to be peripheral. With uremia, uremic pneumonitis complicates the radiographic findings.

Quite striking renal involvement occurs in 80 to 90% of patients. The typical presentation is hematuria. Urinary sediment shows red cells, white cells, red cell casts, and sometimes broad renal failure casts, especially during the stages of active disease. If glomeruli are not involved, the urinary sediment is benign.

Pathologically, the kidney reveals acute inflammation of the medium-sized vessels, particularly the arcuate and interlobar vessels. Glomerular lesions are predominantly those of ischemia with hyperplasia of the juxtaglomerular apparatus, occasional segmental or diffuse proliferation, and accompanying fibrinoid necrosis. Sometimes crescentric glomerulonephritis can occur and it can be associated with immune complex deposition of Ig or complement components.

Polyarteritis nodosa is treated like other forms of vasculitis with corticosteroids. A retrospective survey found a 5 year survival of 48% in steroid treated cases vs. 13% in untreated cases.[36] The addition of cytotoxic drugs, including azathioprine or cyclophosphamide, may be beneficial.[23] More recently, intensive plasma exchange, steroids, and cytotoxic drugs have been employed in patients with vasculitis and rapidly progressive renal failure.[37] These early uncontrolled efforts are encouraging.

F. Subacute Bacterial Endocarditis

Subacute bacterial endocarditis may have hemoptysis, pulmonary infiltrates, and nodules. These occur secondary to septic emboli and pulmonary infarction. Renal disease associated with subacute endocarditis can be due to septic emboli or immune complex disease with Ig and complement deposits in the mesangial or glomerular basement membrane. Crescentric glomerulonephritis may occur.

G. Henoch-Schonlein Purpura

Henoch-Schonlein purpura (HSP) or anaphylactoid purpura is a leukoclastic vasculitis of the small blood vessels of the skin, kidney, gastrointestinal tract, lungs, liver, heart, and spleen. There is a nonthrombocytopenic purpuric rash on the lower extremities and buttocks with joint swelling, diarrhea, hematochezia associated with colicky abdominal pain, and nephritis. It occurs 1 to 3 weeks after an upper respiratory infection. Rarely, pulmonary hemorrhage, perihilar patchy infiltrates, reticulonodular changes and pneumonic processes may be present.[24] Rapidly progressive glomerulonephritis may follow. If chronic renal failure results, signs of uremic pneumonitis appear. IgA deposits in dermal capillaries or renal biopsy support the diagnosis of HSP.

H. Hypersensitivity Angiitis

Hypersensitivity angiitis presents with symptoms similar to periarteritis nodosa, although hypertension is usually mild or absent. Pulmonary involvement may be manifested by asthmatic symptoms and is frequently associated with eosinophilia. The development of pulmonary hemorrhage and rapidly progressive glomerulonephritis may simulate Goodpasture's syndrome.

I. Sarcoidosis

Sarcoidosis classically presents with hilar lymphadenopathy on radiograph which is sometimes accompanied by infiltrates or nodules. It is a rare disease under 10 years of age but occasionally infants under 1 year of age are affected. Renal involvement in sarcoidosis occurs in 4 to 11% of patients. Sarcoid granulomas are often present in the kidneys, although they rarely cause functional impairment.[28] Glomerular involvement is rare and when it occurs the glomerular lesions include membranous, mesangial, proliferative, or intracapillary glomerulonephritis. Very rarely focal or segmental hyalinosis may occur.[38] The underlying lesion may be produced by circulating immune complexes. Renal damage (nephrocalcinosis) from hypercalcemia is often.

J. Allergic Granulomatous (Churg Strauss) Angiitis

Allergic granulomatous angiitis, a syndrome distinct from both periarteritis nodosa and hypersensitivity angiitis, was first described by Churg and Strauss in 1951. This disease, rare in children, appears to be IgE mediated. Patients of various ages present with severe intractable asthma, fever and eosinophilia. Characteristic pathologically is the presence of necrotizing granulomas associated with an arteritis. Small arteries and veins are involved with epitheloid cell granulomas and eosinophilic infiltrates. Clinically one sees hypereosinophilia, increased IgE, skin lesions, and pulmonary parenchymal involvement. Pulmonary involvement varies from patchy infiltrates to nodules and occasional cavitation.[24] Extravascular granulomas may be throughout the body, including the kidneys.

K. Mixed Connective Tissue Disease

Mixed connective tissue disease is characterized by an admixture of features resembling SLE, polymyositis, and scleroderma. Raynaud's phenomenon, arthritis, sausage-shaped fingers, and various cutaneous manifestations are present. Laboratory findings of significance are antibody against ribonucleoprotein (RNP) and speckled antinuclear antibody. Renal manifestations (10 to 40% patients) include interstitial nephritis, membranous glomerulonephropathy (nephrosis) and proliferative glomerulonephritis (nephritis). Pulmonary manifestations are one of the worst and most common late complications in this disease but happen less often than they do in SLE. Response to corticosteroids is generally favorable, although severe renal involvement occasionally requires more aggressive therapy.

L. Sjogren's Syndrome

Sjogren's syndrome is a lymphocyte mediated destruction of exocrine glands. Children or adolescent patients may complain of recurrent mumps. These patients have dry eyes, dry mouths with oral ulceration and dental caries, salivary gland swelling, difficulty in swallowing, vulvovaginitis, and gastrointestinal abnormalities. In 25% of adults the disease extends to the muscles, lung (recurrent pneumonitis, effusion, and pulmonary hemorrhage with thrombocytopenia) nervous system, and the kidney (nephrosis and renal tubular acidosis).

M. Scleroderma

Scleroderma is a slow but relentless progression of fibrosis with hyperplasia of connective tissue involving the major internal organs, most notably the heart, intestine, kidney, and lung. Histologically there is increased thickness and density of dermal collagen with perivascular infiltrates of mononuclear cells. There are two types of scleroderma; progressive systemic sclerosis (PSS), more common in adults, and localized scleroderma, more common in children.

With PSS 50% of patients develop pulmonary calcification. There may be repeated episodes of aspiration pneumonia and eventual chest wall restriction secondary to reduced elasticity. Linear or nodular densities appear most commonly in the lower lung fields. Spontaneous pneumothoracis can occur. Pulmonary fibrosis also develops decreased lung compliance and increased work of breathing. Microscopically, proliferation and medial hypertrophy of small arteries and arterioles are present in the vasculature. Of the patients some 30 to 50% have significant hypertension secondary to renovascular changes, especially prevalent in those with pulmonary vascular involvement. In adults with PSS, proteinuria and azotemia may also be present. Renal involvement in adults is 45%.

N. Macroglobulinemia

Macroglobulinemia has been associated with renal disease in myeloma, lymphoma, malignancy (including lymphoma), and immunodeficiency states. Renal tubular acidosis, nephropathy, and pulmonary infiltrates can occur.

O. Cryoglobulinemia

Cryoglobulinemia (mixed IgG/IgM) has been reported in children. The development of cold precipitable mixed globulins may occur in a variety of disease states, e.g., leukemia, lymphosarcoma, infectious mononucleosis, syphilis, SLE, polyarteritis nodosa, arthritis, post-streptococcal states, and idiopathically. Renal involvement is based on immune complex formation and deposition leading to a small vessel vasculitis and glomerulonephritis. One may see hypertension, proteinuria, hematuria, purpura, anemia, arthralgia, positive ANA, decreased complement, and increased immunoglobulins in the serum. Renal involvement may develop acutely. After transient cold exposure or dehydration acute oliguric renal failure may develop. Pathologic features in the kidney include proliferation and swelling of intracapillary cells with neutrophil infiltration into glomeruli. The causal role of cryoglobulins in glomerulonephritis is still not completely known.[39] Pulmonary infiltrates and hemorrhage can be present. Other pulmonary manifestations depend on the associated underlying disease state.

P. Amyloidosis

Amyloidosis is a disorder characterized by the deposition in various organs of a proteinacious material, amyloid, that causes no inflammatory reaction but produces disease by compressing and replacing normal tissue.[40] Amyloidosis in children is rare and is most often associated with chronic infections (tuberculosis or osteomyelitis), familial mediterranean fever, or rheumatoid arthritis (JRA). Its incidence in JRA is 1 to 4% after the fifth year of life. Most commonly affected organs are the liver, spleen, adrenals, and the kidney. Renal involvement presents as proteinuria, nephrosis, renal vein thrombosis, and hypertension.

Death is usually secondary to renal failure. Pulmonary findings include segmental homogeneous opacities, pulmonary nodules with or without cavitation, reticulonodular infiltrates, and hilar or mediastinal adenopathy.

IV. RADIOLOGIC OUTLINE

When one sees a chest radiograph of someone with a renal disorder, there are a few questions that must be asked: what is the clinical status of the patient? Is there fever? Are there respiratory symptoms? What are the types of lung lesions? What has been the time span of the disease? If it is known that the underlying renal disease is associated with certain chest radiographic patterns, are these patterns consistent with the present pulmonary findings?

In interpreting the radiograph it is important to classify the lesions as being homogenous or nonhomogeneous; segmental or nonsegmental; cystic or cavitary; with or without nodules (size and number); acinar, reticular or mixed pattern; with or without effusion. Table 1 summarizes the renal conditions associated with particular pulmonary findings. This outline is based on a recent summary article which attempts to outline the pulmonary manifestations of renal disease.[26]

Table 1
CHEST RADIOLOGIC PATTERN VS. RENAL DISEASE

Chest radiographic pattern	Infection	Polyarteritis	Lymphoma	Radiation	Amyloidosis	Churg Strauss	GU neoplasm	Systemic lupus	Wegener's	Neoplasm or metastasis	Septic emobli	Renal cell CA	Myeloma	Goodpasture's	Pulmonary edema	Scleroderma	Drug induced	Nephrosis	Nephritis	Uremic pleuritis	Dialysis	Hernia of Bochdalek
Homogenous opacity: nonsegmental	X	X	X	X																		
Homogenous opacity: segmental	X		X		X																	
Inhomogenous opacity: nonsegmental	X			X		X	X			X												
Inhomogenous opacity: segmental	X							X														
Cystic and cavitary	X								X	X	X	X										
Solitary pulmonary nodule <6 cm	X		X		X				X	X		X	X									
>6 cm	X		X						X	X		X	X									
Multiple pulmonary nodules +/− cavities	X	X	X		X	X			X	X		X	X									
Diffuse disease mostly acinar[a]	X									X				X	X							
Diffuse, disease mostly reticular reticulonodular	X		X		X			X						X	X	X	X					
Diffuse disease mixed acinar reticulondular	X													X			X					
Effusion without pulmonary disease	X[b]	X						X		X								X	X	X	X[c]	
Effusion with pulmonary disease	X	X	X					X	X	X		X			X							

| Hilar and mediastinal nodes | X | X | X | | X | | | |
| Mediastinal widening | | | | | X | | X | X |

[a] Acinar = air space filling disease.
[b] Subphrenic abscess.
[c] Peritoneal dialysis — from dissection. Hemodialysis — exudate from anticoagulant.

Data acquired and organized from Reference 26.

V. CONCLUSION

As one can see, the range of kidney disease involved with interstitial lung disease is diffuse. A knowledge of the underlying pathologic mechanism in renal disease is essential in deciding whether a developing pulmonary problem is related to the renal process. Unfortunately, the pulmonary symptomatology or radiologic findings may precede the overt renal manifestations, as for example, in Goodpasture's Syndrome.

Often by a thorough pathophysiologic understanding of disease and thoughtful use of laboratory tests, the patient will be saved from unnecessary tests, pain, and financial distress. Even though infection should most times be first in diagnostic possibilities when considering interstitial lung findings in a patient with renal disease, it is by no means exclusive. All too often, it is easier to state that the pulmonary infiltrate is "probably infection". It is much harder to use clinical knowledge with diagnostic acumen and question whether the pulmonary process is not infectious but is directly related to the basic pathophysiology of a systemic disease in particular that involving the kidney.

REFERENCES

1. **Lee, H. Y. and Stretton, T. B.,** The lungs in renal failure, *Thorax,* 30, 46, 1975.
2. **Swartz, C. and Teplick, J.,** Radiographic considerations in maintenance dialysis, *Radiol. Clin. North Am.,* 10, 511, 1972.
3. **Prakash, U.,** Respiratory manifestations of systemic disease. II. Hematologic, endocrine and metabolic, renal, and gastrointestinal diseases, *Postgrad. Med.,* 76, 1984.
4. **Conger, J. D., Hammond, W. S., Alfrey, A. C., et al.,** Pulmonary calcification in chronic dialysis patients, *Ann. Intern. Med.,* 83, 330, 1975.
5. **Mossey, R. T., Kasabian, A., Wilkes, B., Mailloux, L., Susin, M., and Bluestone, P.,** Pulmonary embolism, low incidence in chronic renal failure, *Arch. Intern. Med.,* 142, 1646, 1982.
6. **Schafer, A.,** The hypercoagulatable state, *Ann. Int. Med.,* 102, 814, 1985.
7. **Hakim, R., Breillatt, J., Lazarus, J., and Port, F.,** Complement activation and hypersensitivity reactions to dialysis membranes, *N. Engl. J. Med.,* 311, 878, 1984.
8. **Michelson, E., Cohen, L., Dankner, R., and Kutezycki, A.,** Eosinophilia and pulmonary dysfunction during cuprophan hemodialysis, *Kidney Int.,* 24, 246, 1983.
9. **Fine, R. N.,** Treatment of end stage renal disease in children, *Pediatr. Ann.,* 10, 65, 1981.
10. Case records of the Massachusetts General Hospital, Case 13-1985, *N. Engl. J. Med.,* 312, 843, 1985.
11. **Ramsey, P., Rubin, R., Tolkoff-Rubin, N., Cosimi, A., Russell, R., and Grenne, R.,** The renal transplant patient with fever and pulmonary infiltrates, etiology, clinical manifestations and management, *Medicine,* 59, 206, 1980.
12. **Schaller, J. and Wedgewood, R.,** Rhuematic and connective tissue diseases of childhood, in *Nelson's Textbook of Pediatrics,* 12th ed., Behrman, R. and Vaughan, V., Eds., W. B. Saunders, Philadelphia, 1983.
13. **Penn, I.,** Tumor incidence in human allograft recipients, *Transplant Proc.,* 11, 1047, 1979.
14. **Cohen, D., Loertscher, R., Rubin, M., et al.,** Cyclosporine: a new immunosuppressive agent for organ transplantation, *Ann. Intern. Med.,* 101, 667, 1984.
15. **Schwartz, E., Teplick, J., Onesti, G., and Schwartz, A.,** Pulmonary hemorrhage in renal disease: Goodpasture's syndrome and other causes, *Radiology,* 122, 39, 1977.
16. **Robinson, T. and Rabinowitz, J.,** The nephrotic syndrome, *Radiol. Clin. North Am.,* 10, 494, 1972.
17. **Jacobs, C., Reach, I., and Degoulet, P.,** Cancer in patients on hemodialysis. Letter to editor, *N. Engl. J. Med.,* 300, 1279, 1979.
18. **Schatz, M., Patterson, R., and Fink, J.,** Immunologic lung disease, *N. Engl. J. Med.,* 300, 1310, 1979.
19. **Buffaloe, G. W., Evans, J. E., McIntosh, R. W., et al.,** Antibodies in human glomerular basement membrane: new methodology for detection in serum, *Clin. Exp. Immunol.,* 39, 316, 1979.
20. **Lockwood, C. M., Rees, A. J., Pearson, T. A., et al.,** Immunosuppression and plasma exchange in the treatment of Goodpasture's syndrome, *Lancet,* 1, 711, 1976.
21. **Neilson, E. G., Phillips, S. M., and Agus, A.,** Plasmapheresis in fulminating crescentric nephritis, *Lancet* 1, 264, 1980.

22. **Ognibene, A. J. and Johnson, D. E.,** Idiopathic pulmonary hemosiderosis in adults; report of case and review literature, *Arch. Int. Med.,* 111, 503, 1963.
23. **Fauci, A., Haynes, B., and Katz, P.,** The spectrum of vasculitis, *Ann. Intern. Med.,* 89, 660, 1978.
24. **Prakash, U.,** Respiratory manifestations of systemic disease. I. Rheumatologic and vascular diseases, *Postgrad. Med.,* 76, 119, 1984.
25. **Hensley, M. J., Feldman, N. T., Lazarus, J. M., and Galvanek, E. G.,** Diffuse pulmonary hemorrhage and rapidly progressive renal failure, *Am. J. Med.,* 66, 894, 1979.
26. **Glorioso, L. W. and Lang, E.,** Pulmonary manifestations of renal disease, *Radiol. Clin. North Am.,* 22, 647, 1984.
27. **Godin, M., Fillastre, J. P., Ducastelle, T., Hemet, J., Morere, P., and Nouvet, G.,** Sarcoidosis-retroperitoneal fibrosis, renal arterial involvement and unilateral focal glomerulosclerosis, *Arch. Intern. Med.,* 140, 1240, 1980.
28. Case records of the Massachusetts General Hospital, Case 16-1981, *N. Engl. J. Med.,* 304, 958, 1981.
29. **Balow, J. E., Austin, H. A., Muanz, L. R., et al.,** Effect of treatment on the evaluation of renal abnormalities in lupus nephritis, *N. Engl. J. Med.,* 311, 491, 1984.
30. **Singsen, B. and Platzker, A.,** Pulmonary involvement in the rheumatic disorders of childhood, in *Disorder of the Respiratory Tract in Children,* 4th ed., Kendigt, E. L. and Chernick, V., Eds., W. B. Saunders, Philadelphia, 1983.
31. **Donadio, J. V., Holley, K. E., Wagoner, R. D., et al.,** Treatment of lupus nephritis with prednisone and combined prednisone and azothioprine, *Ann. Intern. Med.,* 77, 829, 1972.
32. **Donadio, J. V., Holley, K. E., Ferguson, R. H., et al.,** Treatment of diffuse proliferative lupus nephritis with prednisone and combined prednisone and cyclophosphamide, *N. Engl. J. Med.,* 299, 1151, 1973.
33. **Felson, D. T. and Anderson, J.,** Evidence for the superiority of immunosuppressive drugs and prednisone over prednisone alone in lupus nephritis, *N. Engl. J. Med.,* 311, 1528, 1984.
34. **Dornfeld, L., Lacky, J. W., and Peter, J. B.,** Polyarteritis and intrarenal artery aneurysms, *JAMA,* 215, 1950, 1971.
35. **Goeke, D. J., Hsu, K., Morgan, C., et al.,** Vasculitis in association with Australia antigen, *J. Exp. Med.,* 134, 330, 1971.
36. **Frohnert, P. P., et al.,** Long-term follow-up study of periarteritis nodosa, *Am. J. Med.,* 43, 8, 1967.
37. **Rossman, R. D., Hersh, E. M., Sharp, J. T., et al.,** Effect of plasma exchange on circulating immune complexes and antibody formation in patients treated with cyclophosphamide and prednisone, *Am. J. Med.,* 63, 674, 1977.
38. Case records of the Massachusetts General Hospital, Case 16-1985, *N. Engl. J. Med.,* 312, 1042, 1985.
39. **Burke, E.,** Macroglobulinemia, cryoglobulinemia, and dysglobulinemia, in *Pediatric Kidney Disease,* Vol. II, Edelman, C., Ed., Little, Brown and Co., Boston, 1978.
40. **Trainin, E.,** Renal involvement in amyloidosis, in *Pediatric Kidney Disease,* Vol. II, Edelman, C., Ed., Little, Brown and Co., Boston, 1978.
41. Case records of the Massachusetts General Hospital, Case 35-1984, *N. Engl. J. Med.,* 311, 585, 1984.
42. **Hall, S., Miller, L., Duggan, E., Mauer, S., Beatty, E., and Hellerstein, S.,** Wegener granulomatosis in pediatric patients, *J. Pediatr.,* 106, 739, 1985.
43. **Hardie, I. R., et al.,** Skin cancer in Caucasian renal allograft recipients living in a subtropical climate, *Surgery,* 87, 177, 1980.
44. **Leatherman, J., Davies, S., and Hoidel, J.,** Alveolar hemorrhage syndromes: diffuse microvascular lung hemorrhage in immune and idiopathic disorders, *Medicine (Baltimore),* 63(6), 343, 1984.
45. **Lewis, E.,** Pulmonary hemorrhage and glomerulonephritis, in *Pediatric Kidney Disease,* Vol. II, Edelman, C., Ed., Little, Brown and Co., Boston, 1978.
46. **Rosenwasser, L. and Wolff, S.,** The vasculitides-A wide spectrum of disorders, *Drug Therapy (Hospital),* 7(10), 25, 1982.
47. **Schaller, J. and Wedgewood, R.,** Rheumatic and connective tissue disease of children, in *Nelson's Textbook of Pediatrics,* 12th ed., Behrman, R. and Vaughan, V., Eds., W. B. Saunders, Philadephia, 1983.
48. **Segal, A., Calabrese, L., Ahamd, M., Tubbs, R., and White, C.,** The pulmonary manifestations of systemic lupus erythematous, *Semin. Arthrit. Rheumatism,* 14(3), 202, 1985.

Chapter 40

INTERSTITIAL LUNG DISEASE IN CHILDHOOD RHEUMATIC DISORDERS

Bonnie Hepburn

TABLE OF CONTENTS

I. INTRODUCTION

Rheumatic diseases are characterized by chronic inflammation involving multiple tissue sites. Disabilities associated with these diseases are related to the inflammatory response itself, to the effects of tissue destruction and fibrosis, and to the disturbed function of the organs which are affected. The commonly involved organs in rheumatic disorders are the joints, skin, muscle, kidneys, and lungs. In the lungs, the disease may affect the pleura, pulmonary vasculature, airways, alveolar spaces, and supporting tissues. An inflammatory cellular infiltrate in the lungs may clear without residual, or may lead to fibrosis and chronic restrictive ventilatory defects with reduced lung volumes and reduced compliance. These features of interstitial lung disease occurring in the context of rheumatic disorders are thought to account for 1600 deaths per year or 25% of all deaths due to interstitial lung disease.[1] Children with rheumatic disease seem to be affected by chronic pulmonary disability less often than adults. This may be related to a shorter disease duration or fewer confounding factors such as an underlying pneumoconiosis or cigarette smoking. The difference may also stem from the fact that childhood rheumatic diseases are not necessarily identical to adult rheumatic diseases. Pulmonary involvement in children with rheumatic diseases is well recognized and has been the subject of numerous journal articles and an excellent review by Singsen and Platzker.[2]

The purpose of this article is to bring to the attention of the clinicians interested in interstitial lung disease, the experience with this entity in childhood rheumatic disorders. It is hoped that this will lead to earlier recognition of this complication and a better understanding of the disease process. The rheumatic disorders associated with interstitial lung disease are listed in Table 1.

II. SYSTEMIC LUPUS ERYTHEMATOSUS

A. Definition and Prevalence

Systemic lupus erythematosus (SLE) is a multisystem inflammatory disease associated with the presence of antinuclear antibodies. The prevalence of SLE in the general population is about one case in 2000. In black women aged 15 to 64 the prevalence is 1 case per 245 and for all women aged 15 to 64 the prevalence is 1 per 700.[3] In children, SLE may occur at any age, but the incidence is very low under the age of 5. During adolescence the incidence is nearly the same as that in adults.[4] Girls are five times more likely to be affected than boys.

B. Clinical Features of Pulmonary Disease

Joints, skin, kidneys, and the hemopoietic system are all commonly affected in adults and children. Some form of pulmonary disease, most often pleural inflammation, occurs in up to 60% of adults with SLE.[3] Pulmonary involvement in children is less common, affecting

Table 1
RHEUMATIC DISEASES OF CHILDHOOD ASSOCIATED WITH
INTERSTITIAL LUNG DISEASE

Systemic lupus erythematosus
Juvenile rheumatoid arthritis
Dermatomyositis and polymyositis
Scleroderma — progressive systemic sclerosis
Mixed connective tissue disease
Ankylosing spondylitis[a]
Sjögren's syndrome[a]
Behcet's syndrome[a]
Vasculitis

[a] Pulmonary complications have been described in adults but not in children.

about 19% of patients between the onset of SLE and the diagnosis, and 13% after diagnosis.[5] Pulmonary involvement may include pleural inflammation often with effusions, acute pneumonitis, and chronic interstitial lung disease. Pulmonary hypertension has been reported. Pulmonary hemorrhage occurred in 7 of 108 children followed by King et al.,[5] and was a major factor contributing to the death of 4 of these children. Pulmonary compromise of some sort contributes to a majority of SLE related deaths in children. At autopsy, the most common pathologic change is acute bronchopneumonia due to bacterial pathogens.[2]

Acute pneumonitis is characterized by the sudden appearance of pulmonary infiltrates and pleural effusions, and occurs in the setting of active lupus. It is often accompanied by fever, cough, chest pain, and tachypnea. Chronic interstitial lung disease, however, may occur with or without symptoms. The most common symptom is dyspnea on exertion. Physical findings associated with chronic interstitial disease may include poor diaphragmatic movement and basilar rales. Cyanosis and clubbing may occur. Radiographic findings include diffuse or localized infiltrates, plate-like atelectasis, unilateral elevation of the diaphragm, and small pleural effusions. When biopsied, early lesions may show inflammatory changes. Later lesions show thickening of alveolar walls with fibrous tissue, plasma cell infiltration of interstices, histiocyte desquamation, and necrosis of alveoli and bronchioles.[3,6]

When Huang and co-workers[7] studied pulmonary function in adult patients with SLE, diffusing capacity was abnormal in 89%, inspiratory capacity was decreased in 87%, forced vital capacity was abnormal in 79%, and total lung capacity was decreased in 61%. Pulmonary function abnormalities were present in almost two thirds of adult patients without current clinical or roentgenographic evidence of pulmonary disease.

Singsen and associates[2] performed pulmonary function tests in 20 children with SLE at a time when they had no clinical or radiographic evidence of disease. The mean age at testing was 15.5 years. Findings included an abnormal diffusing capacity in 25% and pulmonary restrictive defects in 35%. These results suggest less significant interstitial disease in children than in adults.

C. Management and Prognosis

Acute lupus pneumonitis should be treated with corticosteroids. In the child with rapid onset of fever, cough, and tachypnea, however, an infectious etiology must always be sought and appropriate broad spectrum antibiotics should be given, pending the availability of culture results. A general assessment of the lupus activity will help in making the diagnosis, as acute pneumonitis will be likely to occur with other clinical signs of active lupus such as arthralgia, rash, and other organ involvement together with increasing titers of antinuclear antibodies, anti-DNA antibodies, and falling levels of serum complement. When the dif-

Table 2
JRA SUBTYPES[8-10]

Subtype	% Total JRA population	Median age at onset (Years)[9]	Special characteristics
Systemic	15	4	Fever, rash, pleuritis, pericarditis
Pauciarticular, girls	36	2	Antinuclear antibodies, iridocyclitis
Pauciarticular, boys	16	10	B27 positivity
Polyarticular, RF[a] +	6	12	Girls $\gg$ boys, antinuclear antibodies
Polyarticular, RF −	27	2	Girls > boys

[a] RF = rheumatoid factor.

ferential diagnosis cannot be clearly made or if the child has failed to respond to the chosen course of therapy, it may be necessary to give both antibiotics and corticosteroids. The seriously ill child with pneumonitis should continuously be reassessed by a multi-disciplinary team until the problem is defined and brought under control.

Chronic interstitial lung disease in children is likely to progress with few signs or symptoms and may not be detected unless pulmonary function tests are performed. If the impairment is significant and progressive it may be necessary to determine whether the pulmonary dysfunction is caused by a continuing interstitial inflammation which may be steroid responsive or whether the lesion is essentially fibrotic and nonresponsive to steroid. While a lung biopsy may provide the only definitive information, a short trial of corticosteroid therapy after base line pulmonary function testing, may provide the same information without an invasive procedure. If the lung lesion is steroid responsive, improved volumes, and diffusing capacity may be seen after just a few days of corticosteroid therapy. Use of corticosteroids must always be accompanied by recognition of the growth impairment and other serious side effects of long-term therapy.

III. JUVENILE RHEUMATOID ARTHRITIS

A. Definition and Prevalence

Juvenile rheumatoid arthritis (JRA) also known as juvenile arthritis or juvenile chronic polyarthritis is the most common childhood rheumatic disorder. Approximately 11 of 100,000 children are affected each year and the prevalence of the disease, active and inactive, is slightly more than 100 per 100,000 children under age 16.[8] There are several subtypes of this disease which vary considerably one from the other with respect to serologic abnormalities, age and sex of the children affected, the pattern and severity of joint involvement, and the extra articular manifestations of disease (Table 2).

B. Clinical Features of Pulmonary Disease

Lung involvement of any type is extremely rare in children with juvenile rheumatoid arthritis and is mainly to be found in the group with systemic disease, a subset which comprises only about 15% of JRA. In a series of 191 children with juvenile rheumatoid arthritis reported by Athreya and associates,[11] 8 children had pulmonary involvement. Six patients had evidence of interstitial lung disease. Four of these children had accompanying pericardial and pleural effusions. Four had systemic disease. Typical of the children with systemic involvement is the 4-year-old boy whose serial chest radiographs are shown in Figure 1. This child developed a fever, chest pain, pulmonary infiltrates, pleural effusion,

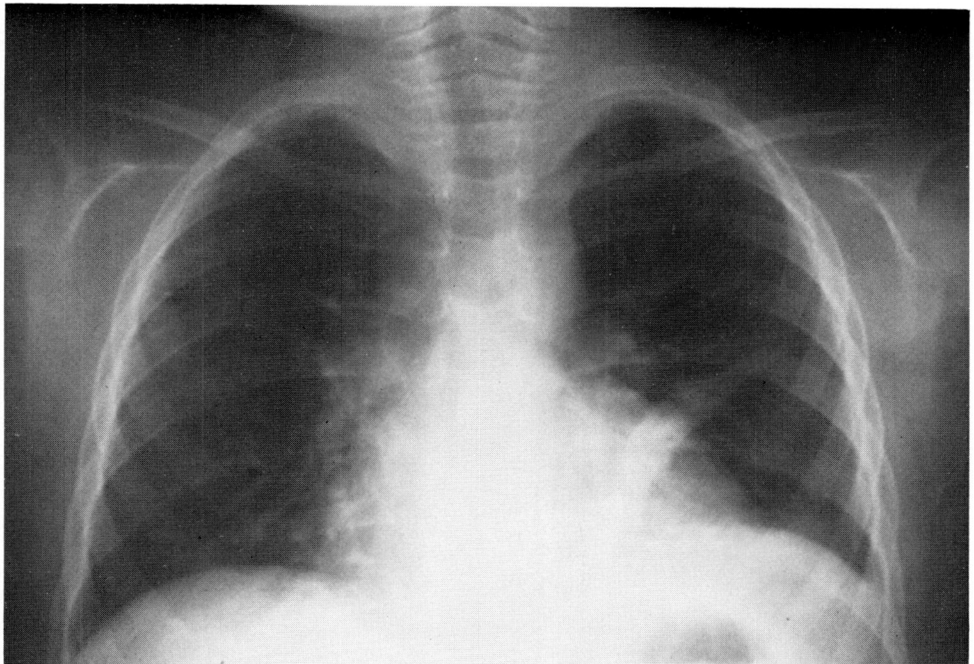

A

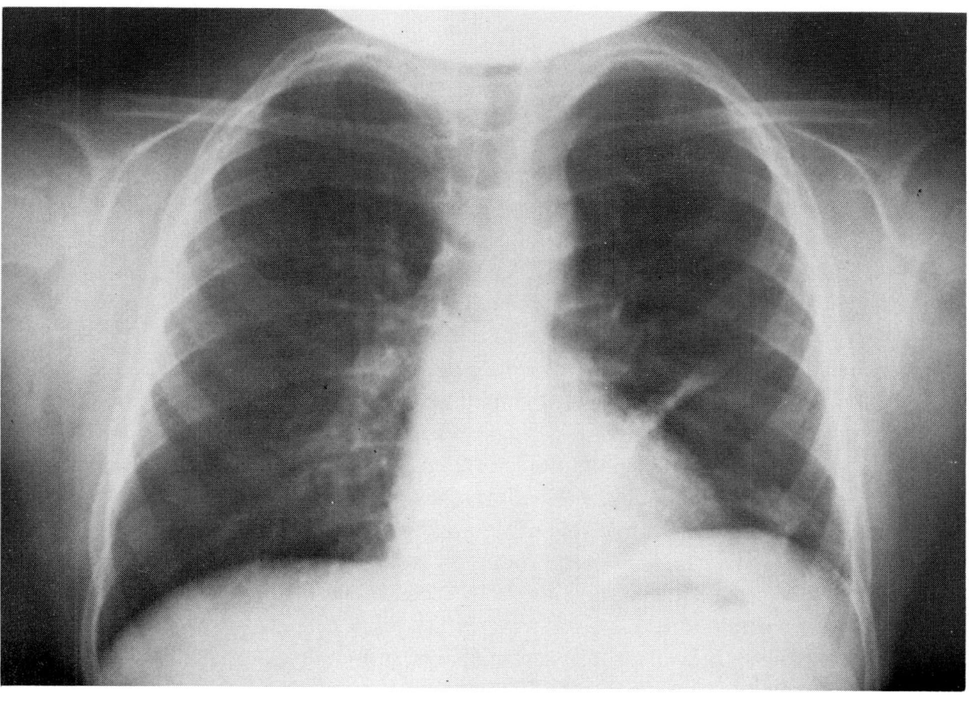

B

FIGURE 1.   Serial radiographs of a 4-year-old boy with systemic juvenile rheumatoid arthritis. (A) Pericardial effusion and pulmonary infiltrate 2 months after initiation of corticosteroid therapy, 7/77[11] (Figure 1A reprinted with permission from W. B. Saunders Co.) (B) Persistence of infiltrate, 9/77. (C) Resolution of infiltrate and all clinical symptoms of disease, 3/78.

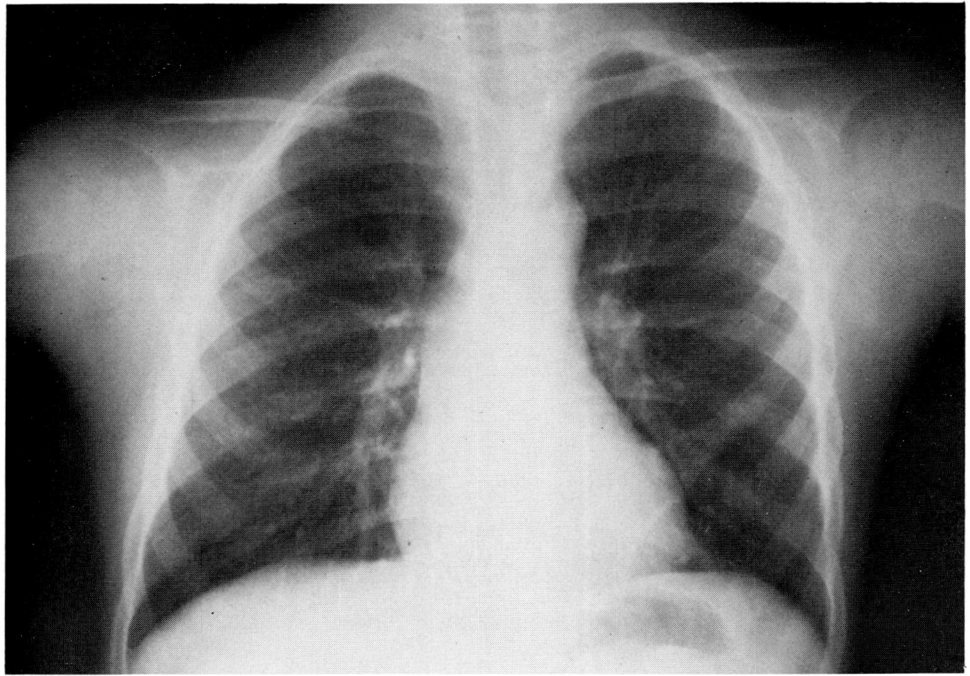

FIGURE 1C

and pericardial effusion during a systemic flare of disease which occurred 20 months after the onset of his arthritis. Tests for rheumatoid factor and antinuclear antibodies were negative. The effusions cleared gradually after initiation of corticosteroid therapy (prednisone 40 mg daily) but infiltrates persisted for at least 4 months. The child was seen in consultation by Athreya during this time and is included in his series of children with JRA and pulmonary disease.[11] One year later the child was well, without clinical evidence of lung disease (Figure 1C). There has been no recurrence of lung or joint disease since, and there has been no need for further corticosteroid. The three children in Athreya's series who had a positive test for rheumatoid factor, however, (one each with systemic, polyarticular, and pauciarticular onset) all had persistent interstitial lung disease with abnormal radiographs after 3 years.

Occasionally scoliosis and chest wall deformities in patients with JRA have led to severe restrictive lung disease. Pulmonary arteritis, pulmonary amyloidosis, and hemosiderosis have also been reported.[2]

Using pulmonary function testing to diagnose unsuspected pulmonary disease in children with JRA, Wagener et al.[12] found abnormalities in two thirds of the patients with polyarticular disease and one half of the children with pauciarticular disease. All of these children were between 6 and 18 years of age. Abnormalities included decreased air flow, decreased lung volume, decreased gas diffusion, and abnormal matching of ventilation to perfusion during exercise. Abnormal diffusing capacity was seen in 45% (7/16) of these patients. Results were compatible with diffuse vascular or parenchymal lung disease. None of these patients had pleural effusions. Lung disease had been previously diagnosed in only one child, and one additional patient had symptoms referrable to the respiratory tract. One child had an abnormal radiograph showing an undiagnosed pulmonary nodule.

In adults, whose arthritis is similar to the polyarticular JRA subtype, chronic interstitial lung disease is common and often is symptomatic. Chest radiographs and measurement of diffusing capacity have revealed abnormalities in 30 to 40% of patients.[2] Decreases in diffusing capacity have been associated with advanced disease.[13] Biopsies have shown interstitial fibrosis.

C. Management and Prognosis

In treating adults with rheumatoid lung disease, an attempt is usually made to reduce the overall activity of the disease by employing remissive or slow acting agents such as gold, penicillamine, or methotrexate. One must be aware, however, that interstitial lung disease is a complication of each of these agents.[14,15] Since these drugs are also used in the treatment of juvenile polyarticular arthritis, they should be considered as a possible cause of interstitial lung disease occurring in this population (see Chapter 31).

Treatment of pulmonary disease related to JRA is generally limited to those patients with active inflammation characterized by fever and pleuritis. The acute process responds well to corticosteroids which should be tapered and replaced by nonsteroidal anti-inflammatory drugs as soon as the disease is under adequate control.

IV. DERMATOMYOSITIS

A. Definition and Incidence

Dermatomyositis (DM) is a chronic inflammatory myopathy which leads to proximal muscle weakness. The myopathy is accompanied by an erythematous rash which occurs primarily on the face and extremities. When not accompanied by rash, the disease is referred to as polymyositis (PM). The incidence of DM-PM in the general population is 5 to 10 cases per million people per year. There is a bimodal distribution to the incidence, with peaks in childhood and in adults over age 45.[16] The mean age of onset in childhood is 6 years.[4] Juvenile DM-PM, unlike the adult form of the disease, is characterized by a diffuse angiopathy which affects the small blood vessels leading to infarction of the gastrointestinal tract, heart, and lungs.

B. Clinical Features of Pulmonary Disease

Pulmonary complications of DM-PM occur in adults and in children. Pulmonary involvement in adults is of three types. Thoracic muscle weakness may lead to hypoventilation and hypostatic pneumonia; esophageal dysmotility may lead to aspiration pneumonia; and parenchymal inflammation may lead to fibrosis.[17] The interstitial pulmonary disease may have an acute or insidious onset and may precede or follow evidence of myopathy. Bibasilar rales are the most common clinical finding. Clubbing is not usually seen. Restrictive defects and diminished diffusing capacity are the most common pulmonary function abnormalities. Increasing interstitial markings may be seen on serial chest radiographs. Of 213 Mayo Clinic patients (adults) with DM-PM reviewed by Frazier and Miller,[18] 5% had radiographic evidence of parenchymal pulmonary disease. Biopsies were performed on 5 of the 10 patients. All showed interstitial pneumonitis and fibrosis.

In a series of 19 children with DM reported by Sullivan and associates,[19] 3 children had dyspnea associated with intercostal muscle weakness. None of these children had evidence of interstitial lung disease. In reviewing the literature, Singsen[2] found just four reported cases of pulmonary fibrosis in childhood dermatomyositis. Two of these patients and a third child with DM but no evidence of pulmonary fibrosis, all developed spontaneous pneumothoraces. Although it has been suggested that the pneumothoraces may be related to the vasculitis of childhood DM, lung biopsies of two children who experienced pneumothoraces showed chronic pneumonitis and fibrosis but no obliterative vascular lesions.[20,21] The increased incidence of pneumothorax in childhood DM, in scleroderma, and in systemic lupus erythematosus may all be related to the interstitial fibrosis seen in these diseases. It is presumed that the pneumothorax results from rupture of subpleural cysts formed by degeneration of alveolar walls.

C. Management and Prognosis

In children and adults with dermatomyositis, the response to corticosteroid therapy is variable. Because steroid therapy may result in a favorable outcome of the pulmonary disease, a trial of therapy is certainly warranted, especially if the pulmonary disease is acute. Azathioprine and methotrexate are effective in treating the muscular inflammation of DM, but there is little experience in using these drugs to treat the pulmonary complications.

V. SCLERODERMA

A. Definition and Incidence

Scleroderma is a rheumatic disease which occurs both in adults and children in systemic and localized forms. Morphea and linear scleroderma are localized forms of disease. It is the generalized disease, progressive systemic sclerosis (PSS), which is associated with severe pulmonary involvement. PSS is characterized by the appearance of Raynaud's phenomenon, skin thickening and tightness, articular disability and involvement of heart, intestines, kidneys and lungs. Singsen et al.,[2] following at least 13 children with PSS, found no significant differences between childhood and adult PSS. The incidence of PSS in the general population is approximately five cases per million people per year.[22] In children, onset has been noted as early as 3 years. The female to male ratio is 6:1.[4]

B. Clinical Features of Pulmonary Disease

The interstitial lung involvement may be the most disabling aspect of the generalized disease. Exertional dyspnea, the most common symptom, may be mild and associated with chronic stable disease; it may be slowly progressive; or it may be extreme and associated with a fulminant disease course. Cough is not common and clubbing is infrequently seen. Basilar rales are a frequent auscultatory finding.

Radiographic abnormalities in the lung may include linear or nodular densities in the lower lung fields, diffuse fibrosis or pleural thickening. Spontaneous pneumothorax, which is an occasional complication, is thought to be due to rupture of subpleural cysts. The most common histologic change found in adult lungs at autopsy is interstitial fibrosis (74%).[23] Vascular lesions are also frequent and may include intimal proliferation and medial hypertrophy of small arteries and arterioles.[23] These lesions may be seen with or without evidence of pulmonary hypertension. Young and Mark[24] noted in an autopsy series that pulmonary fibrosis and pulmonary vascular disease did not correlate well.

Abnormalities of pulmonary function tests may be found early in the disease, sometimes before symptoms of dyspnea or radiographic evidence of disease. Schneider et al.[25] found decreased vital capacity and decreased diffusing capacity with approximately equal frequency when reviewing baseline studies of patients with scleroderma. In 5 years of follow-up there was further loss of forced vital capacity but no difference in diffusing capacity. Other investigators have found a gradual deterioration of diffusing capacity over time.[26]

C. Management and Prognosis

Steen and associates[26] followed 44 patients with PSS treated with a mean dose of 636 mg of D-penicillamine for 2.3 years. They compared these patients with 48 untreated patients who had repeat pulmonary function tests. There was a mean of 3.5 years between sets of pulmonary function tests in the treated group and 4.8 years in the untreated group. There were no significant changes in the vital capacity or forced expiratory volumes in either group but there was a small change in diffusing capacity in penicillamine treated patients, from 76 to 87% of the predicted value. Diffusing capacity in untreated patients changed from 73 to 76% of the predicted value. The improvement in treated patients was associated with no further progression of dyspnea or of fibrosis on chest radiograph. The authors concluded that D-penicillamine might be useful in treatment of PSS involving the lung. Other agents including corticosteroids and immunosuppressive drugs have not been shown to alter the pulmonary outcome although corticosteroids occasionally appear to be of short term benefit when there is evidence of inflammatory disease.

VI. MIXED CONNECTIVE TISSUE DISEASE

A. Definition and Prevalence

Mixed connective tissue disease (MCTD) is an overlap syndrome characterized clinically by features of systemic lupus erythematosus, dermatomyositis, rheumatoid arthritis, and scleroderma. Serologically it is characterized by high titers of antibody to ribonucleic protein. Since it was first described by Sharp et al.[27] in 1972, the disease has been well characterized clinically and there have been numerous reports of children with MCTD. The prevalence of the disease is unknown but it is considerably less common than systemic lupus erythematosus. From 1973 to 1977, 81 adult patients with MCTD were seen at the Mayo Clinic.[28] The mean age of onset was 34 years (range 19 to 67 years). This same report mentions four additional patients seen during this time whose onset occurred prior to age 16. Singsen and associates[29] reported clinical and serologic characteristics of 14 children with MCTD whose disease onset occurred between ages 4 and 16 (median 6 years). Childhood MCTD is similar to MCTD seen in adults.

B. Clinical Features of Pulmonary Disease

In their retrospective study of adult MCTD patients seen at the Mayo Clinic, Prakash and associates[28] found pleuropulmonary involvement in 20 patients (25%). Chest radiographs revealed basilar interstitial processes in 19% and pleural effusions in 5%. The most common symptom was dyspnea (16%). A restrictive pattern was observed in 9 of 13 patients (69%) who had pulmonary function testing. Static lung volumes were reduced and diffusing capacity ranged from 20 to 66% of normal. In a prospective study of adult MCTD patients, with a mean follow-up of 6.3 years, Sullivan et al.[30] found that 85% of patients developed pulmonary disease. Again dyspnea was the most common symptom (58%). Of 11 patients who were asymptomatic, 8 had abnormal pulmonary function testing or chest radiographs or both. The most common abnormality noted on pulmonary function testing was decreased diffusing capacity. The most frequent serious clinical problem in this series was pulmonary disease with the development of pulmonary hypertension associated with proliferative vascular lesions in the lungs and other organs. Pulmonary hypertension contributed to 3 of 4 deaths reported. Of the 14 children with MCTD followed by Singsen et al.,[29] 43% had pulmonary disease. Pulmonary hypertension was a complication in two children and two children had pleural effusions. Pulmonary function testing revealed restrictive lung disease in two children. An additional two children with dyspnea had decreased diffusing capacity. Other studies suggest that testing of asymptomatic patients will reveal a higher incidence of pulmonary disease in this population.[30]

C. Management and Prognosis

The recurrent pneumonitis, pleuritis, and pleural effusions of MCTD which resemble clinical features of systemic lupus erythematosus, usually respond quickly to treatment with corticosteroids. Abnormalities in diffusing capacity may improve after steroid therapy. The progressive pulmonary fibrosis and obliterative vascular lesions associated with pulmonary hypertension, however, are similar in MCTD and scleroderma, and are generally refractory to therapy of any kind. Cytotoxic therapy has been used and may improve the outcome of severe pulmonary manifestations of MCTD.[31]

VII. ANKYLOSING SPONDYLITIS

A. Definition and Prevalence

Ankylosing spondylitis (AS) is the prototype of the seronegative spondyloarthropathies associated with the presence of the HLA-B27 antigen. The prevalence of the disease varies according to the ethnic background of the population, with a prevalence of about 1% in whites and less in blacks.[32] The onset of frequently occurs below age 16 when the disease may be considered a subset of juvenile arthritis. Juvenile ankylosing spondylitis occurs most frequently in boys and may be suspected when an oligoarthritis involves primarily large joints in the lower extremities. Sacroiliac joints are often tender early in the course of disease but radiographic evidence of sacroiliac and spine involvement may not be present until later in the disease, if at all.

B. Clinical Features of Pulmonary Disease

Pulmonary manifestations of AS include chest wall restriction secondary to inflammation and fusion of the thoracic spine and costovertebral joints; apical pleural thickening; and interstitial apical infiltrates which may lead to extensive fibrosis and later to formation of cavities or bullae. Cavities may become secondarily infected with various species of Aspergillus, mycobacteria, and other organisms. Cor pulmonale has been reported as a complication of adult AS.[33]

Perhaps because the pulmonary abnormalities in AS are associated with chronicity of disease, they have not been documented in children. Rosenow and associates,[33] reviewing records of 2080 patients with AS seen at the Mayo Clinic, found pleuropulmonary disease occurring 2 to 38 years (average 21 years) after the onset of AS. Of 26 AS patients with lung disease who were asked, 20 were cigarette smokers.

The fibrobullous lung disease of AS is usually asymptomatic unless secondary infection is present. Abnormalities are usually detected on chest roentgenograms. The fibrous lesions appear as interstitial markings in one or both upper lobes. Bullae became apparent as fibrous tissue breaks down. In patients with normal appearing lung parenchyma on chest roentgenograms, pulmonary function tests have revealed only the restrictive defects associated with low lung volumes. Diffusing capacity has not been significantly reduced.[34]

If not complicated by secondary infection the interstitial lung disease of AS requires no particular treatment. With time the disease may progress with increasing fibrosis, enlarging bullae and the appearance of upper lobe bronchiectasis, or the disease may remain stable for many years.

VIII. SJÖGREN'S SYNDROME

A. Definition and Prevalence

Sjögren's syndrome (SS) is an autoimmune disorder characterized by lymphocyte mediated destruction of the exocrine glands. Decreased secretions and mucosal dryness result. Involvement of the lacrimal and salivary glands leads to the well recognized syndrome of keratoconjunctivitis sicca and xerostomia. Exocrine glands in the gastrointestinal tract, skin, vagina, and respiratory tract may also be affected. The disease may occur alone (primary) or with another autoimmune rheumatic disease (secondary). The true prevalence of the disease is difficult to ascertain but it is more common in adults than any other autoimmune rheumatic disease except rheumatoid arthritis. Women are more commonly affected than men.[35] The disease is known to occur in children. Athreya and associates[36] have described in detail two young girls with SS and SLE. They also reviewed several reported series of patients with SS including other children with SS and SLE, and SS with RA. There were no pulmonary abnormalities described in these children.

B. Clinical Features of Pulmonary Disease

In adults with SS, pulmonary complications are well recognized. In a review of 343 patients with SS at the Mayo Clinic, Strimlan et al.[37] found evidence of pulmonary involvement in 31 (9%). Pulmonary abnormalities included interstitial lung disease, pleural disease, bronchopneumonia, and lymphoma. The most common respiratory symptoms were cough (23 patients) and dyspnea (16 patients). Five patients had no symptoms when an abnormality was first noted on the chest roentgenogram. A diagnosis of SS preceded the onset of respiratory symptoms in all but two patients. The most common radiographic abnormalities included diffuse interstitial infiltrations (16 patients) and reticular or reticulonodular lesions (16 patients). Less commonly seen radiographic features included pleural effusions, coarse nodular lesions, basilar atelectasis, and hilar enlargement. Pulmonary function testing in 18 of these patients showed a restrictive ventilatory pattern or low diffusing capacity or both.

Histologic information was available for 13 patients in Strimlan's series. Lymphocytic interstitial pneumonitis was seen in three patients, two of whom had associated amyloidosis. One patient had a pathologic diagnosis of pseudolymphoma and three patients had malignant lymphoma. Four patients had bronchopneumonia. There was no predominant pathogen.In two patients who were biopsied, and in 11 who were not, the pulmonary diagnosis was diffuse interstitial fibrosis.

C. Management and Prognosis

Respiratory symptoms and pulmonary radiographic abnormalities of SS may regress following treatment with corticosteroids, if treatment is begun early in the course of disease. Failure to respond to therapy suggests the presence of fibrosis or a more advanced lesion. Pseudolymphoma, characterized by infiltrates of mature lymphocytes with true germinal centers, but without histologic criteria for malignancy, may also respond to therapy with corticosteroids or immunosuppressive agents. In other cases pseudolymphoma may progress to malignant lymphoma. A marked decrease in previously elevated IgM level may herald the development of a malignancy.[38]

IX. BEHCET'S DISEASE

A. Definition and Prevalence

Behcet's disease (BD) is characterized by the triad of oral ulcerations, genital ulcerations, and uveitis. These features of disease occur in more than 50% of patients affected. Synovitis and meningoencephalitis occur in 40 and 30% of patients respectively. Serologic markers characteristic of many of the autoimmune rheumatic disorders are missing from this syndrome but immune complexes are found in the sera of 50 to 60% of patients.[39] The prevalence of the disease varies considerably according to the geographic area. In Olmsted County, Minnesota the prevalence is just 1 in 25,000, but it is much more common in eastern Mediterranean countries and in Japan where the prevalence is 1 in 1000.[39] Oshima and associates[40] have reported a series of 85 patients seen at the University of Tokyo, and Chajek and Fainaru[41] have reported a series of 41 patients seen at Hadassah University in Jerusalem. The onset of disease in these series was most often in the third decade but there is an onset before 20 years of age in about 15% of patients. The youngest patient seen was 10 years old at the onset of his disease.[40]

B. Clinical Features of Pulmonary Disease

Pulmonary complications of BD are rare. Cadman et al.[42] have reported a case of hemoptysis and have reviewed 12 patients with BD and pulmonary abnormalities described elsewhere. There have been no reports of children with lung disease. Pulmonary complications in adults have included vasculitis; aneurysms of the pulmonary arterial tree diagnosed by pulmonary arteriography; and pulmonary emboli related to peripheral thrombophlebitis. The vascular problems are not localized to the lung and pulmonary complications generally occur together with active disease elsewhere. Many patients with lung involvement also have thrombosis of the superior vena cava. The hemoptysis associated with the pulmonary lesions may be life threatening. The most common radiographic abnormality in the chest is diffuse infiltration.

C. Management and Prognosis

Treatment of BD has variable and often unsuccessful results. For the severely ill patient, a combination of corticosteroids and chlorambucil may offer the best chance of recovery.[39]

X. VASCULITIS

Polyarteritis nodosa, Wegener's granulomatosis, and Churg-Strauss syndrome, are the primary vasculitides associated with interstitial lung disease. Although rare, juvenile onset of each of these disease entities has been reported.

A. Polyarteritis Nodosa

Polyarteritis nodosa (PAN) in childhood is rare. Infantile polyarteritis resembles Kawaski's disease, but the more common form of disease resembling adult PAN occurs mainly in preadolescent and adolescent children. The most frequently involved organs are kidneys, heart, and liver. Fever, rash, and abdominal pain are common. Pulmonary involvement is rare but reported.[43-45] The pulmonary infiltrates as well as other signs and symptoms of the disease respond to treatment. Corticosteroids and immunosuppressive agents, especially cyclophosphamide have reduced the mortality of this disease.

B. Wegener's Granulomatosis

Wegener's granulomatosis (WG) is a necrotizing granulomatous vasculitis involving upper and lower respiratory tract and kidneys. The disease is particularly rare in children with only 18 reported cases in patients younger than 16 years of age.[2] Clinical signs of fever, cough, chest pain or hemoptysis may be the first evidence of disease. Nodular densities or infiltrates may appear on chest roentgenograms prior to pulmonary symptoms. Pulmonary lesions may progress and cavitate or may be transient. Temporary improvement may be seen with corticosteroid treatment but it is cyclophosphamide which has dramatically improved the outcome of this disease.[46]

C. Churg-Strauss Syndrome

Churg-Strauss syndrome (CSS) is a disorder characterized by eosinophilia, vasculitis, asthma, and allergic rhinitis. Migratory arthralgia or arthritis occur in a majority of patients. Some patients with this syndrome have been reported to have polyarteritis nodosa, or Loeffler syndrome. In a literature review of 138 cases of CSS the mean age of onset was found to be 28 years for rhinitis and 35 years for asthma.[47] Onset of symptoms can occur in childhood.

Pulmonary infiltrates were found in 72% of the patients with CSS reviewed by Lanham et al.[47] In the early or prodromal stage of disease there is extensive eosinophilic infiltration of alveoli and interstitium. In the later vasculitic stage, necrotizing vasculitis and granulomas are seen. Infiltrates are generally transient and patchy without predilection for any one region. Widespread infiltrates may indicate pulmonary hemorrhage. In contrast to Wegener's granulomatosis, cavitation of pulmonary lesions is rare. Pleural effusions have been found in 29% of cases and contain large numbers of eosinophils.

CSS responds well to treatment with corticosteroids. Response is quick and dramatic. Treatment of the vasculitis usually requires several weeks of high doses of prednisone but remissions generally occur without the use of immunosuppressive agents.[47] Immunosuppressive agents may be helpful in treating refractory cases.

XI. SUMMARY

There is considerable overlap with regard to the clinical, roentgenologic, and histologic features of interstitial lung involvement in the varying rheumatic diseases. Hunninghake and Fauci[48] have compared the lung injury which occurs in the rheumatic diseases to that of acute and chronic glomerulonephritis associated with immune complex deposition. The effect of antigen-antibody complexes on the lung has been less clear because lung biopsies are rarely performed early in these diseases and histologic data have not been available. It seems likely, however, that the mechanisms by which immune complexes damage the lung are the familiar ones involving complement activation, release of chemotactic factors, inflammatory cell infiltrates, and cell mediated tissue destruction. The acute processes are often responsive to corticosteroid or immunosuppressive therapy; the more indolent chronic fibrotic changes are often refractory. In early childhood, if only because of the shorter disease course, the pulmonary disease is often responsive to therapy and the outlook is favorable.

REFERENCES

1. **Eisenberg, H.,** The insterstitial lung diseases associated with the collagen-vascular disorders, *Clin. Chest Med.,* 3, 565, 1982.
2. **Singsen, B. H. and Platzker, A. C. G.,** Pulmonary involvement in the rheumatic disorders of childhood, in *Disorders of the Respiratory Tract,* W. B. Saunders, Philadelphia, 1983, chap. 67.
3. **Rothfield, N.,** Clinical features of systemic lupus erythematosus, in *Textbook of Rheumatology,* 2nd ed., Kelley, W. N., Harris, E. D., Jr., Ruddy, S., and Sledge, C. B., Eds., W. B. Saunders, Philadelphia, 1985, chap. 69.
4. **Hanson, V.,** Systemic lupus erythematosus, dermatomyositis, scleroderma, and vasculitis in childhood, in *Textbook of Rheumatology,* 2nd ed., Kelley, W. N., Harris, E. D., Jr., Ruddy, S., and Sledge, C. B., Eds., W. B. Saunders, Philadelphia, 1985, chap. 82.
5. **King, K. K., Kornreich, H. K., Bernstein, B. H., Singsen, B. H., and Hanson, V.,** The clinical spectrum of systemic lupus erythematosus in childhood, *Arthritis Rheumatism,* 20, 287, 1977.
6. **Haupt, H. M., Moore, G. W., and Hutchins, G. M.,** The lung in systemic lupus erythematosus, *Am. J. Med.,* 71, 791, 1981.
7. **Huang, C. T., Hennigar, G. R., and Lyons, H. A.,** Pulmonary dysfunction in systemic lupus erythematosus, *N. Engl. J. Med.,* 272, 288, 1965.
8. **Towner, S. R., Michet, C. J., Jr., O'Fallon, W. M., and Nelson, A. M.,** The epidemiology of juvenile arthritis in Rochester, Minnesota, 1960-1977, *Arthritis Rheumatism,* 26, 1208, 1983.
9. **Schaller, J. G., Ochs, H. D., Thomas, E. D., Nisperos, B., Feigl, P., and Wedgwood, R. J.,** Histocompatibility antigens in childhood-onset arthritis, *J. Pediatr.,* 88, 926, 1976.
10. **Moore, T. L, Osborne, T. G., Weiss, T. D., Sheridan, P. W., Eisenwinter, R. K., Miller, A. V., Dorner, R. W., and Zuckner, J.,** Autoantibodies in juvenile arthritis, *Sem. Arthritis Rheumatism,* 13, 329, 1984.
11. **Athreya, B. H., Doughty, R. A., Bookspan, M., Schumacher, H. R., Sewell, E. M., and Chatten, J.,** Pulmonary manifestations of juvenile rheumatoid arthritis: a report of eight cases and review, *Clin. Chest Med.,* 1, 361, 1980.
12. **Wagener, J. S., Taussey, L. M., De Benedetti, C., Lemen, R. J., and Loughlin, G. M.,** Pulmonary function in juvenile rheumatoid arthritis, *J. Pediatr.,* 99, 108, 1981.
13. **Laitinen, O., Salorinne, Y., and Poppius, H.,** Respiratory function in systemic erythematosus, scleroderma, and rheumatoid arthritis, *Ann. Rheumatic Dis.,* 32, 531, 1973.
14. **Scott, D. L., Bradby, G. V. H., Aitman, T. J., Zaphiropoulos, G. C., and Hawkins, C. F.,** Relationship of gold and penicillamine therapy to diffuse interstitial lung disease, *Ann. Rheumatic Dis.,* 40, 136, 1981.
15. **Cannon, G. W., Ward, J. R., Clegg, D. O., Samuelson, C. O., Jr., and Abbott, T. M.,** Acute lung disease associated with low-dose pulse methotrexate therapy in patients with rheumatoid arthritis, *Arthritis Rheumatism,* 26, 1269, 1983.

16. **Medsger, T. A., Jr., Dawson, W. N., and Masi, A. T.,** The epidemiology of polymyositis, *Am. J. Med.,* 48, 715, 1970.

17. **Hepper, N. G., Ferguson, R. H., and Howard, F. M., Jr.,** Three types of pulmonary involvement in polymyositis, *Med. Clin. North Am.,* 48, 1031, 1964.

18. **Frazier, A. R. and Miller, R. D.,** Interstitial pneumonitis in assocation with polymyositis and dermatomyositis, *Chest,* 65, 403, 1974.

19. **Sullivan, D. B., Cassidy, J. T., Petty, P. E., and Burt, A.,** Prognosis in childhood dermatomyositis, *J. Pediatr.,* 80, 555, 1972.

20. **Park, S. and Nyhan, W. I.,** Fatal pulmonary involvement in dermatomyositis, *Am. J. Dis. Child.,* 129, 723, 1975.

21. **Singsen, B. H., Tedford, J. C., Platzker, A. C. G., and Hanson, V.,** Spontaneous pneumothorax: a complication of juvenile dermatomyositis, *J. Pedatr.,* 92, 771, 1978.

22. **Stallones, R. A.,** The epidemiology of systemic sclerosis, in *Epidemology of Rheumatic Diseases,* Lawrence, R. C. and Shulman, L. E., Eds., Gower Medical Publishing Ltd., New York, 1984, chap. 23.

23. **D'Angelo, W. A., Fries, J. F., Masi, A. T., and Shulman, L. E.,** Pathologic observations in systemic sclerosis (scleroderma): a study of fifty-eight autopsy cases and fifty-eight matched controls, *Am. J. Med.,* 46, 428, 1969.

24. **Young, R. H. and Mark, G. J.,** Pulmonary vascular changes in scleroderma, *Am. J. Med.,* 64, 998, 1978.

25. **Schneider, P. D., Wise, R. A., Hochberg, M. C., and Wigley, F. M.,** Serial pulmonary function in systemic sclerosis, *Am. J. Med.,* 73, 385, 1982.

26. **Steen, V. D., Owens, G. R., Redmond, C., Rodnan, G. R., and Medsger, T. A., Jr.,** The effect of D-penicillamine on pulmonary findings in systemic sclerosis, *Arthritis Rheumatism,* 28, 882, 1985.

27. **Sharp, G. C., Irvin, W. S., Tan, E. M., Gould, R. G., and Holman, H. R.,** Mixed connective tissue disease — an apparently distinct rheumatic disease syndrome associated with a specific antibody to an extractable nuclear antigen (ENA), *Am. J. Med.,* 52, 148, 1972.

28. **Prakash, U. B. S., Luthra, H. S., and Divertie, M. B.,** Intrathoracic manifestations in mixed connective tissue disease, *Mayo Clin. Proc.,* 60, 813, 1985.

29. **Singsen, B. H., Bernstein, B. H., Kornreich, H. K., King, K. K., Hanson, V., and Tan, E. M.,** Mixed connective tissue disease in childhood. A clinical and serologic survey, *J. Pediatr.,* 90, 893, 1977.

30. **Sullivan, W. D., Hurst, D. J., Harmon, C. E., Esther, J. H., Agia, G. A., Maltby, J. D., Lillard, S. B., Held, C. N., Wolfe, F., Sunderrajan, E. V., Maricq, H. R., and Sharp, G. C.,** A prospective evaluation emphasizing pulmonary involvement in patients with mixed connective tissue disease, *Medicine,* 63, 92, 1984.

31. **Wiener-Kronish, J. P., Solinger, A. M., Warnock, M. L., Churg, A., Ordonez, N., and Golden, J. A.,** Severe pulmonary involvement in mixed connective tissue disease, *Am. Rev. Respir. Dis.,* 124, 499, 1981.

32. **Calin, A.,** Spondyloarthropathies, in *Textbook of Rheumatology,* 2nd ed., Kelley, W. N., Harris, E. D., Jr., Ruddy, S., and Sledge, C. B., Eds., W. B. Saunders, Philadelphia, 1985, chap. 64.

33. **Rosenow, E. C., III, Strimlan, C. V., Muhm, J. R., and Ferguson, R. H.,** Pleuropulmonary manifestations of ankylosing spondylitis, *Mayo Clin. Proc.,* 52, 641, 1977.

34. **Citrin, D. L., Boyd, G., and Bradley, G. W.,** Ventilatory function and transfer factor in ankylosing spondylitis, *Scot. Med. J.,* 18, 109, 1973.

35. **Moutsopoulos, H. M., Chused, T. M., Mann, D. L., Klippel, J. H., Fauci, A. S., Frank, M. M., Lawley, T. J., and Hamburger, M. I.,** Sjögren's syndrome (sicca syndrome): current issues, *Ann. Intern. Med.,* 92, 212, 1980.

36. **Athreya, B. H., Norman, M. E., Myers, A. R., and South, M. A.,** Sjögren's syndrome in children, *Pediatrics,* 59, 931, 1977.

37. **Strimlan, C. V., Rosenow, E. C., III, Divertie, M. C., and Harrison, E. G., Jr.,** Pulmonary manifestations of Sjögren's syndrome, *Chest,* 70, 354, 1976.

38. **Anderson, L. G. and Talal, N.,** The spectrum of benign to malignant lymphoproliferation in Sjögren's syndrome, *Clin. Experimen. Immunol.,* 9, 199, 1971.

39. **O'Duffy, J. D.,** Behcet's disease, in *Textbook of Rheumatology,* 2nd ed., Kelley, W. N., Harris, E. D., Jr., Ruddy, S., and Sledge, C. B., Eds., W. B. Saunders, Philadelphia, 1985, chap. 74.

40. **Oshima, Y., Shimizu, T., Yokohari, R., Matsumoto, T., Kano, K., Kagami, T., and Nagaya, H.,** Clinical studies on Behcet's syndrome, *Ann. Rheumatic Dis.,* 22, 36, 1963.

41. **Chajek, T. and Fainaru, M.,** Behcet's disease. Report of 41 cases and a review of the literature, *Medicine,* 54, 179, 1975.

42. **Cadman, E. C., Lundberg, W. B., and Mitchell, M. S.,** Pulmonary manifestations in Behcet's syndrome, *Arch. Intern. Med.,* 136, 944, 1976.

43. **Levin, D. C.,** Pulmonary abnormalities in the necrotizing vasculitides and their rapid response to steroids, *Radiology,* 97, 251, 1970.

44. **Reimold, E. W., Weinberg, A. G., Fink, C. W., and Battles, N. D.,** Polyarteritis in children, *Am. J. Dis. Child.,* 130, 534, 1976.
45. **Melam, H. and Patterson, R.,** Periarteritis nodosa, a remission achieved with combined prednisone and azathioprine therapy, *Am. J. Dis. Child.,* 121, 424, 1971.
46. **Reza, M. J., Dornfeld, L., Goldberg, L. S., Bluestone, R., and Pearson, C. M.,** Wegener's granulomatosis, long term follow-up of patients treated with cyclophosphamide, *Arthritis Rheumatism,* 18, 501, 1975.
47. **Lanham, J. G., Elkon, K. B., Pusy, C. D., and Hughes, G. R.,** Systemic vasculitis with asthma and eosinophilia: a clinical approach to the Churg-Strauss Syndrome, *Medicine,* 63, 65, 1984.
48. **Hunninghake, G. W. and Fauci, A. S.,** Pulmonary involvement in the collagen vascular diseases, *Am. Rev. Respiratory Dis.,* 119, 491, 1979.

Chapter 41

THE INTERSTITIAL PNEUMONIAS

Lourdes R. Laraya-Cuasay

TABLE OF CONTENTS

I. INTRODUCTION

This chapter deals with the clinical, pathologic features, management, and prognosis of the various forms of interstitial pneumonias. Most knowledge of interstitial lung disease (ILD) is derived from adult experience, but emphasis will be drawn to occurrence in children whenever available.

Figure 1 diagramatically presents the etiopathogenesis of the interstitial pneumonias. Lung injury from whatever cause (the stimulus) leads to an alveolitis, peribronchial, and peribronchiolar damage. All these processes could occur simultaneously in varying degrees of severity or intensity in one or more lobes of the lung. Host defense mechanisms influence or modify the response of the lung to injury.[1,2]

Inorganic or organic dusts, gases, fumes, aerosols, drugs, poisons, radiation, infectious agents, cardiac, and metabolic diseases can lead to lung injury. The mechanism of injury could be by direct toxicity to endothelial or epithelial cells, or generation of toxic radicals like superoxide, peroxide, or hydroxyl radicals.[3,4] Neutrophils are recruited to the lungs during complement activation or from release of chemotactic factors that recruit neutrophils after activation of alveolar macrophage.[5] There is incomplete understanding of how neutrophils injure the lung, although studies have shown activated neutrophils to secrete a variety of toxic oxygen radicals, some proteases and other peptides that are capable of initiating and perpetuating lung injury.

An immunologic mechanism may also be involved since immune complexes have been identified in idiopathic pulmonary fibrosis. Lung injury caused by immune complexes results from complement activation and recruitment, activation of neutrophils which injure, and sustain the inflammatory changes as described above.[6-9] Chapter 3 details the cellular response to lung injury.

The derivation of the nomenclature for the interstitial pneumonias is based on the predominant cell in the interstitial infiltrate. When giant cells predominate, it is termed giant cell pneumonia (GIP). When eosinophiles predominate, it is termed pulmonary involvement with eosinophilia (PIE). When obliterative bronchiolitis is associated with interstitial pneumonia, it is called bronchiolitis obliterans with interstitial pneumonia (BIP). When type II pneumonocytes are seen within alveolar spaces, it is termed desquamative interstitial pneumonia (DIP).[10]

Organization of the inflammatory infiltrate with deposition of collagen and fibroblastic proliferation follows.[1,2] Resolution can be partial or complete. The inflammatory cells of the alveolitis can destroy connective tissue. The neutrophil and alveolar macrophage can produce significant amounts of collagenase, elastase, and glycosaminoglycans which attack connective tissue macromolecules.[11] Destruction of connective tissue can also occur by alteration in the antiprotease system. Several of these enzymes have been obtained from bronchoalveolar lavage specimens from patients with idiopathic pulmonary fibrosis.[12] This increase in connective tissue in the lung leads to fibrosis when incompletely resolved. Thereafter, chronic respiratory failure can ensue and progress gradually to ultimate death.

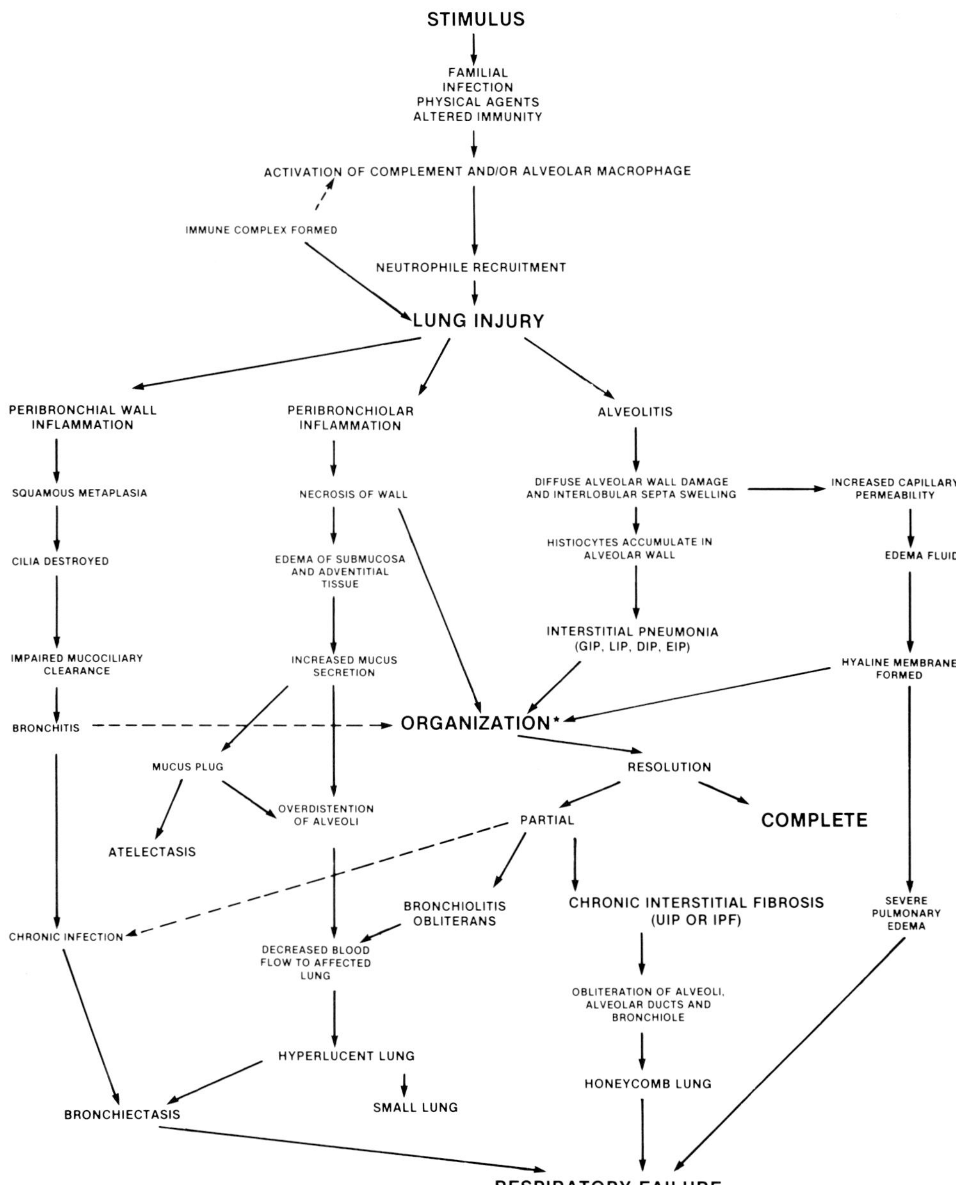

FIGURE 1.   Pathogenesis of the interstitial pneumonias. Organization with incorporation of connective tissue in alveolar wall, reticulin fibrils appear around fibroblast with maturation of reticulin to collagen. GIP — Giant cell interstitial pneumonia, LIP — lymphoid interstitial pneumonia, DIP — desquamative interstitial pneumonia, EIP — eosinophilic interstitial pneumonia, UIP — usual interstitial pneumonia, and IPF — idiopathic pulmonary fibrosis.

II. BRONCHIOLITIS OBLITERANS WITH INTERSTITIAL PNEUMONIA

A. Definition

Bronchiolitis obliterans or obliterative bronchiolitis is defined pathologically as complete or incomplete closure of terminal bronchioles secondary to the development of vascular fibrosis, or granulation tissue.[13]

B. Etiology

Bronchiolitis obliterans can result from complications of pneumonia and bronchiolitis due to bacteria (H. pertussis,[14] *Legionella pneumophila*[15]), virus (rubeola,[14,16] influenza,[17] adenovirus,[18] respiratory syncytial virus[19]), mycoplasma,[20] and inhalation of irritant gases (nitrogen dioxide,[21,22] ozone,[23] ammonia,[24] and some "war gases"). In about one third of cases the cause is unknown.[25] It may be associated with rheumatoid arthritis[26] or with penicillamine used in its treatment.[27] Penicillamine blocks cross linkage of newly synthesized collagen and elastin.[28] In patients with connective tissue disorders who are more prone to bronchiolitis and bronchitis, penicillamine could modify or interfere with the healing process. Bronchiolitis obliterans may also be closely related to eosinophilic pneumonia.[29]

In uremic lung, bronchiolitis obliterans has been described as noninflammatory when young connective tissue extends into and fills the alveoli resulting from organization of intrabronchial exudate containing hemosiderin-laden macrophages. There is always a preceding pulmonary edema followed by organization of fibrinous and protein-rich exudate leading to characteristic plugs of intra-alveolar fibrosis.[30] Also, a bronchiolitis obliterans has been described to occur as a complication of bone marrow transplantation[31] and may possibly be associated with chronic graft vs. host disease.[32,33]

C. Pathogenesis

The pathogenesis of obliterative bronchiolitis is shown in Figure 1. Prominent interstitial mononuclear infiltrate with interstitial fibrosis, honeycombing, and microcyst formation have been found in 10% of bronchiolitis obliterans. These features characterize bronchiolitis obliterans with interstitial pneumonia (BIP).[30] In the newborn, hyaline membranes formed during the acute respiratory distress syndrome, from oxygen toxicity resulting from its therapy, or intrauterine pneumonia acquired during the last week of intrauterine life, may result in bronchiolitis obliterans. Spencer's book shows a remarkable photograph of a stillborn's lung demonstrating obliterative bronchiolitic changes.[30] During the reparative stages of bronchopulmonary dysplasia, obliterative bronchiolitis and cystic bronchiolectasis have been documented.[34]

Bronchiolitis obliterans has been experimentally produced by intratracheal instillation of 1% nitric acid in rabbits.[35] Within 12 hr necrosis and desquamation of epithelium with papillary processes was observed; within 3 days, there was fibroblastic activity, and in 2 weeks, scar formation. These changes were not observed with the use of steroids and antibiotics.

Histologic findings consist of intrabronchiolar and intra-alveolar ductal exudate that undergoes organization in varying degrees. The exudate is mainly lymphocytic in the early stages with some polymorphonuclear leukocytes. Figure 2 illustrates this. Although interstitial inflammation with fibrosis is not the main feature, it can sometimes be the predominant finding. The damaged bronchiole is surrounded by lymphocytes, and other chronic inflammatory cells which may occupy the adjacent peribronchiolar alveoli. Fibroblastic granulation tissue may appear as a polypoid mass leaving a narrow crescentic slit in the intrabronchiolar lumen[13] (see Figure 3). Externally, the lung surface is studded with irregular nodules measuring 1 to 2 mm in diameter. A honeycomb appearance results from air-trapping distal to the obstructed bronchioles. Radiographically, a unilateral hyperlucent lung may be the end-product consequent to air-trapping and over-distention of alveoli with markedly decreased blood flow to the affected lung.

D. Clinical Features

Bronchiolitis obliterans though more usually found in adults has been observed in infants and children. It has no age or sex predilection.[36] In infants and children, bronchiolitis obliterans occurs as a complication of viral, bacterial, or mycoplasmal pneumonia. Adeno-

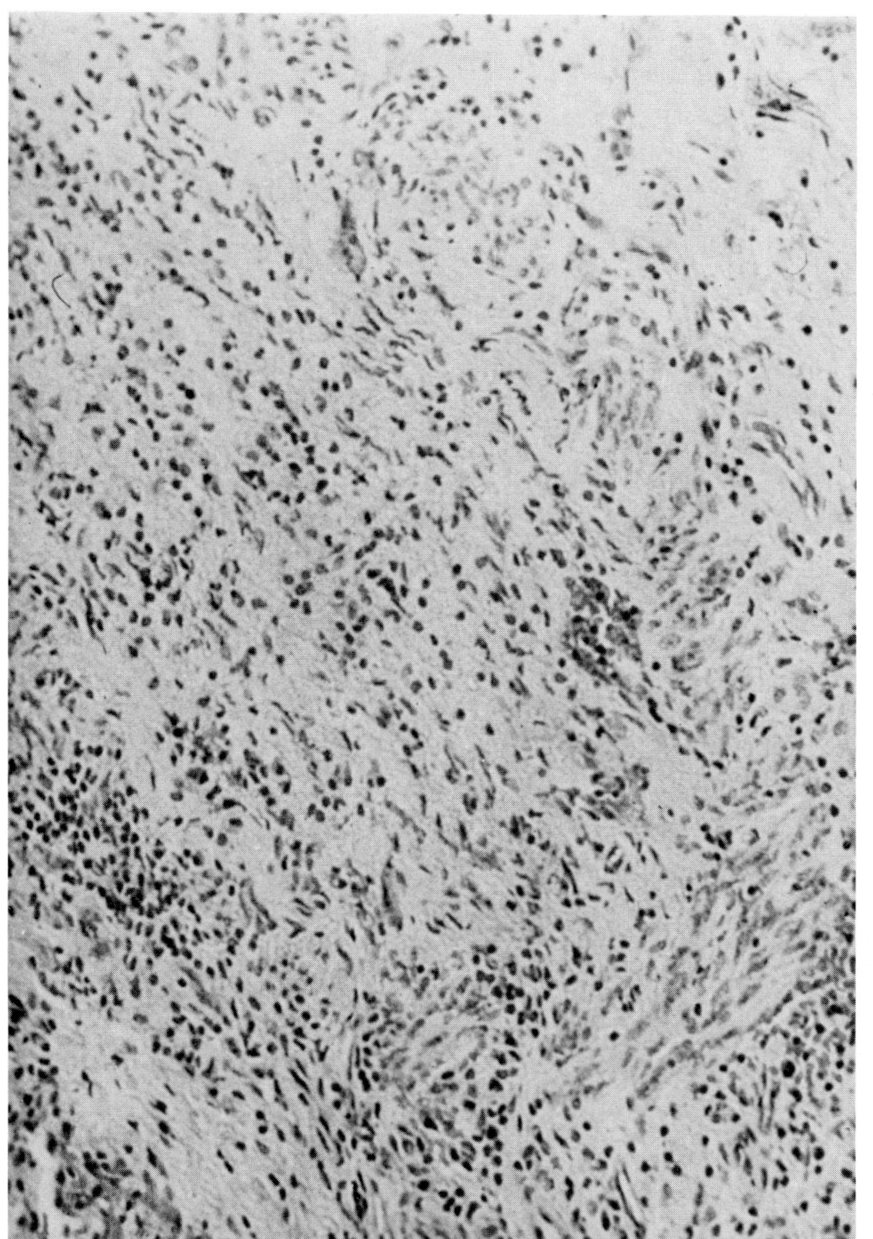

FIGURE 2. Inflammatory exudate made up of lymphocytes, plasma cells and cellular debris occludes the lumen of the bronchiole (lung biopsy specimen, H and E × 142).

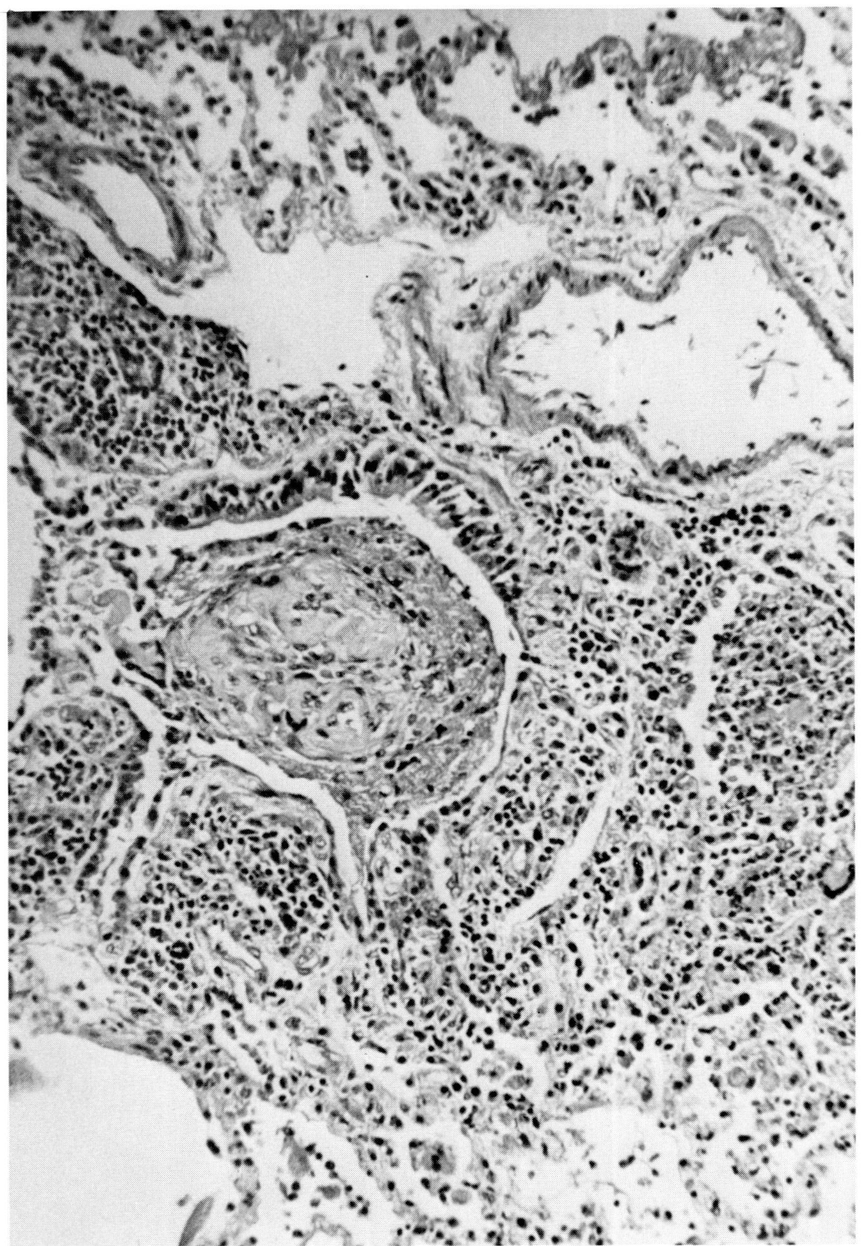

FIGURE 3. Pulmonary biopsy specimen from a patient with influenza A infection showing a polypoid mass of organizing exudate occluding the lumen of a bronchiole with acute inflammatory exudate seen in the surrounding alveoli. (H and E × 125. Courtesy of Dr. Nayere Zaeri, Dept. of Pathology, St. Christopher's Hospital for Children, Philadelphia)

virus is the most commonly involved virus. Persistence of respiratory symptoms way beyond the usual duration of the clinical course of bronchiolitis or pneumonia may indicate that obliterative bronchiolitis has complicated the clinical picture. Localized wheezing may be present. Tachypnea, nonproductive cough, dyspnea, cyanosis, malaise, and chest pain may be present. Diffuse interstitial and alveolar infiltrates may appear radiographically. Pulmonary function documents mixed restrictive and obstructive patterns. A period of relative lack of symptoms or signs can occur for several weeks or months after a lower respiratory tract disease followed by progressive dyspnea, cyanosis, and nonproductive cough in some patients. The three children with post-influenzal A and A$_2$ Hong Kong infection we reported in 1977 persisted to have chronic cough, tachypnea and dyspnea, and diffuse interstitial infiltrates for variable periods of time.[17]

As obliterative changes progress, cicatrization occurs. Episodic obstruction by retained secretions and secondary bacterial infections account for fluctuations in the clinical course. Bronchiolar obliteration may contribute to bronchiectasis by leading to absorption atelectasis, and fibrosis, and by predisposing anatomically and physiologically to stagnation of secretions which result in inflammation.[37]

Unilateral hyperlucent lung develops as progressive air-trapping occurs. The affected lung appears small and mediastinal shift to the unaffected side on expiration is observed.[18,38] This has to be differentiated from unilateral bronchial obstruction by a foreign body or ball-valve mechanism or rarely, congenital absence of the pulmonary artery and branch stenosis of the pulmonary arteries. In infants, congenital lobar hyperinflation, staphylococcal pneumatoceles, and pneumothorax are other considerations. Unilateral absence of the pectoralis muscle, recurrent thromboembolic disease of the pulmonary arteries in adults, and left lower lobe collapse with compensatory upper lobe overaeration need also be excluded.[39]

E. Management

Treatment is conservative and directed towards amelioration of symptoms. When response to bronchodilators is noted, oral and/or nebulized bronchodilating agents are used. Antimicrobials are indicated for pulmonary exacerbations of infectious etiology to prevent further lung damage. Surgical intervention is controversial and is reserved only for cases with hemoptyses, evidence of chronic recurrent infection, or severe impairment of exercise tolerance which is a reflection of ventilation-perfusion inequality in the involved lung. Occasionally, significant improvement in exercise tolerance may be observed after surgery.[39] The advent of more effective anti-infective agents has almost made surgical intervention obsolete except in selected cases.

High-dose steroid therapy is advocated in adults.[15,40] Relapse may occur with discontinuation of steroids.[40] Animal studies have documented response to large doses of steroids,[35] but such experience is not easy to confirm in humans. Timing of administration is crucial and probably should be very early before obliterative changes start to form. It is not possible to predict which infant or child with bronchiolitis or pneumonia will continue to develop obliterative bronchiolitis. In bronchopulmonary dysplasia, use of steroids is being tried but definitive recommendations are still forthcoming.[41]

F. Prognosis

Bronchiolitis obliterans could become fatal within days or weeks of initial symptoms.[42] The more usual course is chronic, a slow progression to bronchiectasis, bronchiolectasis, unilateral hyperlucent lung, and pulmonary fibrosis. Varying degrees of pulmonary impairment is inevitable.

A number of patients have been observed by other authors to be clinically and physiologically stable with no complications for a period of several years.[43] The author has personally followed through 17 years a male patient who has had post-measles interstitial

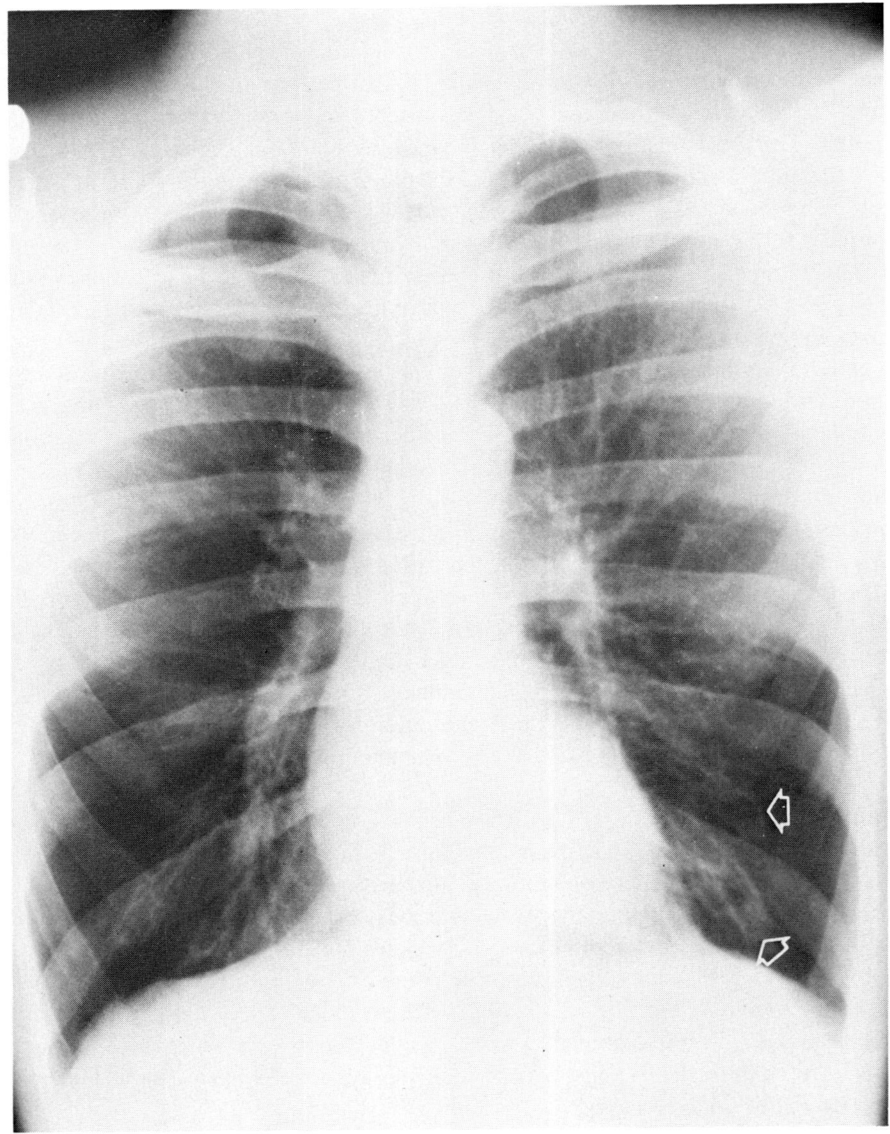

A

FIGURE 4.   (A) Dilated (ectatic) bronchi with peribronchial fibrosis are seen peripherally. (B) The vertically oriented ectatic bronchus is seen on the transverse cross-sectional image as "signet ring" which is due to the bronchial arterial branch traveling along the dilated bronchus. (C) The horizontally traveling ectatic bronchi have a so-called "TRAMLINE" appearance. (Courtesy of Dr. Judy Amorosa, Dept. of Radiology, UMDNJ-Robert Wood Johnson Medical School, New Brunswick, N.J.)

pneumonitis acquired at 6 years of age which complicated into obliterative bronchiolitis, bronchitis, and bronchiectasis.[19] His chest radiograph and computed tomograms are shown in Figures 4A, B, and C. He has not had any complications and has not required any hospitalization in the past 9 years. His pulmonary function shows a moderate restrictive-obstructive pattern and post-exercise arterial hypoxemia. Ventilation-perfusion scans demonstrated poor perfusion and ventilation in all lobes except his left upper lobe. Two of the three children with post-influenzal bronchiolitis obliterans[17] have continued to need bronchodilators and their physiologic findings have been stable.

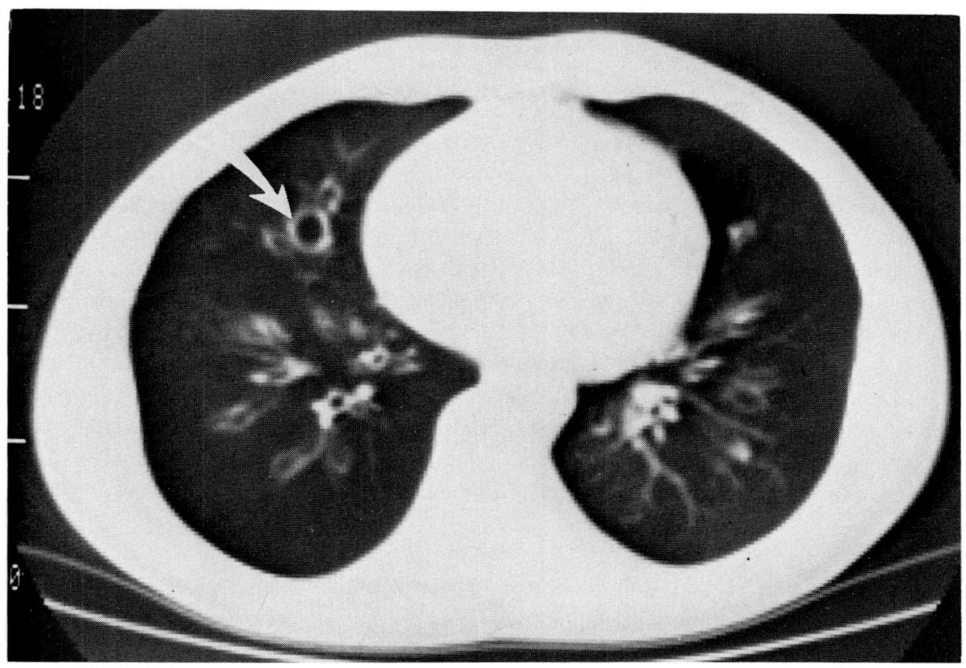

FIGURE 4B

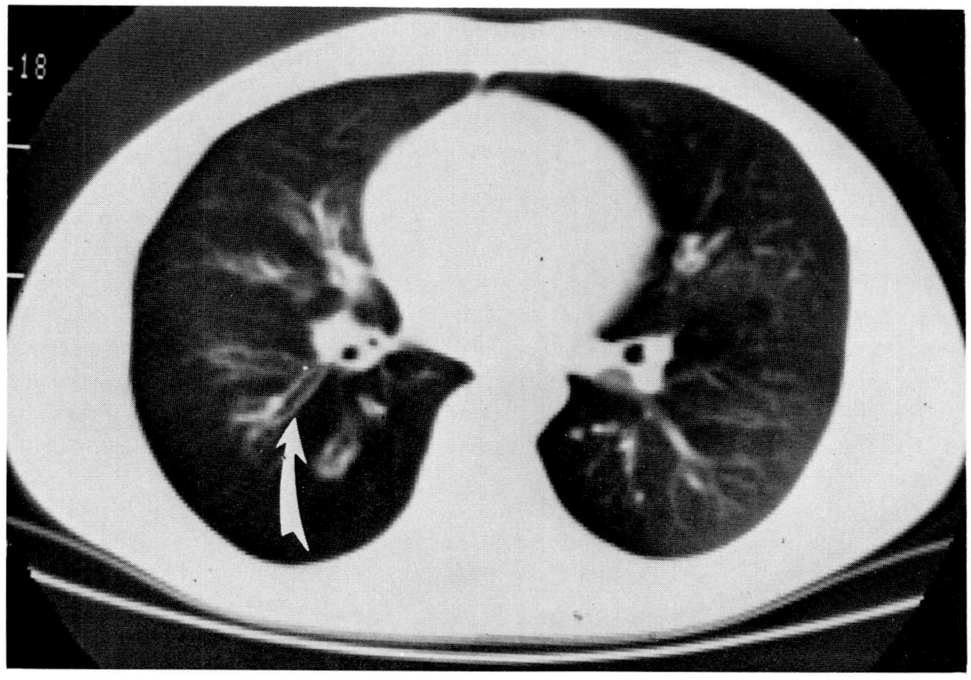

FIGURE 4C

III. DESQUAMATIVE INTERSTITIAL PNEUMONITIS

A. Definition

Histologic criteria established by Liebow and associates.[44] in 1965 to define and diagnose desquamative interstitial pneumonitis (DIP) include: (1) uniform filling of alveolar spaces by large desquamated type II pneumocytes and alveolar macrophages; (2) PAS-positive granules in the cytoplasm of some free alveolar cells; (3) prominent alveolar lining cell population; (4) moderate thickening of alveolar septa from increased connective tissue and mononuclear inflammatory cell infiltrate of histiocytes, lymphocytes, plasma cells, and eosinophils; (5) absence of necrosis or hyaline membranes; and (6) dense collections of lymphocytes and occasional lymphoid follicles (see Figure 5). Focally, there was hyperplasia of smooth muscles in the blood vessels and bronchioles. Eosinophilic intranuclear inclusions described as "virus-like" have been observed in 5 to 80% of cases, occurring in both alveolar lining cells and desquamated cells. Subsequent electron microscopic studies have shown these inclusions to consist of myelin figures derived from degenerative changes. Also, there is clumping of chromatin in the nuclear membrane.[45]

B. Etiology

The exact etiology remains unknown. Among possible factors indicated as contributory[46,47] are rheumatoid factor, antinuclear antibody, lupus erythematosus phenomenon, viral infection, and foreign body reaction. In patients with DIP, UIP, and LIP, circulating immune complexes that have been identified may play a role on pathogenesis.[48] Also, IgM antigen-antibody complexes have been found in two infants with immunoglobulin G deficiency who had congenital rubella.[49] Both infants also had IgM deposits in the alveolar interstitium.

It has long been known that lungs exposed to tungsten carbide dust, asbestos, or nitrofurantoin, show histologic features of DIP. These findings are probably diffuse alveolar damage responses and not responses to those agents as specific etiology for DIP.

The familial occurrences of interstitial lung disease is fully discussed in Chapter 2. Fatal DIP was reported in three infant siblings in 1984.[50] Familial DIP is very rare.[50,51]

C. Pathogenesis

Two infants with congenital rubella presented with DIP at 3 months and 16 weeks of age.[49] Digital clubbing was already present in the 16-week-old infant who had no associated intracardiac lesion. More interstitial fibrosis was noted at post-mortem examination in this infant's lung compared to that seen in the lung of the 3-month-old infant. This probably further documents the newly accepted concept that DIP is an earlier stage of chronic interstitial fibrosis or one type of fibrosing alveolitis.[52,53] Earlier, it was thought that DIP followed other forms of interstitial pneumonia.[54] It is now known that cellular desquamation and mural fibrosis could be present in various proportions in different cases and probably at different stages of the disease.[55]

Necropsy findings resembling both DIP and pulmonary alveolar proteinosis in a 9-month-old infant, and the production experimentally in rabbit's lung of both disorders suggest a common pathogenesis for DIP and alveolar proteinosis.[56]

D. Clinical Features

DIP has been mostly reported in adults until Hewitt's series of 10 cases in 1977[57] and previous isolated case reports of DIP in infants and children. Even as late as 1984, only 33 cases of DIP had been reported in infants and children.[44,49-52,56-71] The youngest patient was a $2^1/_2$-week-old infant.[67]

The onset of DIP is usually insidious. There may be a preceding viral-like illness. Cough has been described, also there is difficulty of breathing, cyanosis, and failure to gain weight

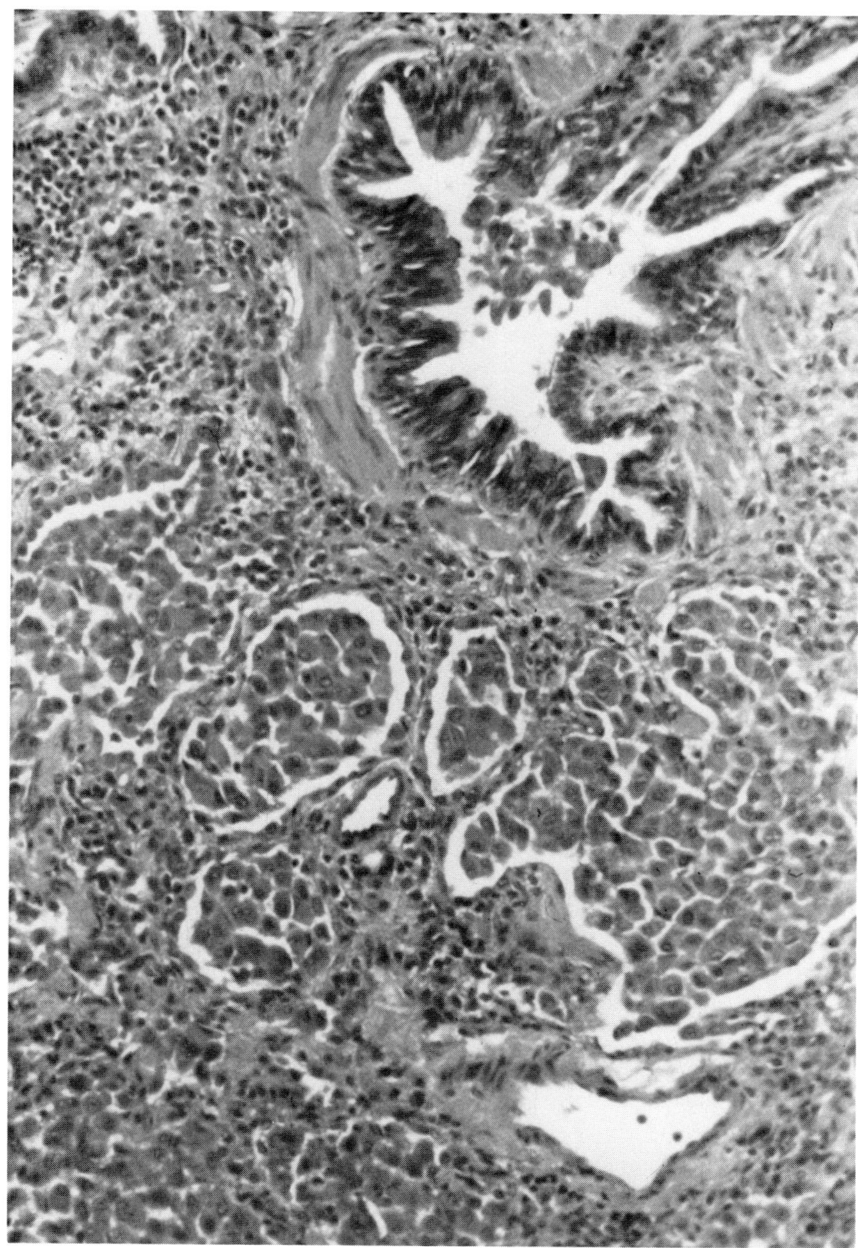

FIGURE 5.   Desquamative interstitial pneumonitis, characterized by compact collections of large mononuclear cells in the alveoli, cuboidal metaplasia of alveolar lining cells, and scanty interstitial lymphoid infiltrate is shown in this lung biopsy specimen. (H. E.; magnification × 100) (From Joshi, V. et al., *Hum. Pathol.*, 16, 241, 1985. Reprinted with permission from W. B. Saunders Co.)

during the first month of life. This is followed by progressive hypoxia and death from respiratory failure before 4 months of age despite intensive drug and supportive treatment.[50] Dyspnea, tachypnea and growth retardation were the prominent findings of 28 patients reviewed by Stillwell and associates.[51] Cough and cyanosis were present in 63% of the patients. The characteristic cough was dry and nonproductive. Clubbing was reported in 26%. Only 11 cases had febrile onset.

Table 1
CLINICAL DATA AT ONSET OF DESQUAMATIVE INTERSTITIAL PNEUMONIA

Data	Group from Mayo Clinic[51,62]	Group reviewed from literature[49-51]
No. of patients	14[a]	19[a]
Sex M/F	5/9	11/8
Age of onset	1—12 years	2½ weeks—16 years
Symptoms and signs		
Dyspnea	12/14	13/15
Cough	8/14	12/16
Growth retardation	11/14	13/13
Febrile onset	6/13	6/15
Tachypnea	14/14	16/17
Rales	6/14	5/18
Cyanosis	9/14	13/18
Clubbing	4/13	3/15
Abnormal chest roentgenogram	14/14[b]	18[c]/19

[a] Different denominators within same group indicate that information was not available or not reported for some patients.
[b] Pulmonary parenchyma was normal radiographically in one patient.
[c] Initially normal in one but 7 days later became abnormal.

Modified from Stillwell, P. C., Norris, D. G., O'Connell, E. J., Rosenow, E. C., III, Weiland, L. H., and Harrison, E. G., Jr., *Chest,* 77, 165, 1980.

Normal physical findings may be found despite functional abnormalities. Tachycardia and tachypnea with dyspnea are prominent in infants. Older children may have dry or nonproductive cough, anorexia, weight loss, and easy fatigability. With progression of the disease, clubbing, more tachypnea, cyanosis with bibasilar rales and end-inspiratory crackles may be heard.[62] Granulomatous lymphadenopathy was present in a 6-year-old black girl.[70] Table 1 shows the clinical features of 33 well documented cases of DIP in children thus far reported.[49-51,62]

The Mayo Clinic experience demonstrated little difference between adults and children with DIP.[51,62] Musculoskeletal complaints and chest pain were more frequently found in adults.

Chest roentgenograms may be normal in DIP.[44,52,72-75] Generally, the pulmonary infiltrates are bilateral and extend from the hilus to the base. The pattern is predominantly interstitial and alveolar but occasionally interstitial or alveolar.[51] The author has seen a 5-year-old girl with acute onset of dyspnea, fever, and cyanosis who rapidly went into cardiac arrest and whose lung at autopsy showed DIP. Chest roentgenograms showed bibasilar densities. No virus was isolated from the lung or other tissues.

Patients may have dyspnea, cough, and reduced diffusion capacity for carbon monoxide. The duration of symptoms may be from 3 months to 9 years. Cor pulmonale can develop. Right ventricular hypertrophy was seen in 50% of Stillwell's 28 cases.[51] Fairly severe restrictive disease may persist.[70]

E. Management
To aid better understanding of the pathologic mechanism of DIP, pulmonary tissue or any other material obtained at biopsy should be sent for culture for viruses, bacteria, Chlamydia, fungi, routine and immunofluorescent staining, and electron microscopic examination. Circulating immune complexes should also be requested.

Corticosteroids have been used to treat DIP after diagnosis is confirmed by open lung biopsy. Spontaneous remissions have been reported.[52,62,76] Therapeutic response to steroids is not predictable and relapses do occur after discontinuation of steroid therapy. Aggressive immunotherapy has been proposed for steroid-resistant cases.[64,67] Three infants reported by Tal[50] and one of two infants reported by Boner[49] did not respond to steroids. Cyclophosphamide was tried but was unsuccessful. Chloroquine was tried in the third infant with the same fatal result. Successful use of chloroquine has since been reported.[77] Quinolone derivatives have been reported to split immune complexes and to inhibit antibody reaction.[78] One of the infants reported with congenital rubella, low IgG and circulating IgM antigen-antibody complex did not respond to immunoglobulin replacement without steroid therapy. Azathioprine was used unsuccessfully in one patient.[68]

F. Prognosis

The ultimate possible courses of DIP had been observed based on second biopsies or autopsy. DIP could progress to honeycomb lung or pulmonary fibrosis[55,65,69] to minimal change in histologic appearance at autopsy after 7, 5, and 3 months of therapy[24-26] or to remission on subsequent biopsy findings 2 months after the start of steroid therapy.[51] With continued steroids at a maintenance dose the latter course was stable at the time of the report. Development of alveolar proteinosis in addition to honeycombing and giant cell pneumonia has also been reported.[56,71]

Mortality is highest when the onset of DIP is in the first 12 months of life. In the Mayo Clinic experience, 35% of deaths occurred 2 months to 4 years after onset.[51] Adults favorably responded to steroids.[76] Steroids should be given a fair trial if the decision for their use has been made.

IV. GIANT CELL INTERSTITIAL PNEUMONIA

A. Defintion

Giant cell interstitial pneumonia (GIP) is a rare type of interstitial pneumonia characterized by the presence of bizarre, multinucleated giant cells and mononuclear cells in the alveolar spaces.[79] When the giant cell pneumonia occurs without clinical measles, it is termed Hecht's pneumonia.

B. Etiopathogenesis

Since 1910, the etiologic relationship between GIP and the measles virus has been strongly considered since 19 of the original 27 children reported aged 6 to 24 months had a history of measles.[1] Inclusion bodies in the giant cells suggested a relationship to distemper and measles virus.[80,81] Measles virus has been isolated from three fatal cases of GIP in patients without clinical manifestations of measles. These children had underlying diseases such as cystic fibrosis, leukemia, and Letterer-Siwe's Disease.[82,83] Since the pulmonary pathology of measles pneumonia and GIP are very similar, a common etiology is possible. Mitus and his associates have shown that measles and GIP had a common etiology when they isolated measles virus after death from two patients 3 to 4 weeks after measles exanthem had disappeared. Both cases showed the histological findings of GIP and both patients had leukemia in the terminal course of their illnesses.[84] An analytical review of the relationship of GIP and measles had served to establish this relationship.[85]

GIP has occurred in young children receiving cyclophosphamide and adrenocorticotrophic hormone therapy. One of these children did not form antibodies to measles. Electronmicroscopic findings have shown fusion of type II alveolar epithelial cells and the intranuclear inclusions consisted of a mass of cross-striated filamentous bodies similar to RNA paramyxovirus of measles.[86] GIP may have been caused by persistent measles virus following depressed antibody formation.[87]

Attempts to define the etiology of GIP in adults have not uncovered any specific cause. Autoimmune studies have been negative. Antilung antibodies have been absent. No infectious agent could be found on histology, microbiology, or viral studies. No inclusion bodies have been found.[88]

C. Pathologic Features

The lungs show an interstitial infiltrate predominantly composed of epithelial giant cells with intranuclear and intracytoplasmic inclusions. The cytoplasm of 10 to 100 adjacent epithelial cells first become eosinophilic with later disappearance of cell walls resulting in giant cell formation.[89] Mononuclear cells may be abundant, mainly consisting of lymphocytes and plasma cells. Squamous metaplasia of the bronchial and bronchiolar epithelium with proliferation of alveolar lining cells have been seen. Hyperplasia of peribronchiolar lymphoid tissue has been found. Discrete desquamated macrophages fill the alveolar spaces, and the alveoli are lined by type II cells. GIP has been considered a variant of DIP.[87] The intra-alveolar cells show a positive reaction to PAS and iron stains. There is no morphologic difference between Hecht's pneumonia and GIP.

The only feature distinguishing measles from GIP is the presence of Warthin-Finkeldey giant cells in measles. These cells are giant reticuloendothelial cells in the lymphoid tissue. They normally appear after the appearance of the measles exanthem, and therefore disappear by the time GIP develops.

D. Laboratory Features

Antibody formation in measles can be measured by the hemagglutination-inhibition test, by measuring complement fixing antibodies which appear within 2 to 3 days, and measurement of neutralizing antibodies which appear as the rash begins to subside, often as early as the fourth day after the rash has appeared. However, antibody formation is depressed in immunosuppressed individuals who are most likely to develop GIP.

Indirect fluorescent antibody technique can show measles antigen within the giant cells.[90] Fluorescent antibody technique may enable early etiologic diagnosis especially when measles is atypical or presents without a rash.[91] Smears of nasal secretions, conjunctival, and buccal tissue may demonstrate typical multinucleated giant cells sometimes containing inclusion bodies. Specific immunofluorescent staining of lung biopsy tissue may confirm the diagnosis.[91]

E. Clinical Features

After an average incubation period of 10 to 12 days, prodromal signs and symptoms appear. These include profuse serous and mucus nasal discharge, excessive lacrimation and photophobia, sneezing and mild irritating cough. As the rash develops, tracheobronchial symptoms and fever increases. A tracheitis may be prominent. Rhonchi and crackles may be heard. If the individual does not recover, a mild cough persists.

GIP may be suspected in children with measles who develop an interstitial pneumonitis especially if the child has an underlying disease that modifies host response to viral injury, such as cystic fibrosis, malignancy on chemotherapy, or malnutrition.[84,85]

Clinical presentation in GIP is similar to that already described in DIP or UIP. Progressive dyspnea, chest pain, cough, fatigue, weight loss, appearance of digital clubbing and bibasilar crackles have been described. Restrictive pattern with resting and post-exercise hypoxemia with normocapnea have been reported.[92,93]

Radiographic findings show bilateral patchy nodular infiltrates involving the midlung fields or upper zones with sparing of the apices and costophrenic angles. Other findings closely parallel those of DIP.[92,93]

The usual criteria for diagnosis of measles may be absent. The children are critically ill and specific diagnosis may need to be established with open lung biopsy. Children on immunosuppressants and on methotrexate when infected with measles can have a fulminating course.[91]

F. Management

Prevention of measles prevents GIP. Constant vigilance in control and surveillance of measles internationally, aggressive response to reported cases, and maintenance of a high immunization status in the communities must be the objectives.[16] Outbreaks in certain communities traceable to unreliable immunization records might be duplicated in other areas and lead to widespread problems.[95] Routine revaccination of children immunized against measles before 15 months of age is necessary.[95] A constant watch for "imported measles" will aid in control.[96]

Administration of Ender's attenuated live measles vaccine to children prevents the occurrence of GIP. However, since the children most likely to develop GIP have altered immunity, such as children with leukemias, the use of large doses of gamma globulin for passive immunization of such children is preferred.[91] The survival of two patients who received large doses of gammaglobulin at the time of exposure has been reported suggesting that this therapy may have value in modifying the course of measles pneumonitis.[85] Use of measles convalescent plasma to administer antibody intravenously may be helpful. Prevention of exposure of susceptibles to measles infection is mandatory.

Steroids have been beneficial in the treatment of GIP in adults. Reduction of digital clubbing, functional, and radiographic improvement and histologic changes on second biopsy showing decrease in numbers of intra-alveolar giant cells and increased number of alveolar pneumocytes have supported the use of steroids in adults.[86]

Symptomatic care, close observation and specific therapy for superimposed infection are requisites of management.

G. Prognosis

GIP is potentially fatal.[79,80,82-88, 97,98] Survival with large doses of gammaglobulin has been reported with modification of the course of the measles pneumonitis. There is a potential for chronic pulmonary disability secondary to sequelae of measles virus infection such as obliterative bronchiolitis, bronchiectasis, and fibrosis.[99,100]

V. PULMONARY INVOLVEMENT WITH EOSINOPHILIA

In 1978, Neva and Hesen described the hypereosinophilic syndromes,[101] (eosinophil counts greater than 3000/mm^3), which presently are thought to be of parasitic, fungal, drug-induced, vasculitic or idiopathic etiology. A clinical classification of pulmonary involvement with eosinophilia was proposed by Crofton.[102] There are five distinct groups based on the duration of pulmonary infiltrates and presence of asthma. Their clinical features are summarized in Table 2.

Pulmonary eosinophilia or pulmonary infiltration with eosinophilia (PIE) both refer to a form of pneumonia characterized by eosinophilic infiltration of lung tissue.

A. Loeffler Syndrome

Loeffler in 1932, reported a group of patients with transient pulmonary infiltrates, moderate eosinophilia of 10 to 20%, mild to absent systemic symptoms and a benign course.[103] Spencer has suggested abandoning the term Loeffler syndrome as pathologic basis is lacking.[104] Eosinophilic pneumonia might be a better term. Blood eosinophilia usually accompanies the pulmonary eosinophilia but this too is not invariably present. *Ascaris lumbricoides* was reported as etiologic in some of Loeffler's original cases. The fleeting nature of the pulmonary infiltrates was attributed to the lung migration phase of parasitic nematodes most notably

Table 2
PULMONARY INVOLVEMENT WITH EOSINOPHILIA

Clinical group[a]	I	II	III	IV	V[b]
Description	Loeffler syndrome simple pulmonary involvement with eosinophilia	Prolonged pulmonary eosinophilia	Tropical eosinophilia (eosinophilic lung, Weingarten syndrome, occult filariasis)	Pulmonary eosinophilia with asthma	Polyarteritis nodosa
Duration of pulmonary infiltrates	Up to 1 month	2 to 6 months (uncommon in children)	Prolonged	Prolonged	Prolonged

Etiologic considerations
Infection
	Parasitic
	Nematodal infestation:
	  Ascaris lumbricoides
	  Ancyclostoma
	  Toxocara canis
	   (visceral larva
	   migrans stage I)
	  Trichuris
		As in I	Reaction to degenerating microfilariae in eosinophilic granuloma in the absence of circulating adult filarial worms (Wuchereria bancrofti, Brugia malayi)	Fungal — May be superimposed on the allergic reactions to causative fungus (allergic bronchopulmonary aspergillosis)	Auto-immune processes resulting in vasculitis syndromes, collagen-vascular diseases and eosinophilic granuloma

Drugs	+ Acetylsalicyclic acid Penicillin Sulfonamide Chlorpromazine Nitrofurantoin Methylphenidate Imipramine	— As in I	None	None	Association with certain collagen-vascular disease
Symptoms/signs	May be asymptomatic, cough or wheeze	Wheeze, cough	Cough, wheeze, chest pain, dyspnea, weight loss, fatigue	Episodic wheezing elevated temperature, wheezing, weight loss, cough, production of brown mucus plugs, clubbing, and anorexia	Multisystemic complaints, simulates viral-like illness in infants arthritis, hypertension

Clinical course	Spontaneous remission and exacerbations, self-limited	Severe and prolonged	Remission and recrudescences common	Chronic	Chronic and may be fatal
Complications	In general, none	Recovery	May result in chronic lung disease	Mucoid impaction Bronchiectasis obliterans Fibrosis	Varying degrees of restrictive lung disease: bronchiolitis obliterans in rheumatoid arthritis
Pulmonary functions If wheezing, $FEV_1 \downarrow$	+	+	+	+	+
Restrictive pattern	+	+	+	+	+
Hypoxemia	+	+	+	+	+
Obstructive pattern	−	−	+	+	+
Elevated IgE levels				+ + + as high as several thousand	
Treatment Specific Rx	Antihelminthics: Thiabendazole 25—50 mg/kg/day doses given 7 to 10 days. Repeat in 4 weeks	Same as Group 1	Diethylcarbamazine (Hetrazan) 5 mg/kg/day for 7 to 10 days	Antifungal agents tried by aerosol but ineffective	Immunosuppressant drugs
Corticosteroids	For severe symptoms	+	For very ill patients	+	+
Bronchodilators	−	−	−	+	+
Physical therapy	−	−	+	+	+

a   As defined by Crofton.[102]

b   Refer to Chapter 40 for details of collagen vascular pulmonary involvement.

Ascaris lumbricoides, Toxocara canis, Ancylostoma duodenale, or *Trichiuris trichiura*. Peripheral unilateral or bilateral pulmonary densities were usual. Infiltration of alveolar septae and alveolar spaces by eosinophils and histiocytes without basement membrane damage has been shown. A family history of atopy or allergy may be present.

Pulmonary infiltrates in simple pulmonary involvement with eosinophilia (Crofton's group I) may last a few days to a month. Symptoms may be mild or absent. Only an occasional cough or wheeze may be present. Rhonchi and scattered rales in one or both lungs may be observed. Clinical pneumonia and/or atelectasis may have to be ruled out depending on the size of the infiltrates on the chest roentgenograms. Elevated eosinophils sometimes up to 50% and a history of pica and/or owning a dog for a pet might favor the diagnosis of visceral larva migrans. This disease is very similar to Loeffler syndrome except for hepatomegaly. Initial examination of stools for ova and parasites are repeated at 2 to 4 week intervals because the pulmonary phase antedates the appearance of ova in the stools. Enzyme-linked immunosorbent assay (ELISA) may demonstrate toxocaral antibodies that differentiate toxocariasis from ascariasis.

Elevated IgE levels as high as 10,000 units/mℓ have been reported. Allergic bronchopulmonary aspergillosis (ABPA or Crofton's group IV) is identified with expectoration of brown mucus plugs containing hyphae, recovery of *Aspergillus fumigatus* on fungal culture, and positive immunologic evidence of allergy to *Aspergillus* antigens. Duration of the clinical illness is longer and central type bronchiectasis is usual.

Various drugs have been reported to cause eosinophilic pneumonia,[105] among them furazolidine, penicillin, para-amino-salicylic acid, hydralazine, chlorpropamide, mephenesin, mecamylamine, and the sulfonamides. Pulmonary edema with hyaline membrane disease and interstitial and intra-alveolar eosinophil and mononuclear cell reaction occur with subsequent interstitial lung fibrosis. Pulmonary interstitial infiltrates disappear after drug withdrawal but reappear promptly with re-exposure to the culprit drug. There is good response to steroid treatment.

The acute form of nitrofurantoin-induced lung disease has a diffuse pulmonary infiltrate simulating noncardiac pulmonary edema. Pleural effusion may be present. It may mimic infectious pneumonitis except that with discontinuation of nitrofurantoin there is dramatic resolution. In contrast, the chronic form of nitrofurantoin lung disease has a presentation and course similar to idiopathic pulmonary fibrosis. Chronic nitrofurantoin lung disease may take 6 months to several years to completely evolve. Progressive cough and dyspnea are usual. It may respond more favorably to steroid treatment than idiopathic pulmonary fibrosis.[106] Cell mediated immune responses to nitrofurantoin have been demonstrated suggesting a possible immune mechanism in its pathogenesis.[107]

Cromolyn sodium and aerosolized steroids (beclomethasone) have been known to induce pulmonary infiltrates with eosinophilia in a few patients with asthma.[108] Demonstration of both humoral and lymphocytic factors in sensitive patients may indicate that some immune mechanism might be operative.

B. Visceral Larva Migrans

The clinical syndrome consists of peripheral eosinophilia, hepatomegaly, and pneumonitis. Nematode larvae cannot mature in the human host and thus migrate through and invade human tissues with resultant pneumonitis, bronchitis, asthma, hepatomegaly, abdominal pain, muscle and joint pain, weight loss, and various neurological and ophthalmological findings. Fever is intermittent, sweating profuse and hyperleucocytosis common even sometimes mistaken for leukemia.[109]

C. Tropical Eosinophilia (Weingarten Syndrome, Eosinophilic Lung)[110,111]

Signs and symptoms resemble those of a chronic upper respiratory infection accompanied by sustained peripheral eosinophilia. Pulmonary eosinophilic infiltrates are of prolonged duration. The etiology is attributed to the reaction of the lung to degenerating microfilariae in the absence of circulating adult filarial worms. The diagnosis is suspected when a person from an endemic area for human filariasis presents with prolonged and severe pulmonary eosinophilia. High titers of antifilarial antibodies can be detected in the patient's serum by enzyme-linked immunoabsorbent assay (ELISA), complement fixation or hemagglutination tests. Immunoglobulin E is also elevated to even as high as 5000 IU/mℓ but generally not as high as in allergic bronchopulmonary aspergillosis.

Tuberculous or suppurative bronchopneumonia may be simulated radiographically and clinically as these patients have a chronic cough, weight loss, and malaise. Densities may be patchy or confluent, radiating from the hilum and associated with confluent patches at the periphery. A severe peripheral eosinophilia is present and may be as high as 50 to 80% of the total white count. Efficacy of the antifilarial diethylcarbamazine (Hetrazan) has been proven. Corticosteroids have been tried for very ill patients.

D. Eosinophilic Pneumonia Associated with Asthma

This is Crofton's group IV disease.[102] Hinson was the first to report severe asthma in England with mainly eosinophilic pulmonary infiltrations and *Aspergillus fumigatus* in sticky mucoid sputum.[112] These characteristic mucus plugs are dead, partially necrotic eosinophils laid down in dense, compact circumferentially disposed layers with degenerated fungal hyphae.[113] Alveolar interstitium, bronchial walls, and peribronchial tissues are heavily infiltrated with eosinophils, lymphocytes, few plasma cells and plasmacytoid cells; the alveoli are filled with eosinophils, macrophages and desquamated alveolar epithelial cells. Spencer[104] described desquamative interstitial pneumonia in one case of severe interstitial eosinophilic pneumonia. As disease progresses, mucus plugs laden with fungi may find their way to smaller and more distal bronchi and are ultimately responsible for causing a central type of bronchiectasis.

Smaller bronchi become dilated and filled with thick, viscid mucus loaded with eosinophils, nuclear debris, and fungal hyphae. Granulation tissue forms in damaged bronchial walls inciting obliterative bronchiolitis. "Eosinophil abscess" may be seen in lung parenchyma as necrotic foci of eosinophils surrounded by histiocytes. In severe allergic pulmonary aspergillosis, "eosinophil abscesses" are prominent in bronchial walls, peribronchial tissues, and alveolar interstitium. Disintegrating eosinophils form eosinophilic granular material which are engulfed by histiocytes. Crystalline bodies resembling Charcot-Leyden crystals may be seen within small giant cells that surround the abscesses.[104]

Aspergillus skin test is positive, an immediate type hypersensitivity. Serum precipitins are present and Ige levels very elevated. Response to steroid treatment is excellent.[114]

E. Polyarteritis Nodosa and Variants[115]

Crofton's group V represents a very prolonged duration of pulmonary infiltrates with eosinophilia associated with autoimmune processes resulting in vasculitis and collagen-vascular diseases, of which polyarteritis nodosa is considered an example. This type apppears to affect older age groups and is progressive despite corticosteroid therapy. A history of asthma is present in one third of the cases. Pulmonary involvement usually occurs before multisystem disease. Symptoms are severe and the disease is usually fatal. Radiographic findings vary from interstitial markings to peripheral infiltrates to total consolidation. Hypersensitivity angiitis is associated with a necrotizing alveolitis.[115]

Discussion of the collagen-vascular diseases and its association with interstitial lung disease is dealt with in Chapter 40 and will not be discussed here.

A careful allergic history and proper investigation of patients with pulmonary involvement with eosinophilia are stressed inasmuch as the use of corticosteroids may be beneficial for lesions persisting for longer than a week or more.

F. Chronic Eosinophilic Pneumonia

Prolonged pulmonary eosinophilia with characteristic clinical and roentgenographic features of unknown etiology is termed chronic eosinophilic pneumonia. This entity has been well described in adults. The characteristic peripheral location of the pulmonary infiltrates rather than central has been referred to by Carrington and his colleagues[116] as the "photographic negative" of the shadow seen in pulmonary edema. The dense pulmonary pattern progresses with time. The progressive pulmonary infiltrates correlate with pathologic changes of eosinophilic exudation in the alveoli and interstitium, and respond dramatically to steroid therapy. Only one case in a 1-year-old child is found in literature.[117]

VI. USUAL INTERSTITIAL PNEUMONIA

A. Synonyms

Cryptogenic or idiopathic fibrosing alveolitis, fibrosing alveolitis, Hamman-Rich syndrome, idiopathic pulmonary fibrosis (IPF), chronic interstitial pneumonia, organizing interstitial pneumonia, idiopathic diffuse interstitial fibrosis of the lung, bronchiolar emphysema, chronic diffuse sclerosing alveolitis, muscular cirrhosis of the lung, honeycomb lung, and familial fibrocystic pulmonary dysplasia.

B. Definition

Usual interstitial pneumonia (UIP) is a syndrome characterized by progressive exertional dyspnea leading to respiratory failure or corpulmonale causing death within 6 months as reported by Hamman and Rich in five patients seen between 1933 and 1944.[118,119] Thickened alveolar walls and inflammatory and connective tissue changes in the distal airspaces were described. A nonfulminant course or a more chronic state lasting several years have been subsequently reported.[120,121]

C. Etiology

Attempts at defining the etiology of Hamman-Rich syndrome in infancy and childhood led to the demonstration of virus-like particles by electron microscopy in one case.[121] Most of the cases reviewed seemed to be related to a preceding infection or some obscure inflammatory reaction (see Figure 6). Influenza A_2 infection can lead to pulmonary fibrosis.[122,123] Mycoplasma pneumonia has been reported to evolve into IPF.[7] An autoimmune etiology has been proposed as IPF is found in many disorders with altered immunity. The circulating T-lymphocytes of patients with UIP appear to be sensitized to type I collagen.[124] Immune complexes found in bronchoalveolar lavage fluid from patients with IPF stimulate alveolar macrophages to secrete a neutrophil chemotactic factor which is believed to sustain the alveolitis.[4,12,125,126] Circulating immune complexes have been found in IPF.[13,14] It appears that a familial background for IPF is present and has a heterogeneous presentation.[128-133] The familial mode of inheritance is autosomal dominant with reduced penetrance.[128] It has been reported in at least 73 cases in 19 families.[129] A significant increase in the frequency of B-cell alloantigen HLA-DR$_2$ in IPF suggest that genes of the major histocompatibility complex may influence susceptibility to this disorder.[134] A coexistence of hypocalciuric hypercalcemia and interstitial lung disease in a family has been shown.[135]

IPF has been associated with tuberous sclerosis,[23] neurofibromatosis,[137] oculocutaneous albinism,[138] and lymphangioleiomyomatosis[139] which are all autosomal disorders.

Most cases of IPF, however, are of unknown etiology. An underlying anatomic or physiologic defect must be uncovered even if the presentation appears to be "classic" for UIP. The coexistence of IPF with unilateral arterial and venous stenosis and arteriovenous occlusion emphasizes this point.[140]

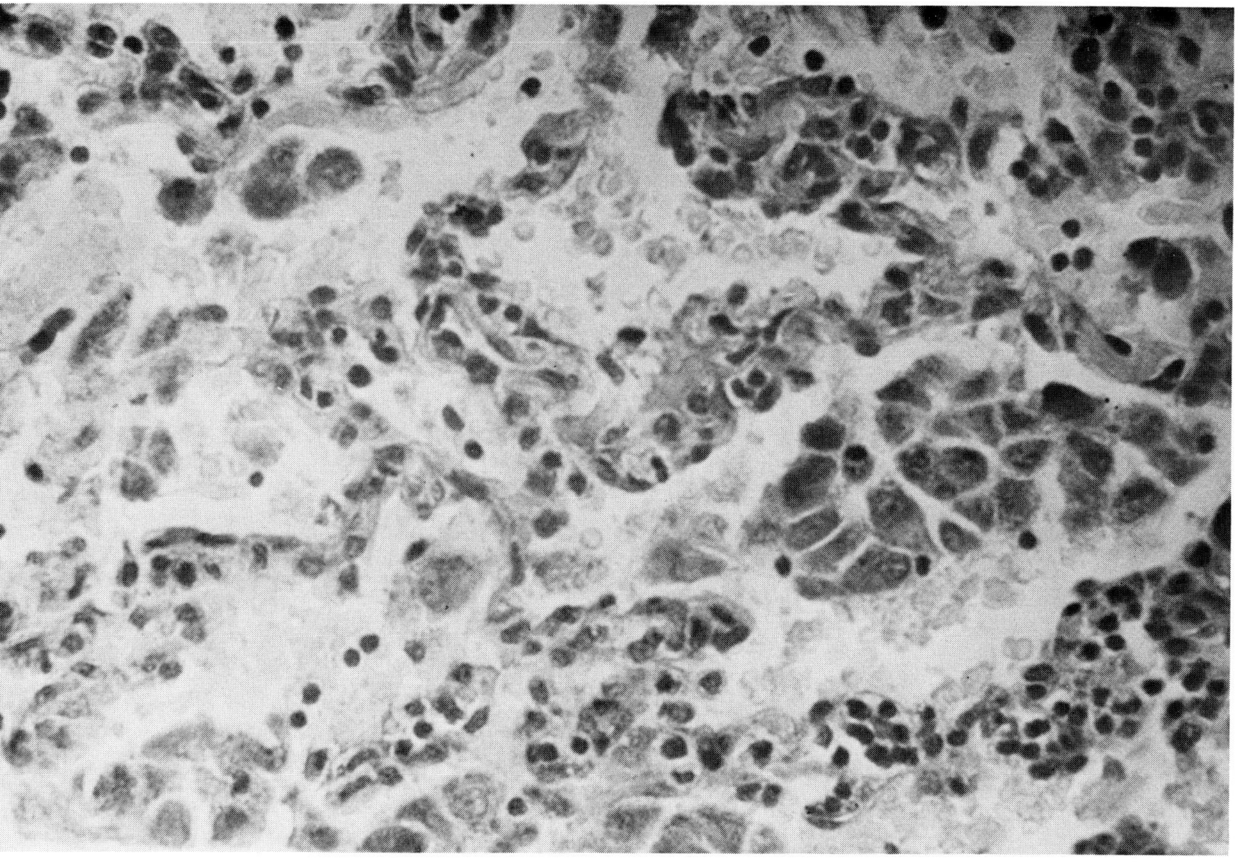

FIGURE 6.   Usual interstitial pneumonia with small cluster of intra-alveolar macrophages from a pulmonary biopsy specimen of a patient with influenza A pneumonia (H and E × 250). Courtesy of Dr. Nayer Zaeri, Dept. of Pathology, St. Christopher's Hospital for Children, Philadelphia).

Table 3
**CLINICAL AND RADIOGRAPHIC FINDINGS IN
USUAL INTERSTITIAL PNEUMONITIS IN
INFANTS, CHILDREN, AND ADOLESCENTS**

Signs and symptoms		Radiographic findings	
Failure to thrive	8	Clear or normal chest	3
Dyspnea	13	at presentation	
Cough	8	Honeycomb lung	2
Cyanosis	8	Streaky or fibrillary	1
Tachypnea	13	in basilar areas	
Wheezing	1	Diffuse fine granular	1
Sputum production	1	pattern	
Tachycardia	2	Ground-glass	1
Cardiac failure	4	Diffuse interstitial	3
Low-grade fever	5	densities	
Pulmonary hypertension	1	Confluent densities	1
Clubbing	4	suggestive of infection	
Recurrent bronchitis	2		

Note: Summary obtained from review of 27 cases reported in literature
with some cases where more than one sign or symptom may be
present in the same patient. Radiographic findings were insuffi-
ciently described in some cases.[121,128,134,140,142-150]

D. Pathogenesis

IPF results from incomplete resolution of lung injury (see Figure 1).[141] A stimulus such
as an infectious agent could cause activation of the complement pathway or activation of
alveolar macrophage (AM) thought to lead to recruitment of neutrophils and production of
alveolitis. Immune complexes may be formed which result in lung injury. Peribronchial and
peribronchiolar inflammatory changes lead to bronchiolitis obliterans with consequent hyperlucent lung. This is complicated by bronchiectasis with pulmonary fibrosis. Alveolar wall
damage causes thickening of the alveolar wall due to inflammatory changes with histiocytes
accumulating in the wall producing an interstitial pneumonia.[10] Organization of the damaged
alveolar wall occurs, connective tissue is incorporated into the alveolar wall and collagen
is deposited. Incomplete or partial resolution leads to UIP or IPF. In time, cystic bronchiolectasis and alveolectasis develop and ultimately progress to end-stage lung. Genetic susceptibility of the patient to IPF, certain abnormal host defenses and the dose of the infecting
agent will all modify the response to lung injury and determine the outcome of the healing
process (see Chapter 4).

E. Clinical Features

Table 3 shows the signs and symptoms of 27 cases of IPF in children that were reviewed
by the author.[121,128,134,140,142,150] There were 7 males and 11 females and 9 others whose sex
was not reported. Ages ranged from birth to 18 years. Twelve cases were from three
families.[15] A preceding pertussis infection has been reported.[149] Failure to gain weight,
cough, and cyanosis were prominent symptoms. Spontaneous pneumothorax occurred in two
cases. One case had persistent diarrhea and rash.[142] Recurrent bronchitis occurred in two
patients who were also poorly nourished. The clinical course was modified by the use of
steroids in eight cases with temporary improvement in three. Death had occurred in 16 cases
at the time the reports were written. Cor pulmonale with evidence of pulmonary hypertension
with four deaths from cardiac failure were noted. In two interesting cases involving female

twins aged 17, one sibling was diagnosed to have IPF 3 years and 3 months before the other. In both, histopathologic findings at the time of diagnosis were identical.[150] The reports did not state whether the girls were identical twins.

The presence of unexplained progressive pulmonary insufficiency associated with a refractory nonspecific failure to gain weight is suggestive but not diagnostic of UIP. In infants, a vigorous search for a familial history suggestive of pulmonary fibrosis must be made as it appears that the incidence of familial background for IPF is high. Dry or paroxysmal cough which may not be impressive occurs. Occasionally, there is sputum production. Dyspnea and tachypnea may be prominent in infants. Low-grade fever may accompany cough, cyanosis, and failure to gain weight. Clubbing of the digits is a late finding and usually appears in adolescence. The pulmonary lesion may be silent and resistant to clinical detection for many years. Digital clubbing may precede obvious pulmonary symptoms. Pathologic, physiologic, and radiographic changes may manifest themselves before the appearance of clinical symptoms.[130]

Very early at the onset of the disease, radiographs may be normal or may show linear, nodular, or "ill-defined" densities or even a ground glass pattern representing the alveolitis of IPF.[152] As symptoms like cyanosis and dyspnea occur, fine streaky or fibrillary patterns may be found in perihilar areas fanning towards the periphery. Progressive involvement of upper and lower lobes persist through weeks or years with development of homogeneous lung density with loss of bronchovascular pattern terminally. Cystic areas may or may not be appreciated radiographically, even in those who eventually develop spontaneous pneumothorax. Emphysematous blebs or bullae may be seen in other cases. In a case described by Donahue, it took 3 months for fine streaks to progress to homogeneous density.[128] Initial radiographs were negative despite intermittent cough for 2 months. Minimal excursion of the diaphragm was observed as the disease progressed. After the lungs were totally opaque roentgenographically, the infant lived for 1 month. The various radiographic findings are summarized in Table 1 from the 27 cases reviewed where radiographic descriptions were available.

As a diagnostic aid, chest radiographs are helpful only in early IPF and in the relatively late stage of the disease.[12] The pulmonary arteries dilate and a coarse reticular pattern develops. The terminal stage shows cystic lesions with severe coarse reticulation of the lung.[12]

The classic physiologic concept of patients with IPF was described by Austrian and his associates.[154] They found that in general, patients have reduced lung volumes, reduced diffusing capacity, normal forced expiratory volume in one second/forced vital capacity ($FEV_1\%$), and arterial hypoxemia which worsened with exercise. The thickened alveolar interstitium was the anatomic barrier that explained the hypoxemia, thus, the term "alveolar-capillary block".

In 1962, the etiology of the hypoxemia was investigated by Finley and his group and they attributed the hypoxemia to ventilation-perfusion mismatch.[155] In 1976, both the ventilation-persfusion imbalance and the diffusion barrier to oxygen during exercise were found present in interstitial diseases.[156]

Zapletal published his studies in 65 children and adolescents with IPF ranging from 5 to 20 years who had been on steroid therapy.[157] Increased lung recoil pressure at maximal inspiratory level and reduced vital capacity, inspiratory capacity and total lung capacity were the most typical abnormalities. Indices of lung elasticity suggested that regions of fibrosis and emphysema had become present. Smaller patients were also noted to have stiffer lungs.

Hypoxemia was a major finding in studies of interstitial lung disease.[1,158-160] The details of the physiologic abnormalities are discussed in Chapter 5. Sleep quality is abnormal in patients with hypoxemic ILD and oxygen saturation falls during rapid eye movement sleep during periods of snoring.[161]

F. Management

Corticosteroids and immunosuppressant therapy have been used in UIP.[1,162-164] Steroid-resistant cases have been reported with good results after alternative use of azathioprine or cyclophosphamide.[162] When 10% or more of the cells obtained by bronchoalveolar lavage are neutrophils, and when there is an associated increase in eosinophils, the response to therapy is poor and prognosis is unfavorable.[125,165] An increased percentage of lymphocytes in lavage fluid is associated with favorable therapeutic response.[165,166] Because IPF occurs in those with connective tissue disorders, immunosuppressants have been used. Oral prednisone at 1 to 2 mg/kg/day for 4 weeks, and then reduced to 5 mg four times a week with 3-day intervals between weekly dosages, or 5 mg every other day was the schedule received by all the children with IPF reported by Zapletal and his associates.[157] Decreased dyspnea, improvement in chest roentgenograms and in pulmonary function will be seen in those who will respond to therapy within 2 weeks from initiation of therapy. There must be a careful watch for the significant side effects of steroid therapy and cyclophosphamide. If stabilization or clinical improvement cannot be achieved, steroid or immunosuppressant therapy should be discontinued because these drugs have significant adverse reactions. Steroid therapy can cause immunosuppression and salt and water retention, hyperglycemia or overt diabetes mellitus, depression and peptic ulcer disease among other complications. Withdrawal of steroids may result in fatigue, weakness, arthralgia, anorexia, orthostatic hypertension and hypoglycemia. Severe hypoxemia at rest and/or exercise should be treated with supplemental oxygen. Diuretic therapy may be indicated in the therapy of cor pulmonale. When pneumothorax occurs, pleurectomy may be effective. This complication is associated with varying degrees of pain that require adequate analgesic medication. Prolonged chest tube drainage with high levels of negative pressure (20 to 40 mm hg) may be required.

G. Prognosis

The clinical course can vary from days to years. In familial IPF cases, obvious carriers of the abnormal gene could remain asymptomatic. Varying degrees of pulmonary impairment and radiographic abnormalities occur. Intercurrent respiratory infections can be disastrous to those with marginal function. With advances in ambulatory oxygen therapy, more patients are living longer and with a better quality of life. Amelioration of dyspnea and improved exercise tolerance may result from successful steroid therapy and/or immunosuppressant treatment. Analysis of survival data in 100 consecutive patients aged 16 to 77 years showed a longer survival of younger patients and in patients with a shorter duration of symptoms before presentation. The most favorable diagnostic sign seemed to be an early response to steroid therapy.[167] Death occurs from chronic respiratory failure.

REFERENCES

1. **Crystal, R. G., Gadek, J. E., Ferrans, V. J., Fulmer, J. D., Line, B. R., and Hunninghake, G. W.,** Interstitial lung disease: current concepts of pathogenesis, staging and therapy, *Am. J. Med.,* 70, 542, 1981.
2. **Fulmer, J. D. and Crystal, R. G.,** Interstitial lung disease, in *Current Pulmonology,* Simmons, D. E., Ed., Houghton-Mifflin Professional Publishers, Boston, 1979.
3. **Fox, R. B., Hoidal, J. R., and Brown, D. M.,** Pulmonary inflammation due to oxygen toxicity: involvement of chemotactic factors and polymorphonuclear leukocytes, *Am. Rev. Resp. Dis.,* 123, 521, 1981.
4. **Hunninghake, G. W., Gadek, J. E., and Lawley, T. J.,** Mechanisms of neutrophil accumulation in the lungs of patients with idiopathic pulmonary fibrosis, *J. Clin. Invest.,* 68, 259, 1982.
5. **Kazmierowski, J. A., Gallin, J. I., and Reynolds, H.Y.,** Mechanisms for the inflammatory response in primate lungs: demonstration and partial characterization of an alveolar macrophage-derived chemotactic factor with preferential activity for polymorphonuclear leukocytes, *J. Clin. Invest.,* 59, 273, 1977.

6. **Ward, P. A.,** Immune complex injury of the lung, *Am. J. Pathol.,* 97, 85, 1979.
7. **Weissman, G., Smolen, J. E., and Korchak, H. M.,** Release of inflammatory mediators from stimulated neutrophils, *N. Engl. J. Med.,* 303, 27, 1980.
8. **Schatz, M., Patterson, R., and Fink, J.,** Immunologic lung disease, *N. Engl. J. Med.,* 300, 1310, 1979.
9. **Fauci, A. S.,** The spectrum of vasculitis: clinical, pathologic, immunologic, and therapeutic considerations, *Ann. Intern. Med.,* 89, 660, 1978.
10. **Liebow, A. A.,** New concepts and entities in pulmonary disease, in *The Lung,* Liebow, A.A. and Smith, D. E., Eds., Williams & Wilkins, Baltimore, 1968.
11. **Crystal, R. G. and Rennard, S. I.,** Pulmonary connective tissue and environmental lung disease, *Chest,* 80, 33S, 1981.
12. **Crystal, R. G., Fulmer, J. D., Roberts, W. C., Moss, M. L., Line, B. R., and Reynolds, H. Y.,** Idiopathic pulmonary fibrosis, clinical, histologic, radiographic, scintigraphic, and biochemical aspects, *Ann. Int. Med.,* 85, 769, 1976.
13. **Barr, H. S. and Galindo, J.,** Bronchiolitis obliterans, *Thorax,* 21, 209, 1966.
14. **Fawcitt, J. and Parry, H. E.,** Lung changes in pertussis and measles in childhood: a review of 1894 cases with a follow-up study of the pulmonary complications, *Br. J. Radiol.,* 30, 76, 1957.
15. **Sato, P., Madtes, D. K., Thorning, D., and Albert, R. K.,** Bronchiolitis obliterans caused by Legionella *pneumophila, Chest,* 87, 840, 1985.
16. **Reid, L., Simon, G., Zorab, R. A., and Seidelin, R.,** The development of unilateral hypertransradiancy of the lung, *Br. J. Dis. Chest,* 61, 190, 1967.
17. **Laraya-Cuasay, L. R., Deforest, A., Huff, D., Lischner, H., and Huang, N. N.,** Chronic pulmonary complications of early influenza virus infection, *Am. Rev. Resp. Dis.,* 116, 617, 1977.
18. **Becroft, D. M. P.,** Bronchiolitis obliterans, bronchiectasis and other sequelae of adenovirus type 21 infection in young children, *J. Clin. Pathol.,* 24, 72, 1971.
19. **Laraya-Cuasay, L. R.,** Pulmonary sequelae of acute respiratory viral infection, *Pediat. Ann.,* 7, 42, 1978.
20. **Stokes, D., Sigler, A., Khouri, N. F., and Talamo, R. C.,** Unilateral hyperlucent lung (Swyer-James syndrome) after severe Mycoplasma *pneumonia* infection, *Am. Rev. Resp. Dis.,* 117, 145, 1978.
21. **Lowry, T., Schuman, L. M.,** "Silo-filler's disease" — a syndrome caused by nitrogen dioxide, *JAMA,* 162, 153, 1956.
22. **Ramirez, R. J., Dowell, A. R.,** Silo-filler's disease: nitrogen dioxide-caused lung injury, *Ann. Int. Med.,* 74, 569, 1971.
23. **Castleman, W. L., Dungworth, D. L., Schwartz, L. W., and Tyler, W. S.,** Acute respiratory bronchiolitis, *Am. J. Pathol.,* 98, 811, 1980.
24. **Murphy, D. M. F., Fairman, R. P., Lapp, N. L., and Morgan, W. K. C.,** Severe airway disease due to inhalation of fumes from cleansing agents, *Chest,* 69, 372, 1976.
25. **Gosink, B. B., Friedman, P. J., and Liebow, A. A.,** Bronchiolitis obliterans: roentgenologic-pathologic correlations, *Am. J. Roentgenol.,* 117, 816, 1973.
26. **Geddes, D. M., Corrin, B., Brewerton, D. A., Davies, R. J., and Turner-Warwick, M.,** Progressive airway obliteration in adults and its association with rheumatoid disease, *Q. J. Med.,* 46, 427, 1977.
27. **Murphy, K. C., Atkins, C. J., Offer, R. C., Hogg, J. C., and Stein, H. B.,** Obliterative bronchiolitis in two rheumatoid patients treated with penicillamine, *Arth. Rheum.,* 24, 557, 1981.
28. **Nimni, M. E., and Bavetta, L. A.,** Collagen defect induced by penicillamine, *Science,* 150, 905, 1965.
29. **Cooney, T. P.,** Interrelationship of chronic eosinophilic pneumonia, bronchiolitis obliterans, and rheumatoid disease, a hypothesis, *J. Clin. Pathol.,* 34, 1828, 1981.
30. **Spencer, H.,** Diseases of the bronchial tree, in *Pathology of the Lung,* Pergamon Press, Oxford, 1985.
31. **Ostrow, D., Buskard, N., Hill, S., Vickars, L., and Churg, A.,** Bronchiolitis obliterans complicating bone marrow transplantation, *Chest,* 87, 1828, 1985.
32. **Link, H., Reinhard, D., and Neithammer, D.,** Obstructive ventilation disorders as a severe complication of chronic graft-versus-host disease after bone marrow transplantation, *Exp. Hematol.,* 10, 92, 1982.
33. **Ralph, D. D., Springmeyer, S. C., and Sullivan, K. M.,** Rapidly progressive airflow obstruction in marrow transplant recipients; possible association between obliterative bronchiolitis and graft-versus-host disease, *Am. Rev. Resp. Dis.,* 129, 641, 1984.
34. **Anderson, W. R. and Engel, R. R.,** Cardiopulmonary sequelae of reparative stages of bronchopulmonary dysplasia, *Arch. Pathol. Lab. Med.,* 107, 603, 1983.
35. **Moran, T. J. and Hellstrom, H. R.,** Bronchiolitis obliterans, *Arch. Pathol.,* 66, 691, 1958.
36. **Azizirad, H., Polgar, G., Borns, P. F., and Chatten, J.,** Bronchiolitis obliterans, *Clin. Pediatr.,* 14, 527, 1975.
37. **Spencer, H.,** Influenzal pneumonitis, in *Pathology of the Lung,* Pergamon Press, Oxford, 1985.
38. **Cumming, G. R., MacPherson, R. I., and Chernick, V.,** Unilateral hyperlucent lung syndrome, *J. Pediatr.,* 78, 250, 1971.
39. **Kogutt, M. S., Swischuk, L. E., and Goldblum, R.,** Swyer-James syndrome, (unilateral hyperlucent lung) in children, *Am. J. Dis. Child.,* 125, 614, 1973.

40. **Morrisey, W. L., Gould, L. A., and Carrington, C. B.**, Silofiller's disease, *Respiration*, 32, 81, 1975.
41. **Avery, G. B., Fletcher, A. B., Kaplan, M., and Brudno, S.**, Controlled trial of dexamethasone in respirator-dependent infants with bronchopulmonary dysplasia, *Pediatrics*, 75, 106, 1985.
42. **Lyle, W. H.**, D-penicillamine and fatal obliterative bronchiolitis, *Br. Med. J.*, 1, 105, 1977.
43. **Figueroa-Cases, J. C. and Jenkins, D. E.**, Unilateral hyperlucency (Swyer-James syndrome): case report with fourteen years observation, *Am. J. Med.*, 44, 301, 1968.
44. **Liebow, A. A., Steer, A., and Billingsley, J. G.**, Desquamative interstitial pneumonia, *Am. J. Med.*, 39, 369, 1965.
45. **McNary, W. F. and Gaensler, E. A.**, Intranuclear inclusion bodies in desquamative interstitial pneumonia, electron microscopic observations, *Ann. Int. Med.*, 74, 404, 1971.
46. **Hilman, B. C.**, Interstitial and hypersensitivity pneumonitis and their variants, *Pediatr. Rev.*, 1, 229, 1980.
47. **Daniele, R. P., Henson, P. M., Fantone, J. C., Ward, P. A., and Dreisin, R. B.**, Immune complex injury of the lung. State of the art, *Am. Rev. Resp. Dis.*, 124, 738, 1971.
48. **Dreisin, R. B., Schwarz, M. I., Theofilopoulus, A. N., and Stanford, R. E.**, Circulating immune complexes in the idiopathic interstitial pneumonia, *N. Engl. J. Med.*, 298, 353, 1978.
49. **Boner, A., Wilmott, R. W., Dinwiddie, R., Jeffries, D. J., Matthew, D. J., Marshall, W. C., Mowbray, J. F., Pincott, J. R., and Rivers, R. P.**, Desquamative interstitial pneumonia and antigen-antibody complexes in two infants with congenital rubella, *Pediatrics*, 72, 835, 1983.
50. **Tal, A., Maor, E., Bar-Ziv, J., and Gorodischer, R.**, Fatal desquamative interstitial pneumonia in three infant siblings, *J. Pediatr.*, 104, 873, 1984.
51. **Stillwell, P. C., Norris, D. G., O'Connell, E. J., Rosenow, E. C., III, Weiland, L. H., and Harrison, E. G., Jr.**, Desquamative pneumonitis in children, *Chest*, 77, 165, 1980.
52. **Scadding, J. G. and Hinson, K. F. W.**, Diffuse fibrosing alveolitis (diffuse interstitial fibrosis of the lungs). Correlation of histology at biopsy with diagnosis, *Thorax*, 22, 291, 1967.
53. **Patchefsky, A. S., Israel, H. L., Hoch, W. S., and Gordon, G.**, Desquamative interstitial pneumonia, relationship to interstitial fibrosis, *Thorax*, 28, 680, 1973.
54. **Liebow, A. A.**, Definition and classification of interstitial pneumonias in human pathology. Alveolar interstitium of the lung, *Prog. Respir. Res.*, 8, 1, 1975.
55. **Mc Cann, B. G. and Brewer, D. B.**, A case of desquamative interstitial pneumonia progressing to "honeycomb lung", *J. Pathol.*, 112, 199, 1974.
56. **Bhagwat, A. G., Wentworth, P., and Conen, P. E.**, Observations on the relationship of desquamative interstitial pneumonia and pulmonary alveolar proteinosis in childhood. A pathologic and experimental study, *Chest*, 58, 326, 1970.
57. **Hewitt, C. J., Hull, D., and Keeling**, Fibrosing alveolitis in infancy and childhood, *Arch. Dis. Child.*, 52, 22, 1977.
58. **Kapanci, Y. and Chauvet, M.**, La pneumonie desquamative interstitielle, *Schwweiz. Med. Worchenschr.*, 97, 1199, 1967.
59. **Schneider, R. M., Nevius, D. B., and Brown, H. Z.**, Desquamative interstitial pneumonia in 4-year old child, *N. Engl. J. Med.*, 277, 1056, 1967.
60. **Radice, C., Conconi, G., Quarti, M. K., et al.**, Pneumopatia interstiziale desquamativa, *Minerva. Pediatr.*, 1, 29, 1969.
61. **Buchta, R. M., Park, S., and Giammona, S. T.**, Desquamative interstitial pneumonia in a 7-week-old infant, *Am. J. Dis. Child.*, 120, 341, 1970.
62. **Rosenow, E. C., III, O'Connell, E. J., and Harrison, E. G., Jr.**, Desquamative interstitial pneumonia in children. Report of two cases, *Am. J. Dis. Child.*, 120, 344, 1970.
63. **Wipf, R.**, Pneumopathie interstitielle desquamative chez un écolier nord-africain vraisemblablement associée à une tuberculose pulmonaire, *Schweiz. Med. Wochenschr.*, 100, 1845, 1970.
64. **Bates, D. V., Macklem, P. T., and Christie, R. V.**, *Respiratory Function in Disease.*, W. B. Saunders, Philadelphia, 1971.
65. **Bolens, M., Mégevand, A., Kapanci, Y.**, Evolution d'une pneumonie desquamative interstitielle en fibrose pulmonaire diffuse, *Helv. Paediatr. Acta.*, 26, 114, 1971.
66. **Neuhauser, E. B. D.**, Desquamative interstitial pneumonia, *Postgrad. Med.*, 49, 65, 1971.
67. **Howatt, W. F., Heidelberger, K. P., Le glovan, D. P., and Schnitzer, B.**, Desquamative interstitial pneumonia. Case report of an infant unresponsive to treatment, *Am. J. Dis. Child.*, 126, 346, 1973.
68. **Barnes, W. E., Godfrey, S., Millward-Sadler, G. H., and Roberton, N. R.**, Desquamative fibrosing alveolitis unresponsive to steroid or cytotoxic therapy, *Arch. Dis. Child.*, 50, 324, 1975.
69. **Larbre, F., Déchelette, E., Gilly, J., et al.**, A propos d'un cas de pneumonie desquamative interstitielle chez un nourrisson, *Pediatrie.*, 30, 305, 1975.
70. **Vlagopoulos, B., Chung, H. T., Fitzmaurice, F. M., Cambell, J. C., and Villacorte, G. V.**, Desquamative interstitial pneumonia associated with granulomatous lymphadenopathy, *Chest*, 72, 780, 1977.

71. **Wigger, H. J., Berdon, W. E., and Ores, C. N.,** Fatal desquamative interstitial pneumonia in an infant. Case report with transmission and scanning electron microscopical studies, *Arch. Pathol. Lab. Med.,* 101, 129, 1977.
72. **Sokolowski, J. W. and Harrer, W. V.,** Desquamative interstitial pneumonia associated with normal chest film, *Postgrad. Med.,* 66, 135, 1979.
73. **Sahn, S. A. and Schwarz, M. I.,** Desquamative interstitial pneumonia with a normal chest radiograph, *Br. J. Dis. Chest,* 68, 228, 1874.
74. **Goldberg, N. M. and Mostyn, E. M.,** Desquamative interstitial pneumonia. A brief review of the literature and discussion of treatment with oxygen and corticosteroids, *Dis. Chest,* 52, 245, 1967.
75. **Epler, G. R. and Gaensler, E. A.,** Normal chest roentgenograms in chronic interstitial and pulmonary vascular disease, *Am. Rev. Resp. Dis.,* 115, 104, 1977.
76. **Carrington, C. B., Gaensler, E. A., Coutu, R. E., Fitzgerald, M., and Gupta, R. G.,** Natural history and treated course of usual and desquamative interstitial pneumonia, *N. Engl. J. Med.,* 298, 801, 1978.
77. **Leahy, F., Pasterkamp, H., and Tal, A.,** Desquamative interstitial pneumonia responsive to chloroquine, *Clin. Pediatr.,* 24, 230, 1985.
78. **Szilagi, T. and Karai, M.,** The effect of chloroquine on the antigen-antibody reaction, *Acta. Physiol. Acad. Sci. Hung.,* 38, 411, 1970.
79. **Hecht, V.,** Die Riesenzellen pneumonie im kindesalter eine historische experimentelle studie, *Beitr. Path. Anat.,* 48, 263, 1910.
80. **Pinkerton, H., Smiley, W. L., and Anderson, W. A. D.,** Giant cell pneumonia with inclusions. Lesion common to Hecht's disease, distemper, and measles, *Am. J. Path.,* 21, 1, 1945.
81. **Adams, J. M. and Imagawa, D. T.,** The relationship of canine distemper to human respiratory disease, *Pediatr. Clin. North Am.,* 4, 193, 1957.
82. **McCarthy, K., Mitus, A., Cheatham, W., and Peebles, T. C.,** Isolation of virus of measles from three fatal cases of giant cell pneumonia, *Am. J. Dis. Child.,* 96, 500, 1958.
83. **Enders, J. F., McCarthy, K., Mitus, A., and Cheatham, W. J.,** Isolation of measles virus at autopsy in cases of giant cell pneumonia, *N. Engl. J. Med.,* 261, 875, 1959.
84. **Mitus, A., Enders, J. F., Craig, J. M., and Holloway, A.,** Persistence of measles virus and depression of antibody formation in patients with giant cell pneumonia after measles, *N. Engl. J. Med.,* 261, 882, 1959.
85. **Janigan, J. T.,** Giant cell pneumonia and measles: ana analytical review, *Can. Med. Assoc. J.,* 85, 741, 1961.
86. **Archibald, R. W. R., Weller, R. O., and Meadow, S. R.,** Measles pneumonia, and the nature of inclusion-bearing giant cells: a light and electron microscopic study, *J. Pathol.,* 103, 27, 1971.
87. **Spencer, H.,** Pneumonias due to rickettsiae, Bedsoniae, viruses and mycoplasma, in *Pathology of the Lung,* Pergamon Press, Oxford, 1985.
88. **Reddy, P. A., Gorelick, D. F., and Christianson, C. S.,** Giant cell interstitial pneumonia (GIP), *Chest,* 58, 319, 1970.
89. **Sherman, F. E., Ruckle, G.,** In vivo and in vitro cellular changes for measles, *Arch. Pathol.,* 65, 587, 1958.
90. **Koffler, D.,** Giant cell pneumonia. Fluorescent antibody and histochemical studies on alveolar giant cells, *Arch. Pathol.,* 78, 267, 1964.
91. **Lewis, M. J., Cameron, A. H., Shah, K. J., Purdham, D. R., and Mann, J. R.,** Giant cell pneumonia caused by measles and methotrexate in childhood leukaemia in remission, *Br. Med. J.,* 1, 330, 1978.
92. **Sokolowski, J. W., Cordray, D. R., and Cantow, E. F.,** Giant cell pneumonia: report of a case, *Am. Rev. Resp. Dis.,* 195, 417, 1972.
93. **Young, L. W. and Ross, D. W.,** Radiological case of the month, Giant cell pneumonia, *Am. J. Dis. Child.,* 134, 511, 1980.
94. **Hull, H. F., Montes, J. M., Hays, P. C., and Lucero, R. L.,** Risk factors for measles vaccine failure among immunized students, *Pediatrics,* 76, 518, 1985.
95. **Bloch, A. B., Orenstein, W. A., Stetler, H. C., Wassilak, S. G., Amler, R. W., Bart, K. J., Kirby, C. D., and Hinman, A. R.,** Health impact of measles vaccination in the United States, *Pediatrics,* 76, 524, 1985.
96. **Amler, R. W., Block, A. B., Orenstein, W. A., Bart, K. J., Turner, P. M., Jr., and Hinman, A. R.,** Imported measles in the United States, *JAMA,* 248, 2129, 1982.
97. **Mawhinney, H., Allen, I. V., and Beare, J. M.,** Dysgamma-globulinemia complicated by disseminated measles, *Br. Med. J.,* 2, 380, 1971.
98. **Breitfeld, V., Hashida, Y., and Sherman, F. E.,** Fatal measles infection in children with leukemia, *Lab. Invest.,* 28, 279, 1973.
99. **Laraya-Cuasay, L. R. and Germon, P.,** Long-term follow-up of post-measles obliterative bronchiolitis, bronchitis and bronchiectasis, submitted for publication.

100. **Fawcitt, J. and Parry, H. E.,** Lung changes in pertussis and measles in childhood. A review of 1894 cases with a follow-up study of the pulmonary complications, *Br. J. Radiol.,* 30, 76, 1957.

101. **Neva, F. A. and Ottesen, E. A.,** Tropical (filarial) eosinophilia, *N. Engl. J. Med.,* 298, 1129, 1978.

102. **Crofton, J. W., Livingston, J. L., Oswald, N. C., and Roberts, A. T. M.,** Pulmonary eosinophilia, *Thorax,* 7, 1, 1952.

103. **Loeffler, W.,** Zur differential-Diagnose der Lungeninfiltrierungen. II. Ueber flectige Succedan-Infiltrate (mit Eosinophilie), *Beitr. Klin. Tuberk.,* 79, 368, 1932.

104. **Spencer, H.,** Pulmonary parasitic diseases, in *Pathology of the Lung,* Pergamon Press, Oxford, 1985.

105. **Wilson, I. C., Gambill, J. M., and Sandifer, M. G.,** Loeffler's syndrome occurring during Imipramine therapy, *Am. J. Psychiat.,* 119, 892, 1963.

106. **Pearsall, H. R., Ewalt, J., Tsoi, M., Sumida, S., and Backus, D.,** Nitrofurantoin lung sensitivity, *J. Lab. Clin. Med.,* 83, 728, 1974.

107. **Rosenow, E. C., III,** Drug-induced pulmonary disease, *Clin. Notes Resp. Dis.,* 16, 3, 1977.

108. **Massie, F. S.,** Hypersensitivity pneumonitis and pulmonary reactions to rugs and chemicals, in *Allergic Diseases of Infancy, Childhood and Adolescence,* Bierman, C. W. and Pearlman, D. S., Eds., W. B. Saunders, Philadelphia, 620, 1980.

109. **Chandra, R. K.,** Visceral larva migrans, *Indian J. Pediatr.,* 30, 338, 1963.

110. **Weingarten, R. J.,** Tropical eosinophilia, *Lancet,* 1, 103, 1943.

111. **Donohugh, D. L.,** Tropical eosinophilia, an etiologic inquiry, *N. Engl. J. Med.,* 269, 1357, 1963.

112. **Hinson, K. F. W., Moon, A. J., and Plummer, N. S.,** Bronchopulmonary aspergillosis. A review and a report of eight new cases, *Thorax,* 7, 317, 1952.

113. **Jelihovsky, T.,** The structure of bronchial plugs in mucoid impaction, bronchocentric granulomatosis and asthma, *Histopathology,* 7, 153, 1983.

114. **Wang, J. L. F., Patterson, R., Roberts, M., and Ghory, A. C.,** The management of allergic bronchopulmonary aspergillosis, *Am. Rev. Resp. Dis.,* 120, 87, 1979.

115. **Citro, L. A., Gordon, M. E., and Miller, W. T.,** Eosinophilic lung disease, (or how to slice P.I.E.), *Am. J. Roentgen. Rad. Ther. Nucl. Med.,* 117, 787, 1973.

116. **Carrington, C. D., Addington, W. W., Goff, A. M., Madoff, I. M., Marks, A., Schwaber, J. R., and Gaensler, E. A.,** Chronic eosinophilic pneumonia, *N. Engl. J. Med.,* 280, 787, 1969.

117. **Rao, M., Steiner, P., Rose, J., Kassner, E. G., Kottmeier, P., and Steiner, M.,** Chronic eosinophilic pneumonia in a one year-old child, *Chest,* 68, 118, 1975.

118. **Hamman, I., and Rich, A. R.,** Fulminating diffuse interstitial fibrosis of the lungs, *Trans. Am. Clin. Climatol. Assoc.,* 52, 154, 1935.

119. **Hamman, I. and Rich, A. R.,** Acute diffuse interstitial fibrosis of the lungs, *Bull. Johns Hopkins Hosp.,* 74, 177, 1944.

120. **Rubin, E. H. and Lubiner, R.,** The Hamman-Rich syndrome; review of literature and analysis of 15 cases, *Medicine,* 36, 397, 1957.

121. **O'Shea, P. A. and Yardley, J. H.,** The Hamman-Rich syndrome in infancy: report of a case with virus-like particles by electron microscopy, *Johns Hopkins Med. J.,* 126, 320, 1970.

122. **Pinkser, K. L., Schneyer, B., Becker, N., and Kamholz, S.,** Usual interstitial pneumonia following Texas A$_2$ influenza infection, *Chest,* 80, 123, 1981.

123. **Haufman, J. M., Cuvelier, C. A., and vanderStareten, M.,** Mycoplasma pneumonia with fulminant evolution into diffuse interstitial fibrosis, *Thorax,* 35, 140, 1980.

124. **Kravis, T. C., Ahmed, A., Brown, T. E., Fulmer, J. D., and Crystal, R. G.,** Pathogenic mechanisms in pulmonary fibrosis, *J. Clin. Invest.,* 58, 1223, 1976.

125. **Rudd, R. M., Haslam, P. L., and Turner-Warwick, M.,** Cryptogenic fibrosing alveolitis, relationship of pulmonary physiology and bronchoalveolar lavage to response to treatment and prognosis, *Am. Rev. Resp. Dis.,* 124, 1, 1981.

126. **Reynolds, H. Y., Fulmer, J. D., and Kazmirowski, J. A.,** Analysis of cellular and protein content of bronchoalveolar lavage fluid from patients with idiopathic pulmonary fibrosis and chronic hypersensitivity pneumonitis, *J. Clin. Invest.,* 59, 165, 1977.

127. **Haslam, P. L., Thompson, B., Mohammed, I., Townsend, P. J., Hodson, M. E., Holborow, E. J., and Turner-Warwick, M.,** Circulating immune complexes in patients with cryptogenic fibrosing alveolitis, *Clin. Exp. Immunol.,* 37, 381, 1979.

128. **Donohue, W. I., Laski, B., Uchida, I., and Mann, J. D.,** Familial fibrocystic pulmonary dysplasia and its relation to the Hamman-Rich syndrome, *Pediatrics,* 24, 786, 1959.

129. **King, T. K. C., and Norum, R. A.,** Unusual inherited pulmonary diseases which provide clues to pulmonary physiology and function, in *Genetic Determinants of Pulmonary Disease,* Lenfant, C., Ed., Marcel Dekker Inc. New York, 1977.

130. **Solliday, N. H., Williams, J. A., Gaensler, E. A., Coutu, R. E., and Carrington, C. B.,** Familial chronic interstitial pneumonia, *Am. Rev. Resp. Dis.,* 108, 193, 1973.

131. **Swaye, P., Van Orstrand, H. S., McCormack, L. J., and Wolpaw, S. E.,** Familial Hamman-Rich syndrome, report of eight cases, *Chest,* 55, 7, 1969.
132. **McKusick, V. A. and Fisher, A. M.,** Congenital cystic disease of the lung with progressive pulmonary fibrosis and carcinomatosis, *Ann. Int. Med.,* 48, 774, 1958.
133. **Bonnani, P., Frymoyer, J. W., and Jacox, R. F. F.,** A family study of idiopathic pulmonary fibrosis, *Am. J. Med.,* 39, 411, 1965.
134. **Libby, D. M., Gobofsky, A., Fotino, M., Waters, S. J., and Smith, J. P.,** Immunogenetic and clinical findings in idiopathic pulmonary fibrosis, *Am. Rev. Resp. Dis.,* 127, 618, 1983.
135. **Auwer, J., Demedts, M., Boiullon, R., and Desmet, J.,** Coexistence of hypocalciuric hypercalcemia and interstitial lung disease in a family: a cross-sectional study, *Eur. J. Clin. Invest.,* 15, 6, 1985.
136. **Malik, S. K., Pardee, N., and Martin, C. J.,** Involvement of the lung in tuberous sclerosis, *Chest,* 58, 538, 1970.
137. **Massaro, D. and Katz, S.,** Fibrosing alveolitis, its occurrence in von Recklinghausen's neurofibromatosis, *Am. Rev. Resp. Dis.,* 93, 934, 1966.
138. **Garay, S. M., Gardella, J. E., Fazzini, E. P., and Goldring, R. M.,** Hermansky-Pudlak syndrome: pulmonary manifestation of a ceroid storage disorder, *Am. J. Med.,* 66, 737, 1979.
139. **Carrington, C. B., Cergell, D. W., Gaensler, E. A., Marks, A., Redding, R. A., Schaaf, J. T., and Tomasian, A.,** Lymphangioleiomyomatosis, *Am. Rev. Resp. Dis.,* 116, 977, 1977.
140. **Diamond, I.,** The Hamman-Rich syndrome in childhood, report of a case with unilateral arterial and venous stenosis and arteriovenous occlusion, *Pediatrics,* 22, 279, 1958.
141. **Fulmer, J. D.,** An introduction to the interstitial lung diseases, *Clin. Chest Med.,* 3, 457, 1982.
142. **Johnston, D. I.,** Persistent diarrhea, eosinophilia, erythema annulare and fibrosing alveolitis in a female infant, *Proc. Roy. Soc. Med.,* 66, 346, 1973.
143. **Fraire, A., Greenberg, S. D., O'Neal, R. M., Weg, J. G., and Jenkins, D. E.,** Diffuse interstitial fibrosis of the lung, *Am. J. Clin. Pathol.,* 59, 636, 1973.
144. **Feinerman, B. and Harris, L. E.,** Unusual interstitial pneumonitis, report of two cases in children, *Proc. Staff Meet. Mayo Cli.,* 32, 637, 1957.
145. **Macmillan, J. M.,** Familial pulmonary fibrosis, *Dis. Chest,* 20, 426, 1951.
146. **Grant, I. W. B., Hillis, B. R., and Davidson, J.,** Diffuse interstitial fibrosis of the lungs (Hamman-Rich syndrome), *Am. Rev. Tuberc.,* 74, 485, 1956.
147. **Bradley, C. A.,** Diffuse fibrosis of the lungs in childhood, *J. Pediat.,* 48, 442, 1956.
148. **Aranson, A.,** Hamman-Rich syndrome, *J. Maine M. A.,* 47, 105, 1956.
149. **Baar, H. S. and Braid, F.,** Diffuse progressive interstitial fibrosis of the lungs in childhood, *Arch. Dis. Child.,* 32, 199, 1957.
150. **Sandoz, E.,** Über zwei Fälle von Fötaler Bronchektasie, *Beitr. Path. Anat.,* 41, 495, 1907.
151. **Genereux, G. P.,** The end-stage lung: pathogenesis, pathology and radiology, *Radiology,* 116, 279, 1975.
152. **Epler, G. R., McCloud, T. C., Gaensler, E. A., Mikus, J. P., and Carrington, C. B.,** Normal roentgenograms in chronic diffuse infiltrative disease, *N. Engl. J. Med.,* 298, 934, 1978.
153. **Lemire, P., Bettez, P., Gelinas, M., and Raymond, G.,** Patterns of desquamative interstitial pneumonia (DIP) and diffuse interstitial pulmonary fibrosis (DIPF), *Am. J. Roentgen. Rad. Ther. Nucl. Med.,* 115, 479, 1972.
154. **Austrian, R., McClement, J. H., Renzetti, A. D., Donald, K. W., Riley, R. L., and Cournand, A.,** Clinical and physiologic features of some types of pulmonary diseases with impairment of alveolar-capillary diffusion. The syndrome of alveolar-capillary block, *Am. J. Med.,* 11, 667, 1951.
155. **Finley, T. N., Swenson, E. W., and Comroe, J. H., Jr.,** The cause of arterial hypoxemia at rest in patients with "alveolar-capillary block syndrome", *J. Clin. Invest.,* 41, 618, 1962.
156. **Wagner, P. D., Dantzker, D. R., and Dueck, R.,** Distribution of ventilation-perfusion ratios in patients with interstitial lung disease, *Chest,* 69, 256, 1976.
157. **Zapletal, A., Houstek, J., Samanek, M., and Paul, T.,** Lung function in children and adolescents with idiopathic interstitial pulmonary fibrosis, *Pediatr. Pulmonol.,* 1, 154, 1985.
158. **Gaultier, C., Chaussain, M., Boule, M., Buvry, A., Allaire, Y., Perret, L., and Girard, F.,** Lung function in interstitial lung disease in children, *Bull. Europ, Physiopathol. Respir.,* 16, 57, 1980.
159. **McCarthy, D. and Cherniack, R. M.,** Regional ventilation-perfusion and hypoxia in cryptogenic fibrosing alveolitis, *Am. Rev. Resp. Dis.,* 107, 200, 1973.
160. **Kornbluth, R. S. and Turino, G. M.,** Respiratory control in diffuse interstitial lung disease and diseases of the pulmonary vasculature, *Clin. Chest. Med.,* 1, 91, 1980.
161. **Perez-Padilla, R., West, P., Lertzman, M., and Kryger, M. H.,** Breathing during sleep in patients with interstitial lung disease, *Am. Rev. Resp. Dis.,* 132, 224, 1985.
162. **Weese, W. C., Levine, B. W., and Kazemi, H.,** Interstitial lung disease resistant to corticosteroid therapy: report of three cases treated with azathioprine or cyclophosphamide, *Chest,* 67, 57, 1975.
163. **Brown, C. H. and Turner-Warwick, M.,** The treatment of cryptogenic fibrosing alveolitis with immunosuppressant drugs, *Q. J. Med.,* XL, 289, 1971.

164. **Scott, D. G. I. and Bacon, P. A.,** Response to methotrexate in fibrosing alveolitis associated with connective tissue disease, *Thorax,* 35, 725, 1980.

165. **Haslam, P. L., Turton, C. W. G., Lukoszek, A., Salsbury, A. J., Dewar, A., Collins, J. V., and Turner-Warwick, M.,** Bronchoalveolar lavage fluid cell count in cryptogenic fibrosing alveolitis and their relation to therapy, *Thorax,* 35, 328, 1980.

166. **Ozaki, T., Nakayama, T., Ishimi, H., Kawano, T., Yasuoka, S., and Tsubura, E.,** Glucocorticoid receptor in bronchoalveolar cells of patients with idiopathic pulmonary fibrosis, *Am. Rev. Resp. Dis.,* 126, 968, 1982.

167. **Tuliairen, P., Taskinen, E., Holsti, P., Korhola, O., and Valle, M.,** Prognosis of cryptogenic fibrosing alveolitis, *Thorax,* 38, 349, 1983.

Chapter 42

LYMPHOPROLIFERATIVE DISORDERS OF THE LUNG

Lourdes R. Laraya-Cuasay

TABLE OF CONTENTS

I. INTRODUCTION

This chapter deals with the lymphoproliferative disorders in children which should be considered in the differential diagnosis of interstitial lung infiltrates.

Lymphoid tissue is found throughout the lung organized into various levels structurally, viz., tracheobronchial and hilar lymph nodes (see Chapter 4). There are lymphoid nodules lacking capsules in the walls of the large and medium-sized bronchi. Lymphoid aggregates and infiltrates are distributed diffusely throughout peripheral lung tissue which includes specialized "lymphoepithelial organs" in the respiratory bronchioles which may act as primary antigen-intake points.[1,2] Blood supply to these lymphoid aggregates come from the pulmonary artery which has an extensive capillary network.

II. FAMILIAL ERYTHROPHAGOCYTIC LYMPHOHISTIOCYTOSIS

A. Definition

Familial erythrophagocytic lymphohistiocytosis (FEL) is a rapidly fatal illness occurring usually in infancy, characterized by fever, hepatosplenomegaly, and central nervous system involvement. Nonmalignant lymphohistiocytic infiltrate with prominent erythrophagocytosis has been observed.[3]

B. Clinical Features

Pneumonitis may be part of the initial presenting manifestations[4,5] with fever and hepatosplenomegaly, without frank anemia or distinct pallor being noted immediately. Lymphadenopathy could also be a prominent feature.[6,7] Elevation of serum triglyceride, normal alpha-lipocholesterol, decreased high density lipoprotein cholesterol and severe decrease in protein, increased pre-beta and decreased beta lipoprotein have all been noted.[4]

The author has seen a unique case of FEL in a 17-month-old black female at Middlesex General-University Hospital in 1979. The infant was born to a heroin-addicted 30-year-old mother who was periodically on methadone maintenance. At 3 months of age, FEL was diagnosed from a lymph node biopsy. Thereafter, she had received chemotherapy consisting of hydrocortisone, cyclophosphamide, and vinblastine. Progressive respiratory failure occurred and she died at 20 months of age. At post-mortem examination, FEL was confirmed. The lung showed lymphohistiocytic infiltrates. This was the second case of FEL in the New Brunswick, New Jersey area. The chest roentgenogram is shown in Figure 1A and photomicrographs of the lung are shown in Figures 1B and 1C.

C. Etiopathogenesis

Defects in humoral and cellular immunity and the presence of a plasma inhibitor of in vitro lymphocyte blastogenesis were the features in four reported cases of FEL also with hyperlipidemia.[8] Whether immunodeficiency is the primary defect or is secondary to some other yet ill-defined primary pathogenic mechanism remains unknown.[9]

Its occurrence is suggestive of autosomal recessive inheritance. FEL has been reported in first cousins,[10] in a child from consanguineous union,[7] in several cases of affected siblings,[8,9,11,12] and in two pregnancies after artificial insemination.[11]

D. Pathology

Parenchymal infiltration by lymphocytes, histiocytes, and erythrophagocytes had been found in the liver, lung, spleen bone marrow, and central nervous system. Hepatic fatty metamorphosis and cellular infiltrates, hypoplastic bone marrow, with hemophagocytosis, splenic and nodal lymphoid depletion, and aseptic meningitis had also been observed. Interstitial pneumonitis was noted in both lungs of one patient.[4]

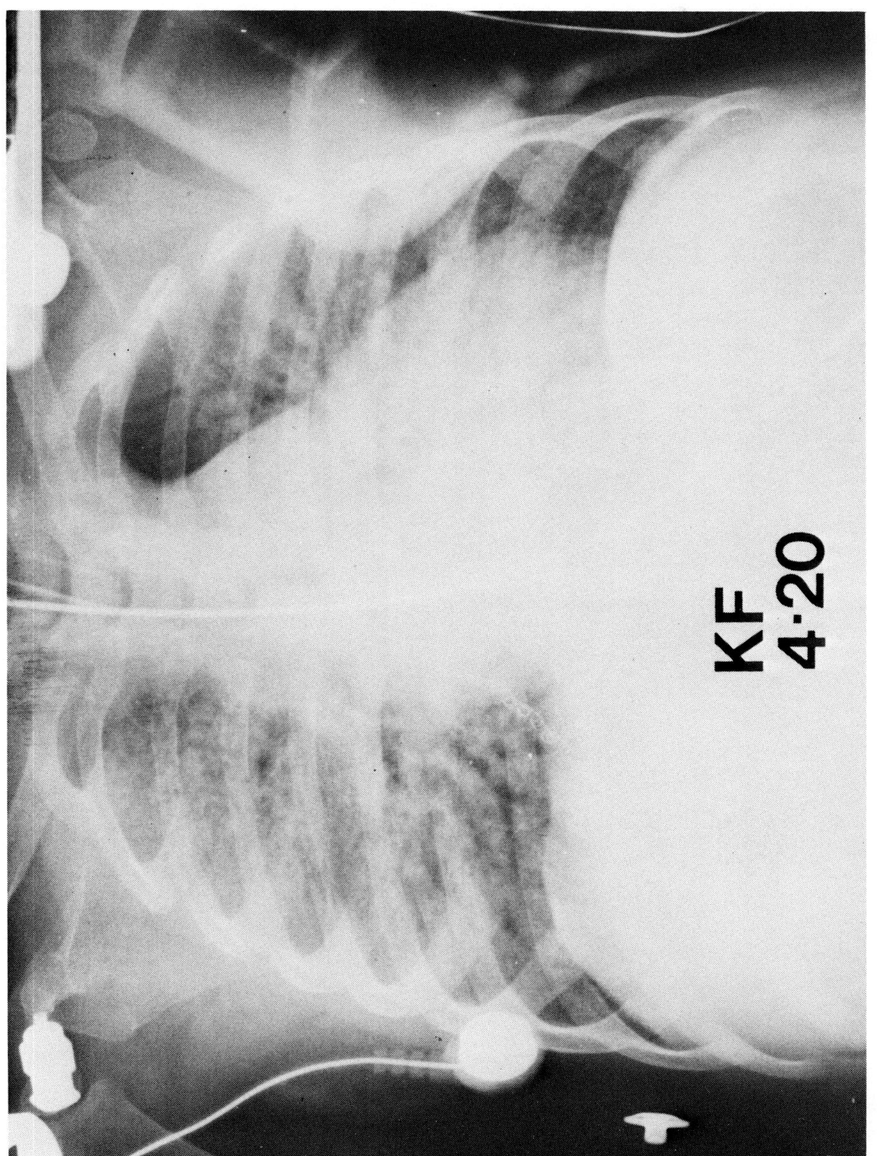

FIGURE 1A.   Chest roentgenogram showing the diffuse interstitial infiltrates in a 20-months-old infant with pulmonary biopsyproven familial erythrophagocytic lymphohistiocytosis.

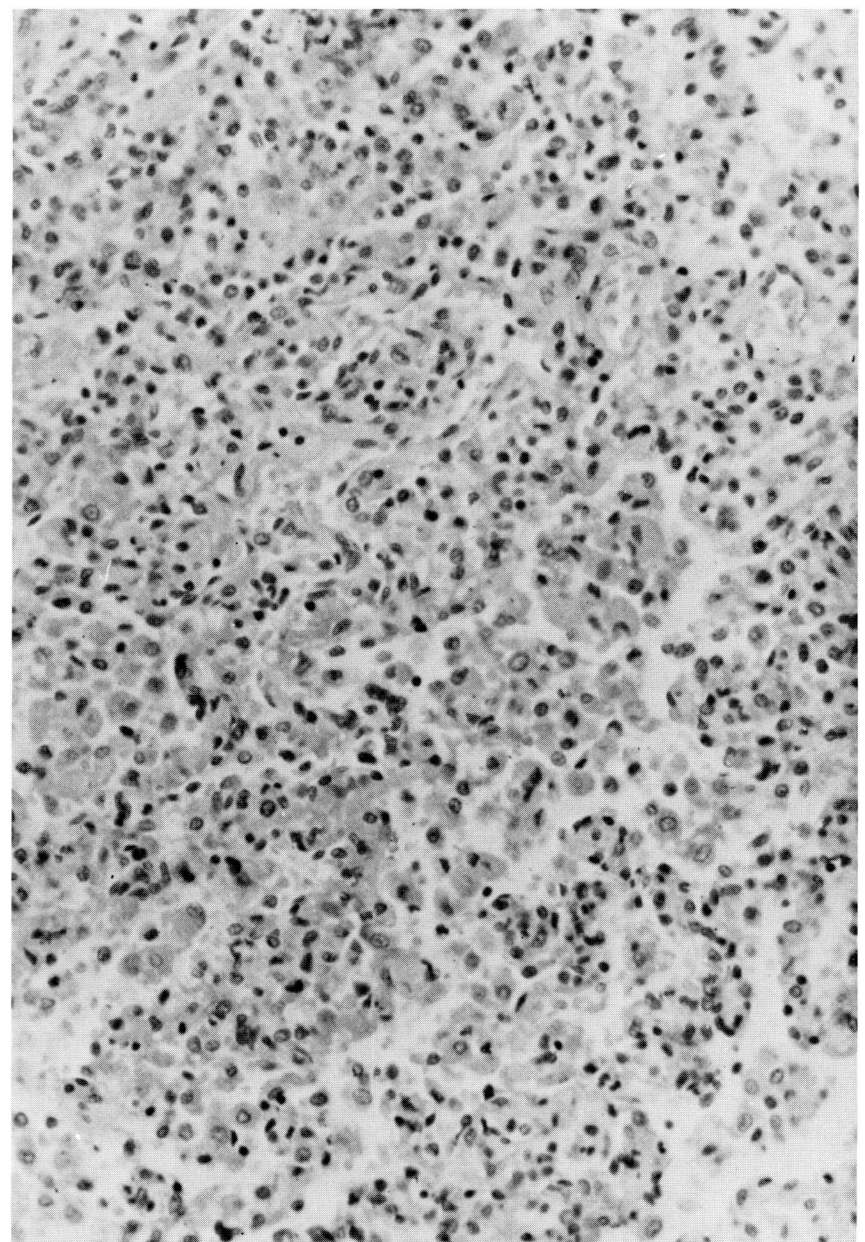

FIGURE 1B.   Photomicrograph of the lung showing extensive interstitial infiltrate. The alveolar spaces are thickened as a result of lymphohistiocytic infiltrate.

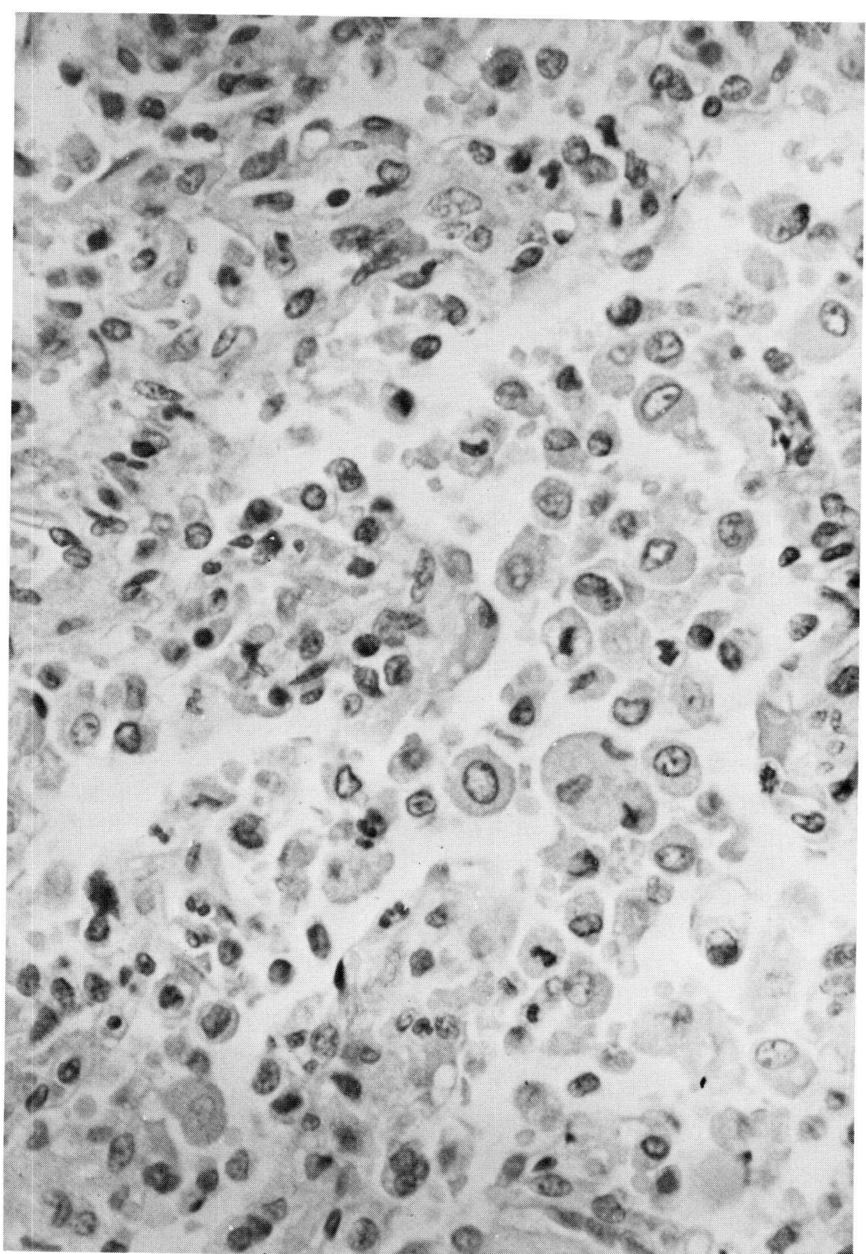

FIGURE 1C. Some histiocytes show the erythrophagocytic phenomenon. There are giant cells with hemosiderin. (H. E. stain, × 142). Courtesy of Department of Pathology, Middlesex General-University Hospital New Brunswick, New Jersey, and Dr. N. Zaeri, Department of Pathology, St. Christopher's Hospital for Children, Philadelphia.)

FEL must be differentiated from malignant histiocytosis, Letterer-Siwe disease and virus-associated hemophagocytic syndrome (VAHS).[14] If abnormal serum lipid values are found, malignant hyperlipidemia (MH) of infancy has to be excluded,[15] since the findings are similar except that erythrophagocytes are not prominent in MH. Whether these two entities represent different stages of the same process remains to be elucidated.

E. Management and Prognosis

Previous attempts to influence its fatal course have been unsuccessful although remission of FEL in two patients after treatment with VP 16-213, a mitotic spindle inhibitor has been reported by Ambruso who found that the drug corrected the serum lipoprotein abnormalities.[16] Four patients with FEL were treated with a combination of epidophyllotoxin, steroids, intrathecal methotrexate, and cranial irradiation, and all four patients had disease-free survival exceeding twelve months and remission of the disease for 27, 20, 16, and 13 months after onset of disease without major setbacks from the treatment.[17] The importance of early diagnosis of FEL in infants with fever, hepatosplenomegaly, central nervous system disease, turbid serum, and pancytopenia, who have hypertriglyceridemia and absent beta-lipoprotein becomes more important in view of these reported successes in treatment.

III. ANGIOIMMUNOBLASTIC LYMPHADENOPATHY

A. Definition

Angioimmunoblastic lymphadenopathy (AILD) is an uncommon, non-neoplastic lymphoproliferative disorder characterized by generalized lymphadenopathy, hepatosplenomegaly, intermittent maculopapular exanthema, frequent fever, weight loss, pruritus, hemolytic anemia, increased frequency of infections and changes in gammaglobulin pattern.[18-20]

B. Etiopathogenesis

The etiology is unknown. Various investigators have suggested a graft-vs.-host reaction,[18] autoimmune disorder,[20] continuing antigenic stimulation,[21] a T-cell deficiency theory or hyperimmune B-cell proliferation.[19] The basic process seems to be a non-neoplastic hyperimmune response and B-cell proliferation involving an exaggeration of lymphocyte transformation to immunoblasts and plasma cells that may be triggered by a hypersensitivity reaction.[19] Functional study of peripheral lymphocytes reveal decreased T-lymphocyte activity consistent with deficient T-cell regulation.[22]

Drugs have been implicated in the causation of AILD. Among these drugs are antibiotics,[18,19,23] primidone,[24] acetylsalicylic acid,[18] chronic liver extract injection,[21] hydroxychloroquine,[25] methyldopa,[26] and insulin.[27] Hydroxychloroquine enhances the expression of the Epstein-Barr virus[28,29] which is believed to be oncogenic in humans and has been incriminated in the development of several lymphoproliferative disorders.[30] Chronic antigenic stimulation by asbestos as predisposing to the development of the immunoproliferative disorder has been seen.[31] Sztern and associates reported AILD and slow-growing squamous cell carcinoma of the lung in a 71-year-old man who refused therapy but who continued to feel well. Their observation raises the possibility that AILD may be secondary to prolonged antigenic stimulation by a slowly growing solid tumor of the lung.[32] Adenocarcinoma of the pancreas has also been reported with AILD.[33]

A high serum Yersinia enterocolitica titer has been found in a 73-year-old man with AILD who was initially treated with trimethoprim-sulfamethoxazole.[34] In at least three cases of chronic relapsing polyneuropathy, an association with AILD has been found.[35]

AILD has been found to be associated with dysproteinemia,[18,23,36,37] including the dysproteinemia in homosexual men with acquired immune deficiency syndrome. Hashimoto's thyroiditis has also been associated with AILD.[38]

Cytogenetic and pathologic studies had been performed on six patients with AILD. None had shown chromosomal abnormalities in their bone marrow cells. Lymph node cells had shown nonrandom acquired clonal chromosomal abnormalities which are consistent features of malignancies.[39] This study suggests that AILD may be a malignant disease despite its original description as a benign proliferative process.

C. Pathologic Features

Histologically, the disease is systemic but lesions in the lymph nodes are specific. The lymph node of AILD presents with the characteristic triad composed of (1) proliferation of arborizing small vessels with thick endothelium; (2) a mixed population of cells, including lymphoid cells of various sizes ranging from small round lymphocytes to immunoblasts, typical plasma cells, eosinophils, neutrophils, and histiocytes; and (3) a small amount of intercellular matrix which is PAS-positive and which ultrastructurally shows to be redundant cell membrane and cytoplasm that only appear to be extracellular by light microscopy.[40,41]

The diagnostic features in bone marrow are focal or relatively circumscribed. Vascular and fibroblastic proliferation with paratrabecular localization and cellular depletion within the lesion surrounded by a hypercellular marrow is usually found. Lymphoid cells of varying sizes may be present.[42] Eosinophilia is not a prominent marrow feature as contrasted with "eosinophilic fibrohistiocytic lesion of bone marrow" where abundant eosinophils is a constant feature, vascular proliferation is absent and scarce immunocytes can be found.[43] When the lymph node biopsy is not definitive for AILD, a bone marrow core biopsy may aid in making the diagnosis.

The spleen, liver, skin, and lung are also involved but changes are less characteristic. Immunofluorescence studies have suggested the presence of cells elaborating a variety of immunoglobulins with an unpredictable pattern.[24]

D. Clinical Features

AILD usually affects elderly patients with average onset of illness at 60 years of age. The onset may be acute or insidious. However, there are very few reports of onset in childhood.[44-47] The clinical description of the disease in children is similar to that in the older age group. Constitutional symptoms, hepatosplenomegaly, skin rashes, anemia with positive Coombs' test and polyclonal hypergammaglobulinemia are present. In the four children described in literature and in one boy whom the author has cared for over 5 years,[48] the clinical findings were generalized lymphadenopathy, hepatosplenomegaly, fever, pruritus, skin rash which was malar usually and intermittent, hyperhidrosis especially at night, and progressive weight loss. All the children were male. The earliest onset was at $2^1/_2$ months in the reported cases. The onset in our patient was at 8 months. Polyclonal hypergammaglobulinemia, anemia and leukocytosis were found in all children. A positive Coombs' test was found in one half of all reported cases. A normochromic normocytic anemia was present in 84% of patients and only one third of these patients had positive Coombs' test. Diagnostic lesions were found in sections of bone marrow core biopsies of spicules closely resembling the lymph node histologically.[42]

Pulmonary infiltrates were present in two children and mediastinal and hilar adenopathy were found in three children.[44,47] Radiographic findings reported in AILD include interstitial pneumonia,[49] pulmonary infiltrates,[50] and combination of parenchymal involvement and hilar and mediastinal lymphadenopathy with or without pleural involvement.[51,52] Pleural effusions have also been found.[53,54] Immunoblasts were identified in pleural fluid. A linear or reticulonodular interstitial pattern is often seen associated with pulmonary fibrosis, and septal lines may be present. Parenchymal infiltrates are frequently seen in the lower lung zones. Alveolar disease may resemble pneumonia or pulmonary edema. Our patient showed interstitial pattern with mediastinal and hilar enlargement[48] (see Figure 2).

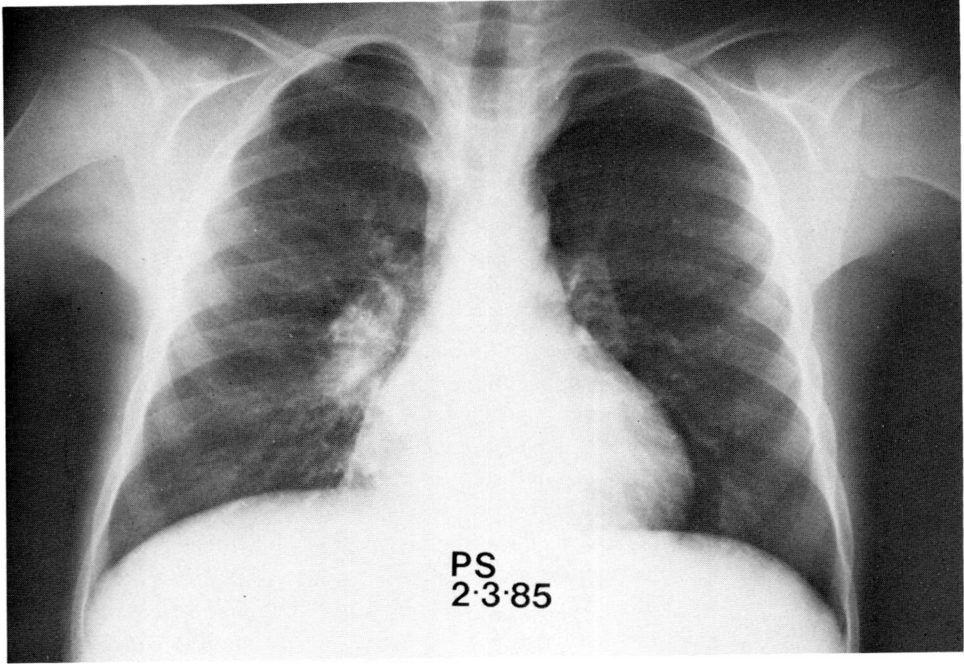

FIGURE 2.   Chest roentgenogram of a 7-year-old male with AILD demonstrating the interstitial infiltrates, mediastinal, and hilar nodal involvement.

AILD may occur together with neurological manifestation as in Fisher syndrome, the ophthalmoplegic variant of Guillain-Barre syndrome (GBS).[55] GBS is also an immunologically mediated disease thought to be caused by delayed hypersensitivity against peripheral myelin or components of myelin.[56] Neurologic complications of AILD include intracerebral hemorrhage, polyneuropathies, spinal cord compression, meningeal infiltration and infection of the central nervous system.[24,34]

Selective myeloid hypoplasia may be associated with AILD.[57] Hypogammaglobulinemia was found in a case of AILD where monocyte suppression may have been implicated in the clinical disease manifested.[58]

Intestinal involvement can be very striking as a result of marked tumorous infiltration of the organ.[59] The gastric involvement may be very prominent.[60] Massive abdominal lymphadenopathy including paraortic and peripancreatic lymph nodes can cause gastrointestinal symptoms to be predominant.

Renal involvement can also be present.[61] Polyarthritis has been reported to occur.[62] Immunoblastic proliferation in the synovium may have occurred such as has been reported in rheumatic diseases.

The clinical course can be very stormy or prolonged and protracted with lymphadenopathy getting more prominent with every acute infection, and regressing in size with steroid therapy.[44] *De novo* disseminated intravascular coagulation in AILD occurred in a nonseptic 80-year-old woman in whom the process reversed after receiving vincristine, methylprednisolone and heparin therapy.[63]

E. Management

Since AILD has been attributed to an abnormal activity of B-lymphocyte, Levamisole has been used as it is a stimulant of the thymus-dependent lymphoid system, and may restore the physiological repression of the T or the B system.[64] The use of levamisole and cytostatics have been studied during sequential therapy in four patients with AILD and the percentage of T-cells tended to fall with increasing disease activity,[65] while the percentage of the B-cells remained almost constant. Improvement in disease status coincided with an improvement of the blast transformation response. Polychemotherapy produced clinical remission and improved blast transformation response without clinical remission.

Synthetic thymic factor could be tried since this approach has been reported to improve cell-mediated immunity and IgA production in three immunodeficient children.[66] Epidophyllotoxin VP 16-213 has been used successfully even after lymphomatous transformation.[67]

AILD has been treated with levamisole, prednisone alone, single-agent chemotherapy and combination chemotherapy with or without prednisone.[67] Prednisone has found best use when an allergen is associated with AILD.[68] The enhancement of severe infections may contraindicate their use.[19] Symptomatic patients are usually treated with steroids. The hemolytic anemia in our patient responded promptly to steroid therapy concomitant with significant regression in the size of his enlarged regional nodes.[48] The two males from Norway were both treated with steroids and one was maintained on small doses daily. Normalization of hematological values and considerable reduction of the lymphadenopathy and hepatosplenomegaly were observed but the T-cell subset proportions and the serum immunoglobulin levels remained unchanged.[44] One boy also received maintenance therapy with methotrexate twice weekly and 6-mercaptopurine daily when steroid was discontinued after 6 weeks. The use of concentrated gammaglobulin appears to decrease the incidence of infection and to stabilize the clinical state.[48] Gammaglobulin substitutes for the nonfunctioning gammaglobulins despite the finding of hypergammaglobulinemia. Our patients had hyper-IgM as high as 2500 mg/dℓ.

Plasmapheresis in one patient with AILD who was resistant to steroids has resulted in 75% reduction in the size of the lymph nodes and disappearance of night sweats.[69] This beneficial result follows removal of antigenic stimulus, antigen-antibody complexes, and other humoral factors which may modulate lymphocyte or macrophage function.

Intensive cytotoxic treatment may be hazardous in some patients, even precipitating their deaths, but long survival after such therapy has been observed by others. Supportive therapy and small doses of steroids appear to be a safe therapeutic approach.[20]

Proof of the efficacy of any specific form of therapy is lacking, hence the need for further research.

F. Prognosis

AILD frequently has a fatal course even in the absence of histologic evidence of malignancy, once the disease has become progressive. The disorder behaves like a malignancy, and experience in the recent years indicates that it is a potentially malignant disease in which the patient is at risk of developing a lymphoma during the clinical course.[69]

Spontaneous remissions can occur.[47,69] The presence of allergies and polyclonal gammopathy are associated with the worst prognosis. Poor prognosis is also associated with hypoalbuminemia, hypogammaglobulinemia (IgG of less than 5 gm/ℓ), disturbance of the peripheral blood leukocyte count and hepatomegaly. Better prognosis was found in drug-induced disease suggesting autoimmune etiology.[71] Total median survival was shorter in patients with diffuse maculopapular rash (4 months with range of 1 to 39 months) whereas those without rash was 3 to 7 months (6 to over 53 months).[72] The predominant cause of death in patients treated with single agents followed by combination therapy was infection associated with neutropenia. In those treated with single agents only, the most frequent cause of death was progressive disease.[43]

Kaposi's sarcoma may complicate AILD.[73,74] Malignant lymphoma can evolve from AILD.[75] Ten to 30% of the cases reported in adults progressed to non-Hodgkin's lymphoma. Rare association with other malignant neoplasms has occurred.[76-78] A substantial number of adult patients with AILD evolved to immunoblastic sarcoma or immunoblastic lymphoma, although many patients died without AILD becoming an immunoblastic sarcoma.[19,69] Progression to immunoblastic lymphoma with prominent gastric involvement has been reported in AILD with dysproteinemia.[60] Ninety percent of individuals in whom remission cannot be induced die within 1 year.[78]

The natural course of AILD in children is unknown as only a few isolated cases have been studied. Spontaneous remission after 1 $\frac{1}{2}$ years has been described in a 7-year-old boy.[47] Our patient[48] and the two males reported from Norway[44] are still alive. No detectable malignant transformation has been observed as yet. Growth retardation was noted in one patient on maintenance steroid therapy.[79] The evolution into an immunoblastic sarcoma has been documented.[45,46]

IV. LYMPHOID INTERSTITIAL PNEUMONIA

A. Definition

Lymphoid interstitial pneumonia (LIP) is an uncommon nonmalignant lymphoproliferative disorder histologically defined as diffuse interstitial infiltration of lung parenchyma with mature lymphocytes, plasma cells, and reticuloendothelial cells.[80] It is less common than desquamative interstitial pneumonia (see Chapter 41).

B. Etiopathogenesis

The etiology is unknown, although it has been associated with hypergammaglobulinemia, hypogammaglobulinemia and autoimmune disorders in adults.[81,82] Only hypogammaglobulinemia was commonly reported in children up to 1981.[83] More recently, however, with the description of the acquired immunodeficiency syndrome (AIDS) in pediatrics, LIP became better recognized since the pneumonitis that accompanies the AIDS complex or prodrome usually proves to be LIP on open lung biopsy.[84] Hypergammaglobulinemia is a common finding. For more discussion on AIDS refer to Chapter 18. Cellular immunity plays an important role in the pathogenesis of LIP. An imbalance of immunoregulatory cells in the lung contributes to hypergammaglobulinemia.[85] The histologic similarity of the lung involvement to Hashimoto's thyroiditis, Waldenstrom's macroglobulinemia and Sjogren's syndrome may suggest that immunologic mechanisms are involved in the induction or expression of this disease.[81,82] In some patients, LIP may be a premalignant state since some histologically proven cases of LIP have been described to have developed into malignant lymphoproliferative disorders.[86] The interstitial infiltrate of lymphocytes lacks true germinal centers and ''active'' mitoses and is distinguised from ''pseudolymphoma'' or malignant lymphoma of the lung by the absence of lymph node and extrapulmonary involvement.[83] Virus-like particles have been seen in the bronchiolar epithelium of a patient with Sjogren's syndrome and LIP.[87] Immunofluorescent studies of a pulmonary biopsy specimen have shown linear deposition of IgG and IgA along the alveolar basement membrane. An autoimmune mechanism has been postulated although the origin of the immunofluorescent deposits was unclear.[88]

Defects in the immune state are common. Monoclonal[89] and polyclonal gammopathy,[90] dysproteinemia[82,91,92] autoerythrocyte sensitization syndrome,[86] agammaglobulinemia with pernicious anemia,[93] chronic active hepatitis with renal tubular acidosis,[94] myasthenia with monoclonal gammopathy,[89] and juvenile rheumatoid arthritis[95] have all been reported with LIP. LIP has been documented to occur after allogeneic bone marrow transplantation and is considered a possible manifestation of chronic graft-vs.-host disease.[96]

C. Clinical Features

LIP is a chronic progressive disease and the diagnosis may not be made until months or years after the onset of symptoms. It was first described 20 years ago by Carrington and Liebow[80] in four women aged 48 to 59 years and a 14-month-old boy whose symptoms included cough, dyspnea, fever, and weight loss. Females are more commonly affected than males. In our experience, the youngest infant with AIDS and pulmonary biopsy-proven LIP was 6 months.[97]

The Mayo Clinic experience reported cases of LIP seen from 1966 to 1976 which involved 12 adult patients, and only one 14-year-old female.[81] All of these patients were white. However, our six patients with LIP associated with AIDS were all black, and a 13-year-old girl with post-measles LIP whom the author managed for 2 years prior to the patient's death from chronic respiratory failure was also black. She lived 10 years post-biopsy-proven LIP. (See Figure 3A to C). LIP has been reported in blacks.[84,90,94] The occurrence in two brothers has been reported.[98] Cough, dyspnea, and significant weight loss were the most common symptoms. As the disease progresses, tachypnea, dyspnea, and orthopnea develop. Hyperhidrosis during sleep is pronounced in all patients with LIP and AIDS. Bibasilar crackles are heard in almost all patients. Digital clubbing ultimately develops in all patients. Hepatosplenomegaly may be found in those with complications. Cardiomegaly in chronic cases develops towards the terminal stage.

Radiographic findings are predominantly basilar, coarse, linear, and nodular interstitial infiltrates. In three of our patients, the infiltrates were diffuse and uniformly distributed throughout the lungs.[97] In advanced stages of LIP, honeycomb lung is seen.[81] Severe bronchiectasis may result in others after a variable number of years.[97]

Restrictive ventilatory function abnormality, diffusion defect and decreased lung compliance, and hypoxemia after exercise without hypercapnia are found in varying degrees during the course of LIP in children.[83,97-99] In contrast, some adults with LIP may have added obstructive ventilatory pattern.[81,82]

D. Management

Response to steroids has been variable and apparently inconsistent in adults.[80,81,97,100] Improvement may not occur. The appropriate treatment is unknown. Some investigators treat the LIP associated with pediatric AIDS with steroids and gammagobulin infusion (see Chapter 18). In our experience, the use of concentrated gammaglobulin infusion alone without steroids can prevent the progress of the LIP in AIDS, and occurrence of superinfection with Candida, Pneumocystis, or Salmonella is prevented.[97] In LIP not associated with pediatric AIDS, use of steroids has shown good results.[98]

When circulating immune complexes are present or when increased cellularity is noted on pulmonary biopsy, potential responsiveness to steroid therapy is indicated.[101] A second biopsy to follow the response to steroid therapy is done in the treatment of adults with LIP.

E. Prognosis

The natural history of LIP in children may not be the same as in adults. Two brothers with LIP were followed for 11 years and their clinical courses were different. The older brother experienced progressive respiratory disability and died 10 years after the onset of symptoms. The younger brother was observed for 11 years, treated with steroids and despite progression of pathological changes in his second lung biopsy, only exercise intolerance was observed and he led an active life. These two cases illustrate the nonmalignant course of disease.[98] LIP ultimately leads to pulmonary fibrosis and bronchiectasis with progressive worsening. Death occurs from respiratory failure usually triggered by complicating intercurrent respiratory viral infection.

Spencer considers LIP a prelymphomatous state that should be considered premalignant or malignant.[102] A 2 $\frac{1}{2}$ year old girl, with LIP and AIDS has been followed for 19 months after she was treated with oxygen, intravenous concentrated gammaglobulin and trimetho-

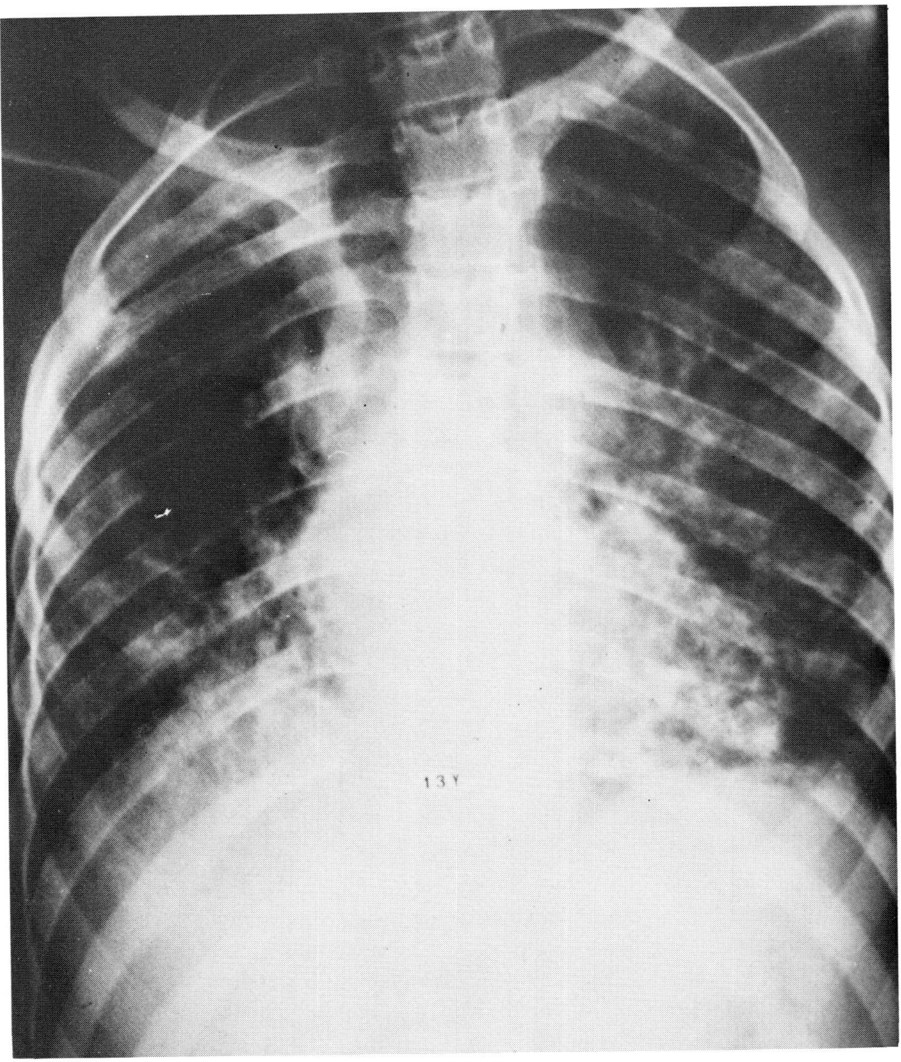

A

FIGURE 3.   (A) Diffuse, bilateral, stringy and patchy parenchymal infiltrate most marked in the bases with more involvement on the left. There is volume loss involving the right upper lobe. Pleural thickening is present and there is narrowing of the interspace between the third and fourth ribs anteriorly. A shift of the mediastinum is present superiorly. The extensive parenchymal infiltrates have caused obliteration of both hemidiaphragms and cardiac silhouettes. Cystic changes are seen in the left and right midlung fields. The pulmonary artery is slightly prominent although the over-all size of the heart is not enlarged. The paucity of subcutaneous tissue is present along the lateral chest wall. Tracheobronchomegaly is identified, particularly in the midportion of the trachea. (B and C) Marked posterior bronchiectasis is shown in the right midlung with difficulty in identifying the bronchopulmonary segments because of previous right upper lobectomy. Both stenosis and ectasia are present with bubbling and pulling in the right midlung posteriorly in the location of the cystic changes in the right midlung. Changes in the right third and fourth ribs secondary to previous surgery are seen. Both obliterative and saccular bronchiectasis are present.

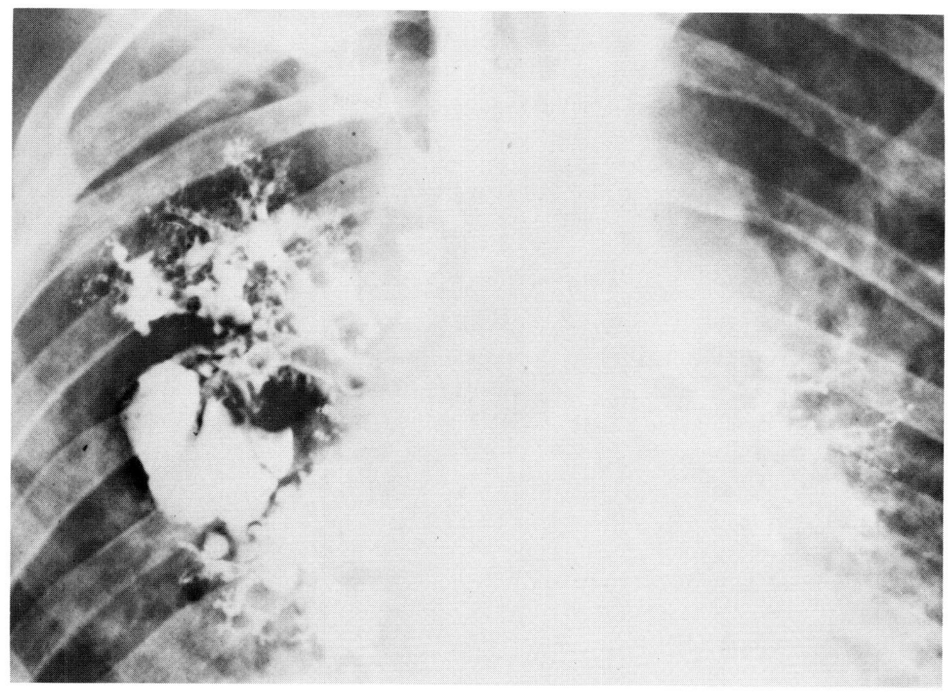

FIGURE 3B

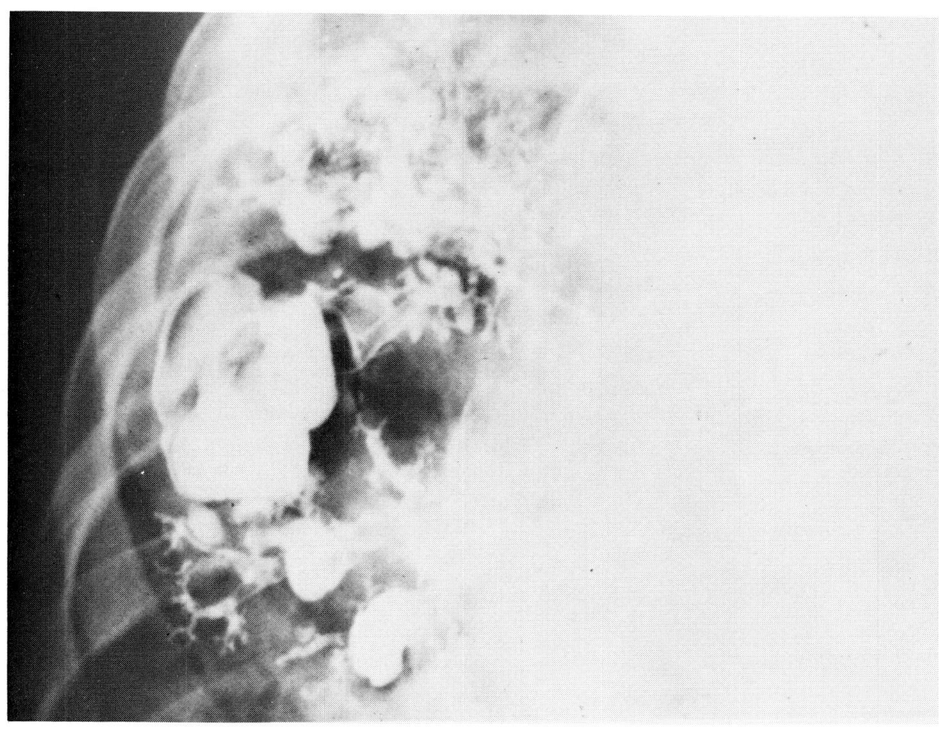

FIGURE 3C

prim-sulfamethoxazole without steroids. Oxygen dependency has decreased, and lymphadenopathy, and hepatosplenomegaly have almost totally disappeared, with significant decrease in tachypnea, dyspnea and increased exercise tolerance. (See Figure 25 of Chapter 6 for her chest radiographic findings.) The clinical course can be very variable in LIP associated with AIDS. Improvement of the lung disease may occur without therapy.[97]

V. PSEUDOLYMPHOMA OF THE LUNG

A. Definition

Pseudolymphoma of the lung (PLL) is a very uncommon condition characterized by the formation of a localized tumour mass with true germinal centers consisting of mixed cellular infiltrate predominantly of mature lymphocytes and plasma cells and without hilar lymph nodal involvement.[103] The latter feature is the most reliable criterion that differentiates this entity from active malignancy. LIP and PLL appear to be two conditions that merge and are identical. Both forms may be seen in the same lung.

B. Etiopathogenesis

Just like LIP, the etiology is unknown. It may be associated with dysproteinemia.[82] A monoclonal macroglobulinemia is usually found.[89]

C. Clinical Features

PLL is usually clinically silent and is a surprise chest radiographic finding. Cough and fever may be the initial symptoms. Older age groups are usually affected but there is a report of PLL in an 11-year-old boy found to have deficient cellular immunity. He underwent right middle lobectomy and removal of surrounding lymph nodes with no recurrence of tumor since surgery, and return of immunologic functions to normal.[104]

D. Radiographic Features

Radiographic findings are usually that of a localized tumor mass usually in one lung but may involve more than one lobe. The mass is usually near the hilar region of the lung. The radiographic features differentiate PLL from LIP as the latter shows nodular and patchy opacities or linear markings in the lower lobes of the lungs.[102]

E. Management

Surgical therapy may be indicated.[103]

F. Prognosis

PLL remains localized in the lung often for a prolonged period before disseminating. It has a slow and locally infiltrative course. Both LIP and PLL frequently develop into malignant lymphoma though this may take several years to occur.[102,103]

REFERENCES

1. **Kaltreider, H. B.,** Expression of immune mechanism in the lungs, *Am. Rev. Resp. Dis.,* 113, 347, 1976.
2. **Bienenstock, J., Johnson, N., and Percy, D. J. E.,** Bronchial lymphoid tissue. I. Morphologic characteristics, *Lab. Invest.,* 28, 686, 1973a.
3. **Farquhar, J. W. and Claireaux, A. E.,** Familial hemophagocytic reticulosis, *Arch. Dis. Child.,* 27, 519, 1952.

4. **Ansbacher, L. E., Singsen, B. H., Hosler, M. W., Grimminger, H., and Herbert, P. N.,** Familial erythrophagocytic lymphohistiocytosis: an association with serum lipid abnormalities, *J. Pediatr.,* 102, 270, 1983.

5. **O'Brien, R. T., Schwartz, A. D., Pearson, H. A., and Spencer, R. P.,** Reticuloendothelial failure in familial erythrophagocytic lymphohistiocytosis, *J. Pediatr.,* 81, 543, 1972.

6. **Scott, R. B. and Robb-Smith, A. H. T.,** Histiocytic medullary reticulosis, *Lancet,* 2, 194, 1939.

7. **Weiss, C. Z. and Norris, D. G.,** Familial erythrophagocytic lymphohistiocytosis, *J. Med. Soc. N. J.,* 74, 39, 1977.

8. **Ladisch, S., Poplack, D. G., Blaese, R. M., and Holiman, B.,** Immunodeficiency in familial erythrophagocytic lymphohistiocytosis, *Lancet,* 1, 581, 1978.

9. **Bell, R. J. M., Brafield, A. J. E., Barnes, N. D., and France, N. E.,** Familial haemophagocytic reticulosis, *Arch. Dis. Child.,* 43, 601, 1968.

10. **Buist, N. R. M., Jones, R. N., and Cavens, T. R.,** Familial hemophagocytic reticulosis in first cousins, *Arch. Dis. Child.,* 46, 728, 1971.

11. **Perry, M. C., Harrison, E. G., Jr., Burgert, E. L., Jr., and Gilchrist, G. C.,** Familial erythrophagocytic lymphohistiocytosis: report of two cases and clinicopathologic review, *Cancer,* 38, 209, 1976.

12. **Botha, J. B. S., Kahn, L. B., and Kaschula, R. O. C.,** Familial haemophagocytic reticulosis: Report of two cases in sibs, *S. Afr. Med. J.,* 49, 1305, 1975.

13. **Shapiro, D. N. and Hutchinson, R. J.,** Familial histiocytosis in offspring of two pregnancies after artificial insemination, *N. Engl. J. Med.,* 304, 757, 1981.

14. **Risdall, R. J., McKenna, R. W., Nesbit, M. R., Krivitt, W., Balfour, H. H., Simmons, R. L., and Brunning, R. D.,** Virus-associated hemophagocytic syndrome, *Cancer,* 44, 993, 1979.

15. **Hagberg, B., Hultquist, G., Scennerholm, L., and Voss, H.,** Malignant hyperlipidemia in infancy, *Am. J. Dis. Child.,* 107, 267, 1964.

16. **Ambruso, D. R., Hays, T., Zwartjes, W. J., Tubergen, D. G., and Favara, B. E.,** Successful treatment of lymphohistiocytic reticulosis with phagocytosis with epipodophyllotoxin, VP 16-213, *Cancer,* 45, 2516, 1980.

17. **Fischer, A., Virelizier, J. L., Arenzana-Seisdedos, F., Perez, N., Nezelof, C., and Griscelli, C.,** Treatment of four patients with erythrophagocytic lymphohistiocytosis by a combination of epipodophyllotoxin, steroids, intrathecal methotrexate, and cranial irradiation, *Pediatrics,* 76, 263, 1985.

18. **Frizzera, G., Moran, E. M., and Rappaport, H.,** Angioimmunoblastic lymphadenopathy with dysproteinemia, *Lancet,* 1, 1070, 1974.

19. **Lukes, R. J. and Tindle, B. H.,** Immunoblastic lymphadenopathy, a hyperimmune entity resembling Hodgkin's disease, *N. Engl. J. Med.,* 292, 1, 1975.

20. **Frizzera, G., Moran, E. M., and Rappaport, H.,** Angioimmunoblastic lymphadenopathy. Diagnosis and clinical course, *Am. J. Med.,* 59, 803, 1975.

21. **Schultz, D. R. and Yunis, A. A.,** Immunoblastic lymphadenopathy with mixed cryoglobulinemia, *N. Engl. J. Med.,* 292, 8, 1975.

22. **Garam, T., Bak, M., and Bakacs, T.,** Angioimmunoblastic lymphadenopathy: a study of lymphocyte populations, *Cancer,* 47, 2850, 1981.

23. **Matz, L. R., Papadimitriou, J. M., Carroll, J. R., Barr, A. L., Dawkins, R. L., Jackson, J. M., Herrmann, R. P., and Armstrong, B. K.,** Angioimmunoblastic lymphadenopathy with dysproteinemia, *Cancer,* 40, 2152, 1977.

24. **Moore, S. B., Harrison, E. G., and Weiland, L. H.,** Angioimmunoblastic lymphadenopathy, *Mayo Clin. Proc.,* 51, 273, 1976.

25. **Schechter, S. L. and Rosenblum, D.,** Immunoblastic lymphadenopathy and hydroxychloroquine, *Arthritis Rheum.,* 23, 256, 1980.

26. **Weisenburger, D. D.,** Immunoblastic lymphadenopathy associated with methyldopa therapy, a case report, *Cancer,* 42, 2322, 1978.

27. **Naparstek, Y., Ben-Charit, E., Okon, E., Estrov, Z., and Eliakim, M.,** Angioimmunoblastic lymphadenopathy in a patient with allergy to insulin: a case report, *Cancer,* 47, 545, 1981.

28. **Seigneurin, J. M., Mingat, J., Lenoir, G. M., Couderic, P., and Micoud, M.,** Angioimmunoblastic lymphadenopathy after infectious mononucleosis, *Br. Med. J.,* 282, 1574, 1981.

29. **Karmali, R. A., Horrobin, D. F., Menezes, J., Patel, P., and Musto, J.,** Chloroquine enhances Epstein-Barr virus expression, *Nature, (London),* 275, 444, 1978.

30. **Pierce, D. A., Stern, R., Jaffe, R., Zulman, J., and Talal, N.,** Immunoblastic sarcoma with features of Sjogren's syndrome and systemic lupus erythematosus in a patient with immunoblastic lymphadenopathy, *Arthritis Rheum.,* 22, 911, 1979.

31. **Maguire, F. W., Mills, C., and Parker, F. P.,** Immunoblastic lymphadenopathy and asbestosis, *Cancer,* 47, 791, 1981.

32. **Sztern, M., Aelion, J. A., Lurie, Y., and Mor, C.,** Angioimmunoblastic lymphadenopathy and squamous cancer of the lung, *Am. J. Med. Sci.,* 287, 21, 1984.

33. **Cibull, M. L., Seligson, G. R., and Mouradian, J. A.,** Immunoblastic lymphadenopathy and adeno-carcinoma of the pancreas, *Cancer,* 42, 1883, 1978.
34. **Karttunen, T., Nevasari, K., Riasianen, O., Taskinen, F. J., and Alavaikko, M.,** Immunoblastic lymphadenopathy with a high serum Yersinia enterocolitica titer. A case report, *Cancer,* 52, 2281, 1983.
35. **Cytowic, R. E., Challa, V. R., Buss, D. H., and Angelo, J. N.,** Chronic relapsing polyneuropathy associated with immunoblastic lymphadenopathy, *Human Pathol.,* 13, 167, 1982.
36. **Koo, C. H., Nathwwani, B. N., Winberg, C. D., Hill, L. R., and Rappaport, H.,** Atypical lympho-plasmacytic and immunoblastic proliferation in lymph nodes of patients with autoimmune disease (autoim-mune-disease-associated lymphadenopathy), *Medicine,* 63, 274, 1984.
37. **Blumenfeld, W. and Beckstead, J. H.,** Angioimmunoblastic lymphadenopathy with dysproteinemia in homosexual men with acquired immune deficiency syndrome, *Arch. Pathol. Lab. Med.,* 107, 567, 1983.
38. **Watanabe, H.,** Association of immunoblastic lymphadenopathy and Hashimoto's thyroiditis, *Ann. Int. Med.,* 87, 62, 1977.
39. **Kaneko, Y., Larson, R. A., Variakojis, D., Haren, M. J., and Rowley, J. D.,** Nonrandom chromosome abnormalities in angioimmunoblastic lymphadenopathy, *Blood,* 60, 877, 1982.
40. **Neiman, R. S., Dervan, P., Handenschild, C., and Jaffe, R.,** Angioimmunoblastic lymphadenopathy, an ultrastructural and immunologic study with review of the literature, *Cancer,* 41, 507, 1978.
41. **Kosmidis, P. A., Axelrod, A. R., Palacas, C., and Stahl, M.,** Angioimmunoblastic lymphadenopathy, a T-cell deficiency, *Cancer,* 42, 447, 1978.
42. **Pangalis, G. A., Moran, E., and Rappaport, H.,** Blood and bone marrow findings in angioimmunoblastic lymphadenopathy, *Blood,* 51, 71, 1978.
43. **Rywlin, A. M., Hoffman, E. P., and Ortega, R. S.,** Eosinophilic fibro-histiocytic lesion of the bone marrow. A distinctive new morphologic finding probably related to drug hypersensitivity, *Blood,* 40, 464, 1972.
44. **Stensvold, K., Brandtzaeg, P., Kval, S., Seip, M., and Lie, S. O.,** Immunoblastic lymphadenopathy with early onset in two boys: immunohistochemical study and indication of decreased proportion of cir-culating T-helper cells, *Br. J. Haematol.,* 56, 417, 1984.
45. **Howarth, D. M. and Bird, C. C.,** Immunoblastic sarcoma arising in a child with immunoblastic lymph-adenopathy, (letter), *Lancet,* 2, 747, 1976.
46. **Morris, J. A., Bird, C. C., Breg, W. R., and Papac, R. J.,** Ultrastructural and immunohistologic study of immunoblastic sarcoma developing in a child with immunoblastic lymphadenopathy, *Cancer,* 44, 171, 1979.
47. **Fiorillo, A., Pettinato, G., Raia, V., Migliorati, R., Angrisani, P., and Buffolano, W.,** Angioim-munoblastic lymphadenopathy with dysproteinemia: report of the first case in childhood evolving toward spontaneous remission, *Cancer,* 48, 1611, 1981.
48. **Laraya-Cuasay, L. R. and Kesarwala, H.,** Angioimmunoblastic lymphadedopathy in a child treated with concentrated gamma globulin, To be published.
49. **Iseman, M. D., Schwarz, M. I., and Stanford, R. E.,** Interstitial pneumonia in angioimmunoblastic lymphadenopathy with dysproteinemia. A case report with special histopathologic studies, *Ann. Int. Med.,* 85, 752, 1976.
50. **Weisenberger, D., Armitage, J., and Dick, F.,** Immunoblastic lymphadenopathy with pulmonary infil-trates, hypocomplementemia, and vasculitis, *Am. J. Med.,* 63, 849, 1977.
51. **Myers, T. J., Cole, S. R., and Pastuszak, W. T.,** Angioimmunoblastic lymphadenopathy, pleural-pulmonary disease, *Cancer,* 40, 266, 1978.
52. **Bradley, S. L., Dines, D. E., Banks, P. M., and Hill, R. W.,** The lung in immunoblastic lymphade-nopathy, *Chest,* 80, 312, 1981.
53. **Lopez-Berenstein, G., Cabanillas, F., Osborne, B. M., Libshitz, H. I., and Bodey, G. P.,** Study of the natural history of immunoblastic lymphadenopathy and atypical immunoproliferative disorders, *Cancer Inv.,* 1, 293, 1983.
54. **Limpert, J., Macmahon, H., and Variakojis, D.,** Angioimmunoblastic lymphadenopathy: clinical and radiological features, *Radiology,* 152, 27, 1984.
55. **Monteiro, M. L. R., Coppeto, J. R., Greco, P., and Pittard, G.,** Angioimmunoblastic lymphadenopathy with Fisher syndrome, *Arch. Neurol.,* 41, 456, 1984.
56. **Lisak, R. P., Mitchell, M., and Qweiman, B.,** Guillain-Barre syndrome and Hodgkin's disease: three cases with immunological studies, *Ann. Neurol.,* 1, 72, 1977.
57. **Snustad, D. G., Koss, W., Fontana, J. A.,** Angioimmunoblastic lymphadenopathy with associated se-lective myeloid hypoplasia, *Cancer,* 53, 2129, 1984.
58. **Rice, L., Abramson, S. L., Laughter, A. M., Wheeler, T. M., and Twomey, J. J.,** Angioimmunoblastic lymphadenopathy with hypogammaglobulinemia, possible role of monocyte suppression, *Am. J. Med.,* 72, 998, 1982.

59. **Moreb, J., Okon, E., Matzner, Y., and Polliack, A.,** Angioimmunoblastic lymphadenopathy, a case with an unusual clinical course with marked tumorous infiltration of multiple organs and striking intestinal involvement, *Cancer,* 51, 487, 1983.

60. **Bauer, T. W., Mendelsonn, G., Humphrey, R. L., and Mann, R. B.,** Angioimmunoblastic lymphadenopathy progressing to immunoblastic lymphoma with prominent gastric involvement, *Cancer,* 50, 2089, 1982.

61. **Wood, W. G. and Harkins, M. M.,** Nephropathy in angioimmunoblastic lymphadenopathy, *Am. J. Clin. Pathol.,* 71, 58, 1979.

62. **Raskin, R. J., Resar, J. T., and Lawless, D. J.,** Polyarthritis in immunoblastic lymphadenopathy, *Arth. Rheum.,* 25, 1481, 1982.

63. **Minerbrook, M., Budman, D. R., Schulman, P., Vinciguerra, V., Degnar, T. J., and Coffey, E.,** De novo disseminated intravascular coagulation in angioimmunoblastic lymphadenopathy (AILD), *Cancer,* 1927, 1983.

64. **Bensa, J. C., Faure, J., Martin, H., Sotto, J. J., and Schaerer, R.,** Levamisole in angioimmunoblastic lymphadenopathy, *Lancet,* 1, 1081, 1976.

65. **Brincker, H. and Birkeland, S. A.,** The relationship between disease activity, treatment response, and immunologic reactivity in immunoblastic lymphadenopathy: a longitudinal study of treatment with levamisole and cytostatics, *Cancer,* 47, 266, 1981.

66. **Bordigioni, P., Bene, M. C., Bach, J. F., Faure, G., Dardenne, M., and Duhelle, J.,** Improvement of cellular immunity and IgA production in immunodeficient children after treatment with synthetic syrum thymic factor, *Lancet,* 2, 293, 1982.

67. **Jacobs, P., Kahn, L. B., and King, H. S.,** Angioimmunoblastic lymphadenopathy, *S. Afr. Med. J.,* 62, 200, 1982.

68. **Newcom, S. R. and Kadin, M. E.,** Prednisone in treatment of allergen-associated angioimmunoblastic lymphadenopathy, *Lancet,* 1, 462, 1979.

69. **Pangalis, G. A., Moran, E. M., Nathwani, B. N., Zelman, R. J., Kim, H., and Rappaport, H.,** Angioimmunoblastic lymphadenopathy, long term follow-up study, *Cancer,* 52, 318, 1983.

70. **Gordon, B. R., Suthanthiram, M., Saal, S., Stenzel, K. H., and Rubin, A. L.,** Plasmapheresis in a patient with angioimmunoblastic lymphadenopathy, *Cancer,* 51, 829, 1983.

71. **Blanchard, F., Brianson, S., Cohen, J. H., Bethevenot, G., and Reyes, F.,** Prognostic factors in angioimmunoblastic lymphadenopathy, (letter), *Lancet,* 1, 1449, 1983.

72. **Archimbaud, E., Coiffier, B., Bryon, P. A., Brizard, C. P., and Viala, J. J.,** Rash implies poor prognosis in angioimmunoblastic lymphadenopathy, (letter), *Lancet,* 1, 998, 1983.

73. **Tosi, P., Auteri, A., and Cintorino, M.,** Angioimmunoblastic lymphadenopathy with dysproteinemia complicated by Kaposi's sarcoma, *Tumor,* 65, 363, 1979.

74. **Kluin-Nelemans, H. C., Elbers, H. R. J., and Ramselaar, C. G.,** Angioimmunoblastic lymphadenopathy followed by Kaposi's sarcoma, *Arch. Dermatol.,* 120, 958, 1984.

75. **Nathwani, B. N., Rappaport, H., Moran, E. M., Pangalis, G., and Kim, H.,** Malignant lymphoma arising in angioimmunoblastic lymphadenopathy, *Cancer,* 41, 578, 1978.

76. **Fayemi, A. D., Ali, M., Braun, E. V., and De Ceio, T.,** Angioimmunoblastic lymphadenopathy: termination as diffuse lymphosarcoma with plasmacytoid features, *Mt. Sinai J. Med. (NY),* 46, 39, 1979.

77. **Knecht, H. and Lennert, K.,** Verlauf, therapie und maligne tranformation der lymphogranulomatosis X (einschliesslich [angio] immunoblasticher Lymphadenopathie), *Schweiz Med. Wochenscher,* 111, 1122, 1981.

78. **Cullen, M. H., Stansfield, A. G., Oliver, R. T. D., Lister, T. A., and Malpas, J. S.,** Angioimmunoblastic lymphadenopathy; report of ten cases and review of the literature, *Q. J. Med.,* 48, 151, 1979.

79. **Brandtzaeg, P. and Stensvold, K.,** Personal communication.

80. **Carrington, C. B. and Liebow, A. A.,** Lymphocytic interstitial pneumonia (abstr), *Am. J. Pathol.,* 48, 36, 1966.

81. **Strimlan, C. V., Rosenow, E. C., Weiland, L. H., and Brown, L. R.,** Lymphocytic interstitial pneumonitis, a review of 13 cases, *Ann. Int. Med.,* 88, 616, 1978.

82. **Liebow, A. A. and Carrington, C. B.,** Diffuse pulmonary lymphoreticular infiltrations associated with dysproteinemia, *Med. Clin. North Am.,* 57, 809, 1973.

83. **Church, J. A., Isaaca, H., Saxon, A., Keens, T. G., and Richards, W.,** Lymphoid interstitial pneumonitis and hypogammaglobulinemia in children, *Am. Rev. Resp. Dis.,* 124, 491, 1981.

84. **Joshi, V. V., Oleske, J. M., and Minnefor, A. B.,** Pulmonary pathology in suspected acquired immunodeficiency syndrome, *Lab. Invest.,* 50, 5P, 1984.

85. **Yoshizawa, Y., Ahdama, S., Ikeda, A., Ohtsuka, M., Masuda, S., and Tanaka, M.,** Lymphoid interstitial pneumonia associated with depressed cellular immunity and polyclonal gammopathy, *Am. Rev. Resp. Dis.,* 130, 507, 1984.

86. Case records of the Massachusetts General Hospital. Case 13-1900, *N. Engl. J. Med.,* 302, 795, 1980.

87. **Sutinen, S. and Huhti, E.,** Ultrastructure of lymphoid interstitial pneumonia: virus-like particles in bronchiolar epithelium of a patient with Sjogren's syndrome, *Am. J. Clin. Pathol.,* 67, 328, 1977.
88. **De Coteau, W. E., Tourville, D., Ambrus, J. L., Montes, M., Adler, R., and Tomasi, T. B., Jr.,** Lymphoid interstitial pneumonia and auto-erythrocyte sensitization syndrome: a case with deposition of immunoglobulins on the alveolar basement membrane, *Arch. Intern. Med.,* 134, 519, 1974.
89. **Montes, M., Tomasi, T. B., Jr., Noehren, T. H., and Culver, G. J.,** Lymphoid interstitial pneumonia with monoclonal gammopathy, *Am. Rev. Resp. Dis.,* 98, 277, 1968.
90. **Young, R. C., Jr., Tillamn, R. L., Burton, A. F., and Sampson, C. C.,** Lymphoid interstitial pneumonia with polyclonal gammopathy. A case report, *J. Natl. Med. Assoc.,* 61, 310, 1969.
91. **Greenberg, S. D., Haley, M. D., Jenkins, D. E., and Fischer, S. P.,** Lymphoplasmacytic pneumonia with accompanying dysproteinemia, *Arch. Pathol.,* 96, 73, 1973.
92. **Moran, T. J. and Totten, R. S.,** Lymphoid interstitial pneumonia with dysproteinemia: report of two cases with plasma cell predominance, *Am. J. Clin. Pathol.,* 54, 747, 1970.
93. **Levinson, A. I., Hopewell, P. C., Stites, D. P., Spitler, L. E., and Fudenberg, H. H.,** Coexistent lymphoid interstitial pneumonia, pernicious anemia, and agammaglobulinemia: comment on auto-iommune pathogenesis, *Arch. Intern. Med.,* 136, 213, 1976.
94. **Helman, C. A., Keeton, G. R., and Benatar, S. R.,** Lymphoid interstitial pneumonia with associated chronic active hepatitis and renal tubular acidosis, *Am. Rev. Resp. Dis.,* 115, 161, 1977.
95. **Lovell, D., Lindsley, C., and Langston, C.,** Lymphoid interstitial pneumonia in juvenile rheumatoid arthritis, *J. Pediatr.,* 105, 947, 1984.
96. **Perreault, C., Cousineau, S., D'Angelo, G., Gyger, M., Nepveu, F., Boileau, J., Bonny, Y., Lacombe, M., and Lavallee, R.,** Lymphoid interstitial pneumonia after allogeneic bone marrow transplantation, a possible manifestation of chronic graft-vs.-host disease, *Cancer,* 55, 1, 1985.
97. **Laraya-Cuasay, L. R., Liscano, M., and Frenkel, L. D.,** Pulmonary manifestations of acquired immunodeficiency syndrome in children, in preparation.
98. **O'Brodovich, H. M., Moser, M. M., and Lu, L.,** Familial lymphoid interstitial pneumonia: a long-term follow-up, *Pediatrics,* 65, 523, 1980.
99. **Hewitt, C. J., Hull, D., and Keeling, J. W.,** Fibrosing alveolitis in infancy and childhood, *Arch. Dis. Child.,* 52, 22, 1977.
100. **Liebow, A. A. and Carrington, C. B.,** The interstitial pneumonias, in *Frontiers of Pulmonary Radiology,* Simons, M., Potchen, E. J., Lemary, M., Eds., Grune and Stratton, New York, 1969.
101. **Dreisin, R. B., Schwarz, M. I., Theofilopoulos, A. N., and Stanford, R. E.,** Circulating immune complexes in the idiopathic interstitial pneumonias, *N. Engl. J. Med.,* 298, 353, 1978.
102. **Spencer, H.,** Pulmonary reticuloses, in *Pathology of the Lung,* Pergamon Press, Oxford, 1985.
103. **Saltzstein, S. L.,** Pulmonary malignant lymphomas and pseudolymphomas. Classification, therapy, and prognosis, *Cancer,* 16, 928, 1963.
104. **Reich, N. E., McCormack, L. J., and Van Ordstrand, H. S.,** Pseudolymphoma of the lung, *Chest,* 65, 424, 1974.

Chapter 43

FUTURE THERAPY OF INTERSTITIAL LUNG DISEASES

David J. Riley

TABLE OF CONTENTS

I. INTRODUCTION

As has been described in previous chapters of this book, there has been considerable progress in the past 15 years in understanding the cellular and biochemical processes involved in the interstitial lung diseases. The ultimate goal of this research is to discover effective, safe therapy for patients with diseases such as sarcoidosis and idiopathic pulmonary fibrosis. So far, there have been no major breakthroughs in the treatment of these disorders. This failure is attributable to our incomplete understanding of basic disease processes such as inflammation, granuloma formation, and fibrogenesis which underlie these diseases.

What are the future propects for treating these diseases? Are there promising new drugs or therapies? A number of agents have been found to be useful in animal models and clinical trials are being started on a few of these agents. The purpose of this chapter is to summarize these results and highlight those approaches which appear to have potential application for treating interstitial lung diseases.

II. GENERAL APPROACHES

The pathogenesis of interstitial lung diseases can be broadly divided into inflammatory and fibrotic phases. Therapeutic approaches can also be classified into those which alter inflammatory events and those which act directly on collagen biosynthesis. In order to understand the sites of therapeutic intervention, it is important to briefly review the mechanisms of interstitial inflammation and excess collagen formation.

The mechanisms of alveolar inflammation ("alveolitis") and granuloma formation overlap.[1] The initial lesion develops in response to an inciting factor. The most prominent cells found in alveolitis are activated macrophages and T-lymphocytes, although polymorphonuclear leukocytes also are found in early inflammation. It appears that the alveolar macrophage plays a major role in granuloma formation. The phagocytic cells in the lung parenchyma appear to cause injury by releasing destructive enzymes, reactive oxygen species (free radicals), and metabolites of arachidonic acid. The presence of alveolar inflammation and granuloma formation leads to progressive injury and fibrosis.

Interstitial fibrosis is a consequence of a variety of disease processes. The fibroblast is the central cell in fibrogenesis because of its capacity to secrete collagen. Mediators released from activated macrophages may trigger fibroblasts to divide and secrete collagen. The hallmark of fibrosis is an excess amount of collagen, and the regulation of the biosynthesis of collagen is known in considerable detail. The steps involve intracellular assembly of procollagen, secretion, extracellular processing, fiber formation, and cross-linking which leads to deposition of insoluble collagen fibers in the interstitium of the lung. Little is known about control of collagen degradation in pulmonary fibrosis. Some of these biosynthetic steps may be useful sites for therapeutic agents which block collagen synthesis or processing.

In considering potential agents which block inflammation or fibrosis, it must be kept in mind that the majority of agents discussed below have been tested to see if a particular process or biosynthetic step might be involved in experimental interstitial lung disease. This approach must be distinguished from testing potential therapeutic agents in which toxicity, dose, and route of administration are considered. The number of agents of this latter type which are being considered for therapy are few.

III. AGENTS WHICH ACT ON INFLAMMATION

There is considerable evidence to suggest that immune and inflammatory factors influence progression toward fibrogenesis. This influence is believed to be modulated by products secreted from inflammatory cells which influence fibroblast proliferation and collagen secretion. Two potential sites of anti-inflammatory intervention are, first, to reduce the number of inflammatory cells such as lymphocytes and neutrophils and second, to block the effect of secreted products of inflammation.

Corticosteroids have broad anti-inflammatory properties and have been shown to be effective in preventing experimental pulmonary fibrosis.[2-4] In humans, corticosteroids slow the progress of idiopathic pulmonary fibrosis and improve most patients with sarcoidosis although long-term survival in both diseases appears to be unaffected by steroid therapy.[5] The generally poor clinical response, coupled with the frequent serious side effects, has led investigators to other approaches to suppress inflammation.

Attempts have been made to specifically deplete T-lymphocytes and neutrophils using anti-lymphocyte or anti-neutrophil antibodies. Anti-lymphocyte globulin was partially effective in ameliorating bleomycin-induced fibrosis.[6] Neutrophils are thought to contribute to lung damage, but experiments in animals have shown that neutrophil depletion with specific antiserum results in increased fibrosis in bleomycin-treated animals.[7,8] These results suggest that the neutrophil may actually serve to limit the extent of fibrosis. It is difficult to draw conclusions from these limited studies, but suppression of T-lymphocytes in chronic interstitial lung disease may be a potential treatment of this disorder. The use of anti-lymphocyte antibodies, however, has severe limitations in a disease which requires year of treatment. Immunosuppressive drugs currently in use, such as azathioprine, cyclophosphamide, and chlorambucil, either alone or in combination with corticosteroids, have limited usefulness in the treatment of idiopathic pulmonary fibrosis and are associated with serious side effects.[5] Although suppressing T-lymphocytes may be a reasonable approach to treating intersitial lung diseases, there are currently no agents that are effective and safe for patients.

A number of secreted products from inflammatory cells have been identified and attempts have been made to block their production to treat interstitial lung diseases. Products which have been thought to play a role include enzymes, oxygen-derived free radicals, prostaglandins, macrophage-derived growth factor, and interleukin-1. Suppression of proteolytic enzymes may be detrimental since collagenolytic enzymes may be needed to reduce collagen accumulation. The generation of oxygen-derived free radicals by agents such as bleomycin may cause injury by way of a ferrous ion-molecular oxygen mechanism. Attempts to block free radical formation by using a chelator of ferric ion, deferoxamine, are conflicting since results in animals have shown an amelioration of bleomycin-induced fibrosis[9] and no benefit.[10] Other agents thought to be involved in inflammation are metabolites of arachidonic acid, macrophage-derived growth factor, and interleukin-1. Too little is known about these products at present to develop strategies for therapeutic intervention. In conclusion, cellular inflammation and their mediators appear to modify fibrogenesis in interstitial lung disease, but not enough is known about these processes to develop useful therapeutic approaches. It appears, therefore, that corticosteroids will continue to be the major anti-inflammatory agent for the foreseeable future.

IV. AGENTS WHICH AFFECT COLLAGEN BIOSYNTHESIS

There has been considerable expansion of knowledge in collagen biochemistry in the recent past, and considerable effort has been made in developing agents which block collagen synthesis and processing. Several reviews on this topic have been published,[11,12] including one recent review on antifibrotic agents in pulmonary fibrosis.[13] Although no agent is currently available for patient use, it is apparent that collagen deposition in organs undergoing fibrosis can be controlled by pharmacologic agents. This section will describe the current status of antifibrotic agents that have been used in experimental pulmonary fibrosis and their potential application to treating human pulmonary fibrosis.

One therapeutic approach to reduce collagen synthesis is to interfere with the ability of gene transcription for collagen. It has recently been shown that corticosteroids reduce the transcription of a number of genes, including that for type I procollagen.[14] Steroids, which are thought to prevent fibrosis by inhibiting inflammation, appear also to have a specific action on suppressing collagen gene expression. It has been shown, for example, that administration of dexamethasone to bleomycin-treated lung fibroblasts results in selective reduction in procollagen type I mRNA levels and procollagen synthesis.[15] Although more needs to be learned about controlling biosynthesis at the level of gene transcription, these findings with corticosteroids suggest it might be possible to control collagen biosynthesis at a very early stage of regulation.

One of the first processing steps required in collagen biosynthesis is the hydroxylation of prolyl and lysyl residues by the enzymes prolyl and lysyl hydroxylase. Hydroxylation is a critical step in collagen biosynthesis because unhydroxylated collagen cannot assume a helical conformation at physiological temperatures. The disease scurvy is a well-recognized example of lack of procollagen hydroxylation caused by dietary deficiency of ascorbic acid, an essential cofactor for prolyl hydroxylase. Analogues have been developed which inhibit prolyl hydroxylase,[16] but it is not known whether these agents act in vivo.

There are other enzymes involved in collagen processing, such as the enzymes which transfer carbohydrate moieties and those which cleave the nonhelical extension peptides on the two ends of the procollagen molecule. Interfering with the latter enzyme might be useful therapeutically since collagen with the carboxy-terminal extension peptides attached cannot be packed into fibrils, presumably because of the size of the extension peptides. Unfortunately, the enzymes that cleave the extensions have not been sufficiently well characterized to allow for development of inhibitors.

Collagen is an unusual peptide since it contains a high percentage of the amino acids prolines and hydroxyproline. The frequent proline groups are considered to be important in determining the distinctive triple helical arrangement of the pro-alpha chains to form the collagen molecule. Collagen which cannot form a triple helix cannot be properly secreted from cells, and collagen fibril formation cannot occur. These unique features of collagen metabolism have been used to develop analogues of proline designed to interfere with collagen triple helical formation. It has been demonstrated that proline analogues are incorporated into collagen polypeptides. The presence of proline analogues in newly synthesized polypeptide chains prevents the chains from folding into a triple helix. Because the chains cannot fold into a triple helix, they remain as totally nonfunctional polypeptides and are catabolized.

There are several theoretical limitations to the use of proline analogues. The first is that they may decrease general protein synthesis since the analogue is incorporated into all proteins in place of proline. Although the effects of proline analogues are relatively specific for collagen in short-term studies, it is likely that changes occur in the function and conformation of all proteins as a result of this substitution. The second objection is that giving an antifibrotic agent over a long time is likely to cause significant side effects in other organs such as normal bones where collagen production is likely to be greater than in fibrotic lungs. Examining the toxicologic effects of proline analogue becomes critical in assessing their therapeutic potential.

Proline analogues have shown to be effective in inhibiting collagen accumulation in several models of fibrosis.[17] There have been several studies showing proline analogues prevent collagen accumulation in experimental pulmonary fibrosis. Using a rat oxygen toxicity model, Riley and associates showed that *cis*-hydroxyproline, L-azetidine-2-carboxylic acid, and L-3,4-dehydroproline were effective in preventing lung collagen accumulation.[18,19] Collagen accumulation in bleomycin-induced fibrosis in rodents was shown to be prevented by *cis*-hydroxyproline[20] and L-3,4-dehydroproline.[21] In addition to the biochemical changes, administration of these agents partially prevented the decreased lung volume found in fibrosis.[20,21] There were no overt toxic effects identified during the 2- to 4-week treatment periods, but the toxic effects of longer treatment periods have not been studied. These animal experiments suggest that short-term treatment with proline analogues is effective in preventing rapid accumulation of lung collagen in doses which do not cause overt toxicity.

One limited trial has been reported of treating patients with the proline analogue L-2,3-dehydroproline. Twelve patients with ARDS who had clinical evidence of rapidly developing pulmonary fibrosis have been administered the analogue intravenously for 1 to 21 days with no untoward effects attributable to the analogues.[22] Of nine patients treated for more than 4 days, seven met criteria which predicted a mortality of 92%. Five of the nine patients treated for more than 4 days survived.[13] The number of patients treated is too few to determine whether this drug had any benefit. Nevertheless, the results of animal studies and the absence of untoward effects in humans would suggest that more extensive clinical trials should be conducted in patients who have evidence of rapidly progressing pulmonary fibrosis.

Intact procollagen molecules are packaged into a vacuole prior to secretion from cells. Drugs such as colchicine and vinblastine which disrupt the assembly of microtubules and therefore inhibit the transport of secretory vesicles have been shown to inhibit the extracellular deposition of collagen. For example, colchine has been shown to be effective in preventing radiation-induced pulmonary fibrosis.[23] The therapeutic application of these drugs is limited, however, since they are not specific for collagen and might interfere with other cell functions such as chemotaxis, phagocytosis, and secretion of all exported proteins.

Covalent crosslinking between adjacent collagen molecules stabilizes the fibrillar structure of collagen and contributes to the high tensile strength of mature collagen fibers. The type of crosslinking which occurs is found only in collagen and elastin. Interference with crosslink formation affects the quality of the fibers formed by making them more soluble and more readily degradable by collagenase. The effect of a crosslink inhibitor is to decrease the net accumulation of collagen in tissue.

It has long been established that lathyrogens such as β-aminopropionitrile (BAPN) inhibit collagen formation. In experimental pulmonary fibrosis, BAPN has been shown to be effective in preventing collagen accumulation in silica,[24] bleomycin,[25,26] radiation,[27] and cadmium chloride-induced fibrosis.[28] There are many published reports on the toxic effects of BAPN on growing animals, a syndrome termed osteolathyrism, characterized by dislocations of joints, spinal deformities, and hind limb paralysis. It is less clear whether osteolathyrism develops in adult animals after a prolonged exposure; most reports suggest no effect or a milder disorder. The use and toxicity of BAPN has been evaluated in a few human trials of fibrosing diseases.[13] Although some serious side effects such as rash, abnormal liver function tests, fever, and anemia were noted, the drug was well tolerated by most patients when given for a few weeks. Eight patients with severe ARDS and rapidly developing pulmonary fibrosis have been given BAPN intravenously for up to 2 weeks.[13] The drug was well tolerated, but there was no obvious clinical benefit.

The other major drug used to inhibit collagen crosslinking is D-penicillamine. The mechanism of action of D-penicillamine is more complex than BAPN, and the agent chelates copper which is a required cofactor for the enzyme mediating crosslinking. D-penicillamine is currently approved for use in humans to treat Wilson's disease and severe, active rheumatoid arthritis. It has been used to treat several fibrosing disorders in humans, including hepatic cirrhosis, progressive systemic sclerosis, and morphea.[12] In regard to pulmonary fibrosis, D-penicillamine has been shown to modify the accumulation of collagen in the lung in radiation-[29] and bleomycin-induced[30] pulmonary fibrosis. Several reports on the use of D-penicillamine in patients with idiopathic pulmonary fibrosis have appeared.[31-33] In most cases, treatment was started late in the diseases, and in about one fourth to one third of patients there appeared to be stabilization of the disease.

V. CONCLUSION

The complexity of inflammation and fibrogenesis, coupled with ignorance of the initiating events in human interstitial lung diseases, accounts for the lack of substantial progress in developing therapeutic agents. With the exception of the antifibrotic proline analogues, there are no new drugs which would appear to be available in the near future. Nevertheless, the continued expansion of our knowledge of the pathogenesis of these diseases holds hope for the future development of effective treatment.

ACKNOWLEDGMENT

This work is supported by PHS Grant HL24262.

REFERENCES

1. **Hunninghake, G. W., Garrett, K. C., Richerson, H. B., Fantone, J. C., Ward, P. A., Rennard, S. I., Bitterman, P. B., and Crystal, R. G.,** Pathogenesis of the granulomatous lung diseases, *Am. Rev. Respir. Dis.,* 130, 476, 1984.
2. **Sterling, K. M., Jr., DiPetrillo, T., Cutroneo, K. R., and Prestayko, A.,** Inhibition of collagen accumulation by glucocorticoids in rat lung after intratracheal bleomycin instillation, *Cancer Res.,* 42, 405, 1982.
3. **Hesterberg, T. W. and Last, J. A.,** Ozone-induced acute pulmonary fibrosis in rats. Prevention of the increased rates of collagen synthesis by methylprednisolone, *Am. Rev. Respir. Dis.,* 123, 47, 1981.
4. **Phan, S. H., Thrall, R. S., and Williams, C.,** Bleomycin-induced pulmonary fibrosis. Effect of steroid on lung collagen metabolism, *Am. Rev. Respir. Dis.,* 124, 428, 1981.
5. **Crystal, R. G., Gadek, J. E., Ferrans, V. J., Fulmer, J. D., Line, B. R., and Hunninghake, G. W.,** Interstitial lung disease: current concepts of pathogenesis, staging and therapy, *Am. J. Med.,* 70, 542, 1981.
6. **Thrall, R. S., Lovett, E. J., III, Barton, R. W., McCormick, J. R., Phan, S. H., and Ward, P. A.,** The effect of T-cell depletion on the development of bleomycin-induced pulmonary fibrosis in the rat, *Am. Rev. Respir. Dis.,* 121, 99, 1980.
7. **Thrall, R. S., Phan, S. H., McCormack, J. R., and Ward, P. A.,** The development of bleomycin-induced pulmonary fibrosis in neutrophil-depleted and complement-depleted rats, *Am. J. Pathol.,* 105, 76, 1981.
8. **Clark, J. G. and Kuhn, C., III,** Bleomycin-induced pulmonary fibrosis in hamsters: effect of neutrophil depletion on lung collagen synthesis, *Am. Rev. Respir. Dis.,* 126, 737, 1982.
9. **Chandler, D. B. and Fulmer, J. D.,** The effect of deferoxamine on bleomycin-induced lung fibrosis in the hamster, *Am. Rev. Respir. Dis.,* 131, 596, 1985.
10. **Cross, C. E., Warren, D., Gerriets, J. E., Wilson, D. W., Halliwell, B., and Last, J. A.,** Deferoxamine injection does not affect bleomycin-induced lung fibrosis in rats, *J. Lab. Clin. Med.,* 106, 433, 1985.
11. **Fuller, G. C.,** Perspectives for the use of collagen synthesis inhibitors as antifibrotic agents, *J. Med. Chem.,* 24, 651, 1981.
12. **Uitto, J., Ryhänen, L., Tan, E. M. L., Oikarinen, A. I., and Zaragoza, E. J.,** Pharmacological inhibition of excessive collagen deposition in fibrotic diseases, *Fed. Proc.,* 43, 2815, 1984.
13. **Salvador, R. A., Fiedler-Nagy, C., and Coffey, J. W.,** Biochemical basis for drug therapy to prevent pulmonary fibrosis in ARDS, in *Acute Respiratory Failure,* Zapol, W. M., and Falke, K. J., Eds., Marcel Dekker, New York, 1985, 477.
14. **Cutroneo, K. R., Rokowski, R., and Counts, D. F.,** Glucocorticoids and collagen synthesis: comparison of in vivo and cell culture studies, *Collagen Rel. Res.,* 1, 557, 1981.
15. **Sterling, K. M., Jr., Harris, M. J., Mitchell, J. J., and Cutroneo, K. R.,** Bleomycin treatment of chick fibroblasts causes an increase of polysomal type I procollagen mRNAs. Reversal of the bleomycin effect by dexamethasone, *J. Biol. Chem.,* 258, 14438, 1983.
16. **Günzler, V., Majamaa, K., Hanuske-Abel, H. M., and Kivirikko, K. I.,** Inhibition of prolyl-4-hydroxylase by structure analogues of 2-oxoglutarate, *Collagen Rel. Res.,* 3, 71, 1983.
17. **Fuller, G. C.,** The pharmacology and toxicology of antifibrotic agents, in *Connective Tissue of the Normal and Fibrotic Human Liver,* Gerlach, U., Pott, G., and Rauterberg, J., Eds., G. Thieme Verlag, Stuttgart, 1982, 219.

18. **Riley, D. J., Berg, R. A., Edelman, N. H., and Prockop, D. J.,** Prevention of collagen deposition following pulmonary oxygen toxicity in the rat by *cis*-4-hydroxy-L-proline, *J. Clin. Invest.,* 65, 643, 1980.
19. **Riley, D. J., Kerr, J. S., and Yu, S. Y.,** Effect of proline analogues on oxygen toxicity-induced pulmonary fibrosis in the rat, *Toxicol. Appl. Pharmacol.,* 75, 554, 1984.
20. **Riley, D. J., Kerr, J. S., Berg, R. A., Ianni, B. D., Pietra, G. C., Edelman, N. H., and Prockop, D. J.,** Prevention of bleomycin-induced pulmonary fibrosis in the hamster by *cis*-4-hydroxy-L-proline, *Am. Rev. Respir. Dis.,* 123, 388, 1981.
21. **Kelley, J., Newman, R. A., and Evans, J. N.,** Bleomycin-induced pulmonary fibrosis in the rat. Prevention with an inhibitor of collagen synthesis, *J. Lab. Clin. Med.,* 96, 954, 1980.
22. **Zapol, W. M., Quinn, D., Coffey, J., and Salvador, R. A.,** L-3,4-Dehydroproline suppression of fibrosis in ARDS: early clinical results, *Am. Rev. Respir. Dis.,* 129, A102(Suppl.), 1984.
23. **Dubrawsky, C., Dubravsky, N. B., and Withers, H. R.,** The effect of colchicine on the accumulation of hydroxyproline and on lung compliance after irradiation, *Radiat. Res.,* 73, 111, 1978.
24. **Levene, C. I., Bye, I., and Saffiotti, U.,** The effect of B-aminopropionitrile on silicotic pulmonary fibrosis in the rat, *Br. J. Exp. Pathol.,* 49, 152, 1968.
25. **Zuckerman, J. E., Hollinger, M. A., and Giri, S. N.,** Evaluation of antifibrotic drugs in bleomycin-induced pulmonary fibrosis in hamsters, *J. Pharmacol. Exp. Ther.,* 213, 425, 1980.
26. **Riley, D. J., Kerr, J. S., Berg, R. A., Ianni, B. D., Pietra, G. G., Edelman, N. H., and Prockop, D. J.,** Beta-aminopropionitrile prevents bleomycin-induced pulmonary fibrosis in the hamster, *Am. Rev. Respir. Dis.,* 125, 67, 1982.
27. **Percarpio, B. and Fischer, J. J.,** Beta-aminopropionitrile as a radiation reaction preventive agent, *Radiology,* 121, 737, 1976.
28. **Chichester, C. O., Palmer, K. C., Hayes, J. A., and Kagan, H. M.,** Lung lysyl oxidase and prolyl hydroxylase: increases induced by cadmium chloride inhalation and the effect of B-aminopropionitrile in rats, *Am. Rev. Respir. Dis.,* 124, 709, 1981.
29. **Ward, W. F., Shih-Hoellwarth, A., and Tuttle, R. D.,** Collagen accumulation in irradiated rat lung: modification by D-penicillamine, *Radiology,* 146, 533, 1983.
30. **Fedullo, A. J., Karlinsky, J. B., Snider, G. L., and Goldstein, R. M.,** Lung statics and connective tissues after penicillamine in bleomycin-treated hamsters, *J. Appl. Physiol. Respirat. Environ. Exercise Physiol.,* 49, 1083, 1980.
31. **Cegla, U. H., Kroidl, R. F., Meier-Sydow, J., Thiel, C., Czarnecki, G., and Schreiber, F.,** Therapy of idiopathic fibrosis of the lung. Experiences with three therapeutic principles: corticosteroids in combination with azathioprine, D-penicillamine and K-paraaminobenzoate, *Pneumonologie,* 152, 75, 1975.
32. **Costobel, U. and Matthys, H.,** Different therapies and factors influencing response to therapy in idiopathic diffuse fibrosing alveolitis, *Respiration,* 42, 141, 1981.
33. **Turner-Warwick, M.,** Future possibilities of therapeutic intervention, in *Lung Cells in Disease,* Bouhuys, A., Ed., Elsevier/North-Holland, Amsterdam, 1976, 329.

INDEX

A

for usual interstitial pneumonia, 144
for Wegener's granulomatosis, 95, 116
Cyclosporin A toxicity, 90—92
Cylindruria, 94
Cystic fibrosis (CF)
    allergic bronchopulmonary aspergillosis in, 29—30
    allergic bronchopulmonary nonaspergillosis
        pneumonia in, 30
    anatomic and physiologic considerations in, 27—
        28
    bronchial hyperreactivity in, 28—29
    clinical presentations in, 28
    drugs used in therapy of, 30
    in giant cell interstitial pneumonia, 133
    hypersensitivity to airway flora in, 30
    ILD associated with, 26—31
    immune complex disease in, 30—31
Cysts, bone, 41
Cytomegalic inclusion virus, 33
Cytosine arabinoside, 7, 11
Cytotoxic agents
    for Goodpasture's syndrome, 93
    for mixed connective tissue disease, 113
    for polyarteritis nodosa, 97
    for Wegener's granulomatosis, 95
Cytoxan, see Cyclophosphamide

D

Dactinomycin, 2
Deferoxamine, 171
Degenerative disorder associated with ILD, 32—33
L-3,4-Dehydroproline, 172—173
Dermatitis, 28, 54
Dermatomyositis (DM), 111—113
Desquamative interstitial pneumonitis (DIP), 130—
    133
Destructiveness, 41
Dexamethasone, 172
Dextroamphetamine, 42
Diabetes insipidus, 83
Diabetic nephropathy, 93
Diarrhea, 95
Diethylcarbamazine, 137
Digital clubbing
    in desquamative interstitial pneumonitis, 130—132
    in giant cell interstitial pneumonia, 134
    in Hermansky-Pudlak syndrome, 23
    in idiopathic pulmonary fibrosis, 143
    in lymphoid interstitial pneumonia, 161
    in neurofibromatosis, 44
    in pulmonary alveolar microlithiasis, 32
    in systemic lupus erythematosus, 107
DIP, see Desquamative interstitial pneumonitis
DM, see Dermatomyositis
Doxorubicin, 2
Drooling, 46
Drug-induced interstitial pneumonitis, see Pulmonary
    toxicity
Dysproteinemia, 156, 160, 164

E

Edema
    in Loeffler syndrome, 138
    in nephrotic syndrome, 89
    in renal failure, 88
    in renal transplant, 91
    in systemic lupus erythematosus, 96
    type II pneumocyte damage and, 3
ELISA, see Enzyme-linked immunosorbent assay
Emphysema, 140, 143
Endocarditis, subacute bacterial, 97
Endocrine disorders, 44, 45
Enzyme-linked immunosorbent assay (ELISA), 138,
    139
Eosinophiles, 68
Eosinophilia
    in allergic granulomatous angiitis, 98
    asthma and, 136
    in Churg-Strauss syndrome, 116
    in CF, 28
    in hypersensitivity angiitis, 97
    in idiopathic pulmonary hemosiderosis, 72
    in Loeffler syndrome, 135, 138
    in polyarteritis nodosa, 139
    prolonged pulmonary, 136
    pulmonary involvement with, 135—140
    tropical, 136, 138—139
    in visceral larva migrans, 138
Eosinophilic abscess, 139
Eosinophilic lung, 138—139
Eosinophilic pneumonia, 135, 139, 140
Epididymitis, 96
Epidophyllotoxin, 156, 159
Episcleritis, 95
Epitheloid cell granulomas, 94, 98
Ergotamine, 7
Erythema nodosum, 54
Esophagitis, 16—17
Esophagoscopy, 18
Esophagram, 17
Ewings sarcoma, 80
Exanthema, 156
Exocrine glands, 114
Exophthalmos, 43
Extrinsic allergic alveolitis, see Hypersensitivity
    pneumonitis

F

Facial nerve palsy, 55
Facies, mask-like, 46
Familial erythrophagocytic lymphohistiocytosis
    (FEL), 152—156
    clinical features of, 152—155
    definition of, 152
    etiopathogenesis of, 152
    management and prognosis of, 156
    pathology of, 152, 156
Familial fibrocystic pulmonary dysplasia, 140